ULTIMATE GUIDE TO
STRETCHING

Thunder Bay Press
An imprint of Printers Row Publishing Group
10350 Barnes Canyon Road, Suite 100, San Diego, CA 92121
www.thunderbaybooks.com • mail@thunderbaybooks.com

Thunder Bay Press
Publisher: Peter Norton
Associate Publisher: Ana Parker
Senior Development Editor: April Graham Farr
Editor: Vicki Jaeger
Senior Product Manager: Kathryn C. Dalby
Production Team: Jonathan Lopes, Rusty von Dyl

Produced by Moseley Road Inc., www.moseleyroad.com
President: Sean Moore
Art and Editorial Director: Lisa Purcell
Editor: Audra Avizienis
Production Director: Adam Moore
Designer: Adam Moore
Photography: Naila Ruechel, www.nailaruechel.com

Library of Congress Control Number: 2019943734

ISBN: 978-1-64517-046-4

Printed in China

23 22 21 20 19   1 2 3 4 5

ULTIMATE GUIDE TO
STRETCHING

WITH DETAILED INSTRUCTIONS AND ANATOMICAL ILLUSTRATIONS FOR 160 STRETCHES

Sophie Cornish-Keefe

THUNDER BAY
P·R·E·S·S

San Diego, California

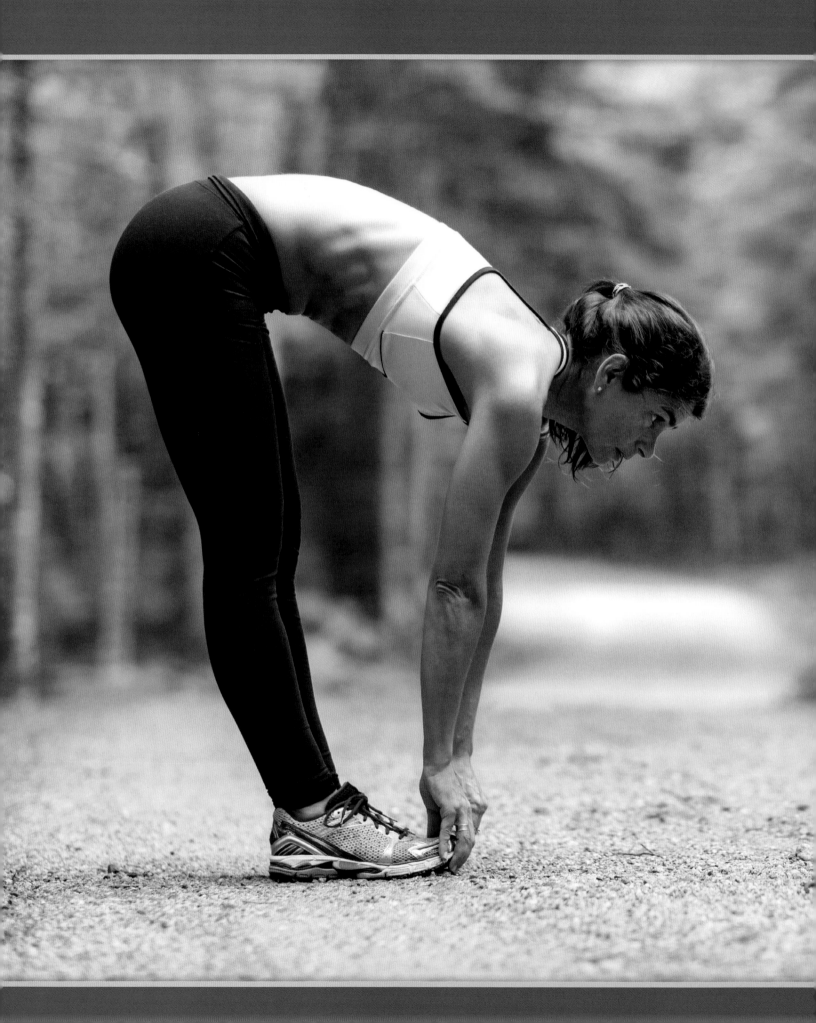

CONTENTS

What Is Stretching?

Stretching is the purposeful lengthening of your muscles to increase your flexibility and improve the range of motion in your joints. Performing stretches is an important part of any exercise or rehabilitative regimen. Stretching helps warm up the body prior to an activity, thus decreasing the risk of injury and muscle soreness. Regular stretching can also be an effective and relaxing antidote to a sedentary workday.

FLEXIBILITY FOR ALL

Flexibility, in a technical sense, can be understood as the complete range of motion of a specific limb or joint. Most of us think of flexibility as a skill possessed only by professional dancers or accomplished yogis. However, maintaining a degree of flexibility is important for everyone. Poor flexibility can lead to sore or stiff joints, poor body alignment and posture, and the potential for chronic pain. Improving, and then maintaining, flexibility is quite simple. Spend a few minutes several times a week moving each of your limbs and joints through their range of motion, making sure to focus on particular problem areas.

WHY STRETCH?

Stretching and regular yoga practice can improve flexibility as well as relieve pain in your body. People who regularly stretch tend to experience less lower-back pain. Stretching your neck seems to be as effective at reducing neck pain as manual therapy. Also, stretching your Achilles tendon can relieve persistent heel pain. New research indicates that within minutes after stretching, there is increased activation of the parasympathetic nervous system (the system in charge of relaxation). This may account, in part, for the feeling of well-being that yogis experience after a stretching session.

WHEN TO STRETCH?

Regular and safely practiced stretching can benefit individuals of all ages and physical abilities. Athletes and those who work out often should make stretching an integral part of both their warm-up and cooldown routines. However, even if you are not a gym-goer, stretching should become an everyday practice in your life. If you work in an office or spend most of your day sitting at a desk, it is highly recommended that you take regular breaks to stretch your legs, shoulders, and chest muscles. Stretching is also incredibly important for those who have suffered an injury or are undertaking rehabilitative treatment for their physical health. A physical therapist can help determine the best stretching exercises for your specific recovery needs.

HOW TO STRETCH?

Stretching should not cause pain. Pain is a sign that you are stretching the muscles, tendons, or ligaments beyond their range of motion. This can lead to injury, a buildup of scar tissue, or a decrease in flexibility. When stretching, you should focus on stretching muscles and tendons (the tissue that attaches muscle to bone), not ligaments (tissue that attaches bone to bone). If the stretch doesn't feel good, you are probably practicing it incorrectly or pushing your body beyond its capability.

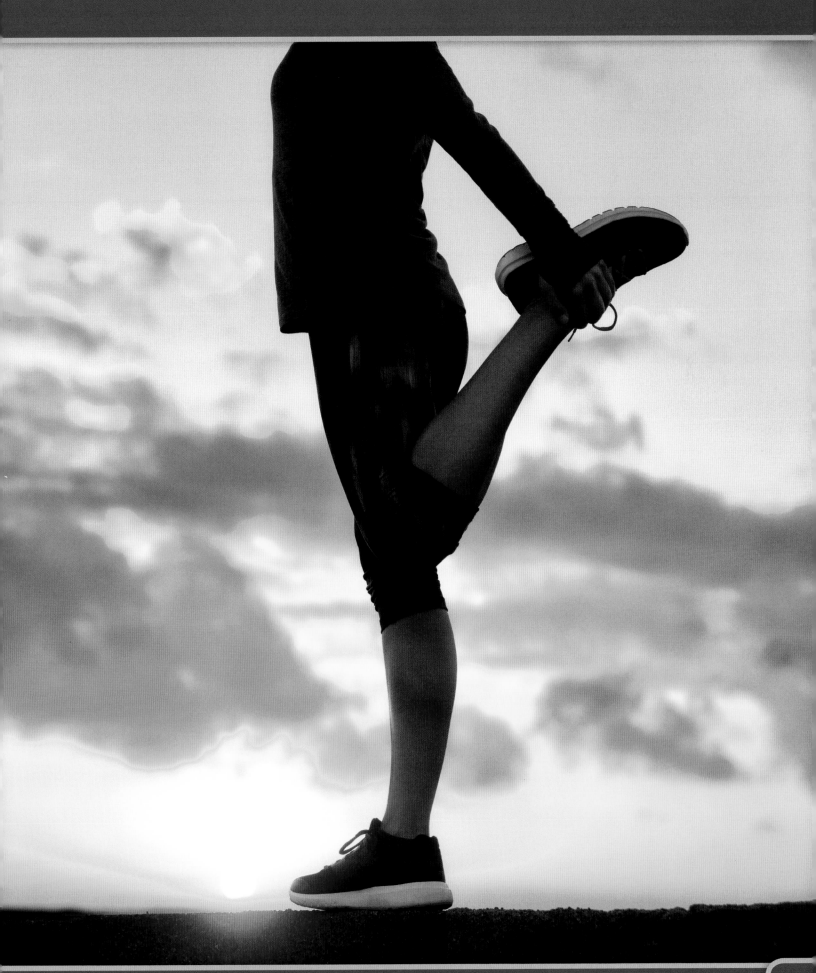

Types of Stretching

All stretching exercises can be broadly classified into one of several categories, based on the techniques they employ. Knowing the differences between the various stretching techniques is essential for determining which stretch is best for your individual physical goals. Understanding the process and intended outcome of a given technique will also help you understand the correct execution so you can perform each stretch safely and effectively.

STATIC AND DYNAMIC STRETCHING

Static Stretching:

Static stretching is the most common form of stretching, under which most exercises can be categorized. Static stretches help to elongate and loosen the targeted muscle, relieving tightness and improving flexibility. These *stretches* are performed by extending the targeted muscle to its maximal point and then holding the body in this position for a particular length of time. The length of time in which a static stretch position is held depends on your age and current ability, as well as any conflicting pain or injuries. Static stretches do not involve any bouncing, repetitive, or rapid movements. They should result in a mild, painless pulling sensation along the targeted muscle while holding the position. They are commonly regarded as the safest and most accessible stretches for beginners.

Types of Static Stretches:

Active stretches: Added force is applied by the person stretching for greater intensity.

Passive, or isometric, stretches: Added force is applied by an external force (e.g., a partner or an assistive device) to increase intensity. For example, have a partner hold your leg up while you resist the pressure and try to force your leg in the opposite direction.

Dynamic Stretching

Unlike static stretching, dynamic stretching requires the use of continuous movement patterns. In general, dynamic stretches are designed to improve the flexibility required to perform a specific sport or activity. For this reason, dynamic stretches often mimic the movements that are practiced in the given activity for which they are designed; for instance, a sprinter might warm up for a race with long, exaggerated lunges. Dynamic stretching involves a series of movements using momentum and active range of motion as opposed to holding a position in a static stretch. These types of exercises help loosen and activate the muscles without overstretching them, as static stretching runs the risk of doing.

BALLISTIC STRETCHING

Ballistic stretching forces a part of your body to go beyond its normal range of motion, by bouncing to a stretched position. It is an active form of stretching that increases your range of motion and triggers your muscle's stretch reflex. This type of stretching is typically used for athletic drills. It utilizes repeated, bouncing movements to stretch the targeted muscle group. While these bouncing movements may lead to an increased risk of injury, they can be safely performed if preceded by static stretching and gradually accelerated from a lower velocity to a higher velocity. Generally, they are practiced only by highly conditioned and competent athletes.

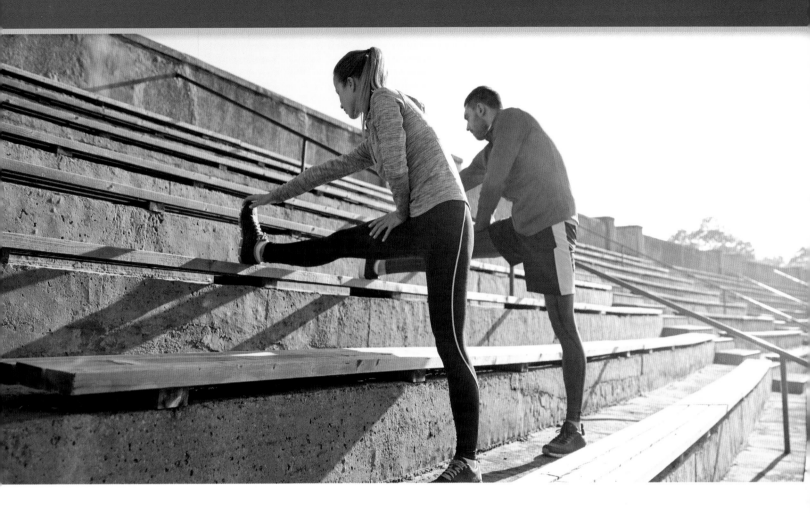

ACTIVE ISOLATED STRETCHING (AIS)

This stretching technique is held for only a couple of seconds at a time. It is performed in several repetitions with the goal of exceeding the previous point of resistance by a few degrees in each ensuing repetition. Much like a strength-training regimen, AIS is performed in several sets, each incorporating a specific number of repetitions. Active isolated stretching is most commonly used by professionals: athletes, trainers, and massage therapists, among others. The goal of an AIS stretch is to reach a certain position that you can hold without any assistance, and then push your body to increase the range of motion of that position in each ensuing attempt. For example, in Seated Forward Bends, you would push your fingertips farther and farther toward your toes in a series of quick, successive attempts. These stretches work with natural physiological processes to increase muscle and fascia elasticity and improve circulation.

MYOFASCIAL RELEASE STRETCHING

This category of exercises involves the use of applied force or an external stretching device, to apply gentle, sustained pressure to specific points of muscle tightness or discomfort. Through the aid of a foam roller or similar device, myofascial release relieves tension and improves flexibility in the fascia (the densely-woven specialized system of connective tissue that covers and connects muscles and organs), and the underlying muscle. Massage therapy is another form of myofascial release, in which the therapist applies gentle pressure to locate any areas of muscle tightness and then addresses those areas through careful, deliberate muscle-stretching techniques. Small, continuous back and forth movements are performed over a small, localized area of the body for 30 to 60 seconds at a time. The individual's pain tolerance will determine the correct amount of pressure to apply to the target area.

Benefits of Stretching

You can experience immediate and long-term benefits from practicing regular stretching. The short-term benefits of stretching include maintaining and increasing your range of motion and boosting the blood supply to your soft muscle tissue, as well as reducing muscle tightness or pain. Improving your flexibility and range of motion can enhance your athletic ability and prevent exercise-related injuries. A regular stretching regimen can also help you maintain your range of motion as you age. Beyond the many physical benefits, stretching is a relaxing form of exercise that calms your mind and elevates your mood.

INCREASED FLEXIBILITY

Greater muscle flexibility can vastly improve the quality of your daily life. Common tasks such as lifting heavy packages, bending to tie your shoes, or hurrying to catch a bus become easier and less taxing. Flexibility training can help strengthen weaker muscles, leading to greater balance in your body and thus improving your posture. Having limber muscles and better body alignment is associated with fewer aches and pains later in life.

IMPROVED CIRCULATION

Stretching enhances blood flow to your muscles. As blood flows into your muscles, it provides oxygen and nutrients and then eliminates waste products from your muscle tissue. Better circulation can help shorten your recovery time if you're healing from a muscular injury. Revving up your circulation and nutrient flow through your body also boosts your energy level.

BETTER POSTURE

The ligaments and tendons in your chest and shoulders can tighten from years of sitting hunched over at a desk, resulting in poor posture. This can lead to severe pain in your lower back and between your shoulder blades. Frequent stretching can help keep your muscles from

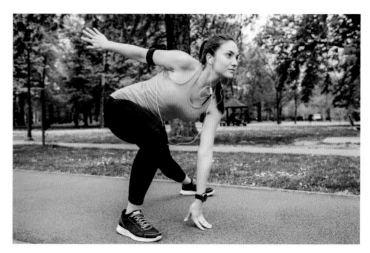

getting tight, allowing you to maintain proper body alignment. With better posture, the muscles surrounding your spine are more balanced and support the body more symmetrically, creating a world of benefit for your body.

STRESS RELIEF

Stretching not only benefits your body but also eases your mind. Stretching relaxes tight muscles that often accompany stress. The feeling of stress often leads to tense muscles in various parts of the body, restricting blood flow and resulting in discomfort. Stretching stimulates receptors in the nervous system that decrease the production of stress hormones. By learning to release and relax your muscles, you will be able to use your body to alleviate stress.

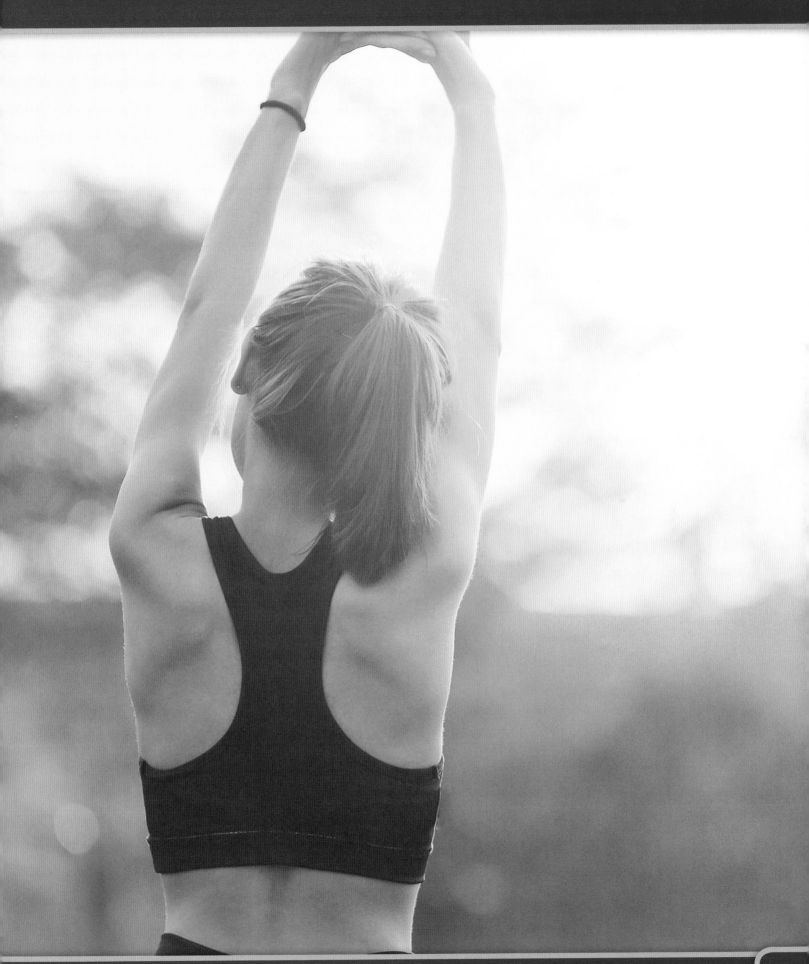

Proper Stretching Technique

It is essential to practice proper stretching techniques. Doing so will allow you to avoid injury. Tips to proper stretching technique include the following:

Warm up first: Stretching muscles when they're cold increases your risk of pulling a muscle. Warm up by walking while gently pumping your arms, or do a favorite exercise at low intensity for five minutes.

Hold each stretch for at least 30 seconds: It takes time to lengthen tissues safely. Hold your stretches for at least 30 seconds—and up to 60 seconds for really tight muscles or problem areas. That can seem like a long time, so wear a watch or keep an eye on the clock to make sure you're holding your stretches long enough. For most of your muscle groups, if you hold the stretches for at least 30 seconds, you'll need to do each stretch only once.

Don't bounce: Bouncing as you stretch can cause microtears, or small tears, in your muscle, which can leave scar tissue as the muscle heals. The scar tissue further tightens the muscle, making you even less flexible—and more prone to pain.

Focus on a pain-free stretch: If you feel pain as you stretch, you've gone too far. Return to the point where you don't feel any pain, then hold the stretch.

Relax and breathe freely: Don't hold your breath while you're stretching. Inhale and exhale slowly and deliberately.

Stretch both sides: Make sure the range of motion in your joints is as equal as possible on both sides of your body.

Stretch before and after activity: Your best bet is to perform light stretching before a strenuous workout, followed by a more thorough stretching regimen after your workout.

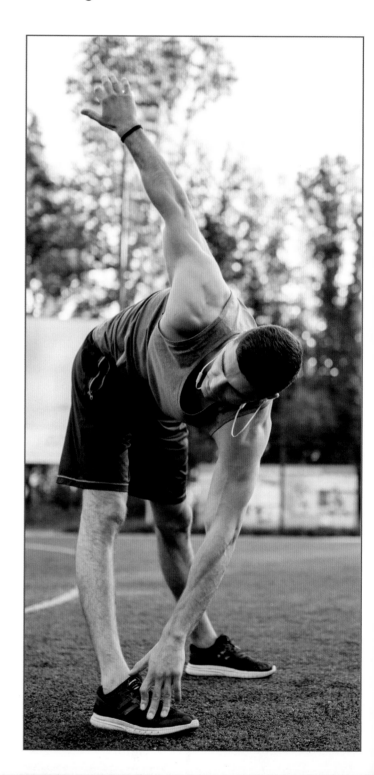

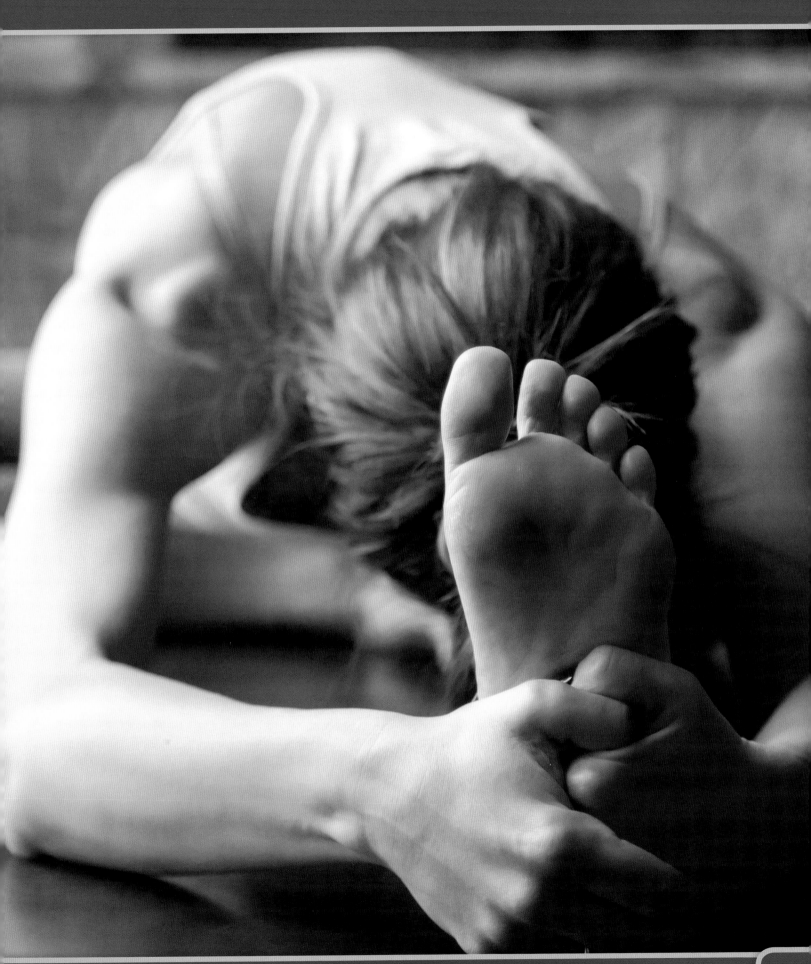

Stretching by Body Part

When you think of flexibility, a common example that might spring to mind is the ability to touch your toes. However, flexibility should be a goal for muscles throughout your body, from your head to your toes. When you design a comprehensive stretching routine for your specific physical needs and areas of muscle discomfort or tightness, it is important to consider each part of your body and make sure that you are engaging muscles in a balanced way throughout your body.

NECK: We have all woken up at one time or another with a stiff neck. The lack of movement during sleep is a common cause of tightness in the neck. Tightness in your neck also occurs from tension that builds up in your middle and upper back as a result of poor posture. Lengthening the larger muscles in your neck helps relieve tension in your back and helps your whole body to relax. Work these muscles gently, however, in this sensitive area of your body.

SHOULDERS: If you tend to keep your shoulders tilted forward in a hunched position, your shoulder muscles are probably quite tight. The more you slouch, the more likely you are to compromise the full range of motion in your shoulders. In order to combat the loss of shoulder mobility, practice regular shoulder stretches. Try some wall-assisted stretches throughout your day to wake up your upper body and relax your shoulders.

BACK: So much of our daily movement depends on a strong and stable back, yet our spines are extremely delicate. Keeping your back limber can help reduce the risk of injury and can alleviate tension that may build up in your lower back. You can improve your posture and reduce back pain by adding back stretches to your daily routine.

GLUTES: Our gluteus, or posterior, muscles are easily the heaviest part of our bodies as well a prime movement complex that helps us to walk, run, and jump efficiently.

Since we use our glutes so frequently, they can get tight and sore easily, and are important to stretch regularly.

HIP FLEXORS: Hip flexor muscles allow your legs to move. Whether you're walking, running, or cycling, you are engaging your hip flexors. However, when you sit at a desk all day, your hip flexors tend to become tight, compromising your day-to-day mobility and pulling on your lower back. In order to combat this, make sure to practice hip flexor stretches frequently.

ADDUCTORS: Your inner thighs might not be the most powerful muscle group, but that doesn't mean they can't get tight. Whether from underutilization, lack of functional movement, or just sitting in a chair with your legs crossed, your inner thighs can get just as tight as your more active muscle groups. Ignoring them can create other muscle imbalances, so make sure to target these muscles as part of your daily routine.

FEET: For such a small body part, your feet contain an incredible number of intricate bones and muscles. All of this anatomical complexity is essential for supporting the weight of your entire body as you move around throughout the day. It's easy to neglect your feet or to strain them, especially if you tend to wear shoes that don't provide enough support. Having a repertoire of basic foot stretches can help you avoid pain in your feet, heels, and ankles while improving your balance and coordination.

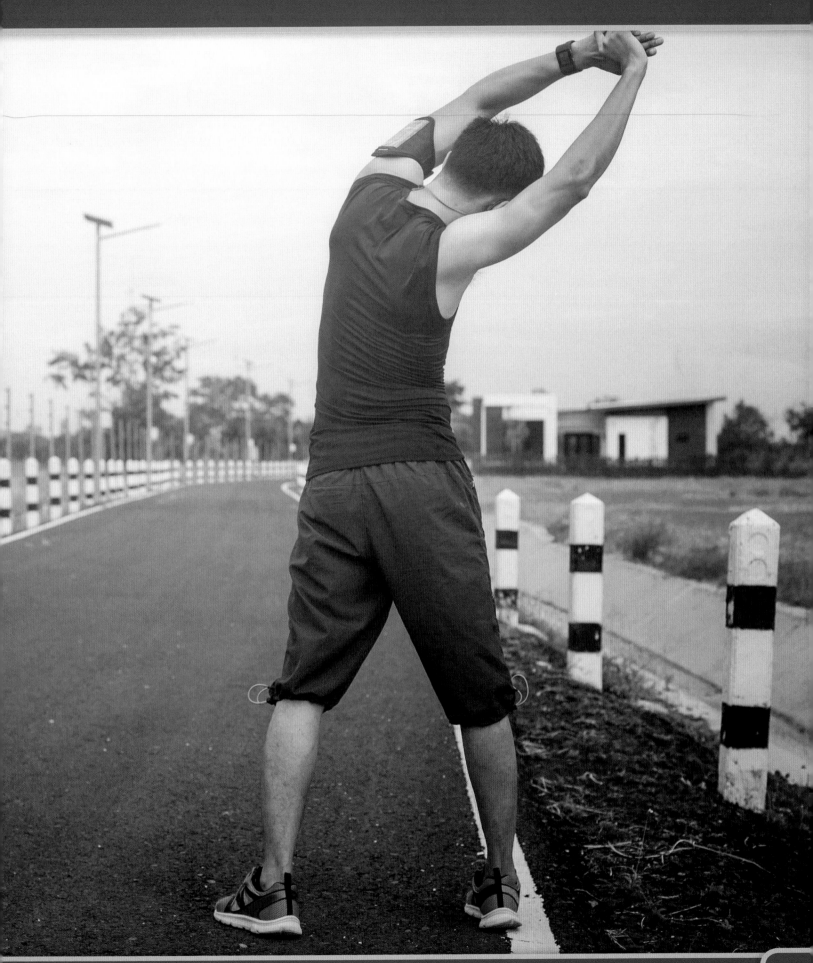

Stretch Safely

Stretching offers innumerable physical benefits, but it is not without certain risks. In order to maximize the positive effects of stretching, it must be practiced safely and correctly. The best way to make sure you are stretching safely is to understand the correct steps and desired outcome of a specific stretch as well as the basic anatomy involved in the exercise.

UNDERSTANDING STRETCHING

To understand stretching, you must realize that your muscles are not actually in charge of your range of motion. Skeletal muscle facilitates bone and joint actions, which dictate the full potential range of motion. When you stretch a muscle, it is actually the joint and ligaments being moved across these various contact surfaces. Each joint has a distinct contact surface that determines its mobility and limitations.

Lengthening the muscles surrounding a specific joint will increase the potential range of motion for that particular body part, but it is important not to attempt to push any joints or ligaments to extremes. Normal range of motion is part of healthy joint movements, but it is very unhealthy for individuals to stretch past their limitations. Stretching should not cause pain or soreness. Studies have shown that people who continuously perform intense stretches that exceed their physical limitation create uneven mechanical wear on the joints and ligaments, which can lead to osteoarthritis.

STRETCH WITHIN REASON

You should never force your body into a stretch. Stretching should feel natural and comfortable. Some people are born with an innate ability to stretch their bodies to extreme limits, but most people have to work at maintaining a normal range of motion. Listen to your body, and progress gradually.

Without question, yoga and Pilates have revolutionized the way many Americans exercise by eschewing the "no pain, no gain" mentality for a more holistic approach to working out the body. However, even these forms of exercise can alter body alignment, muscular balance, and posture when students are pushed to extremes.

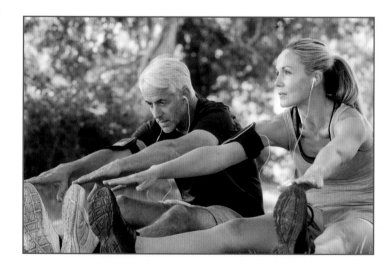

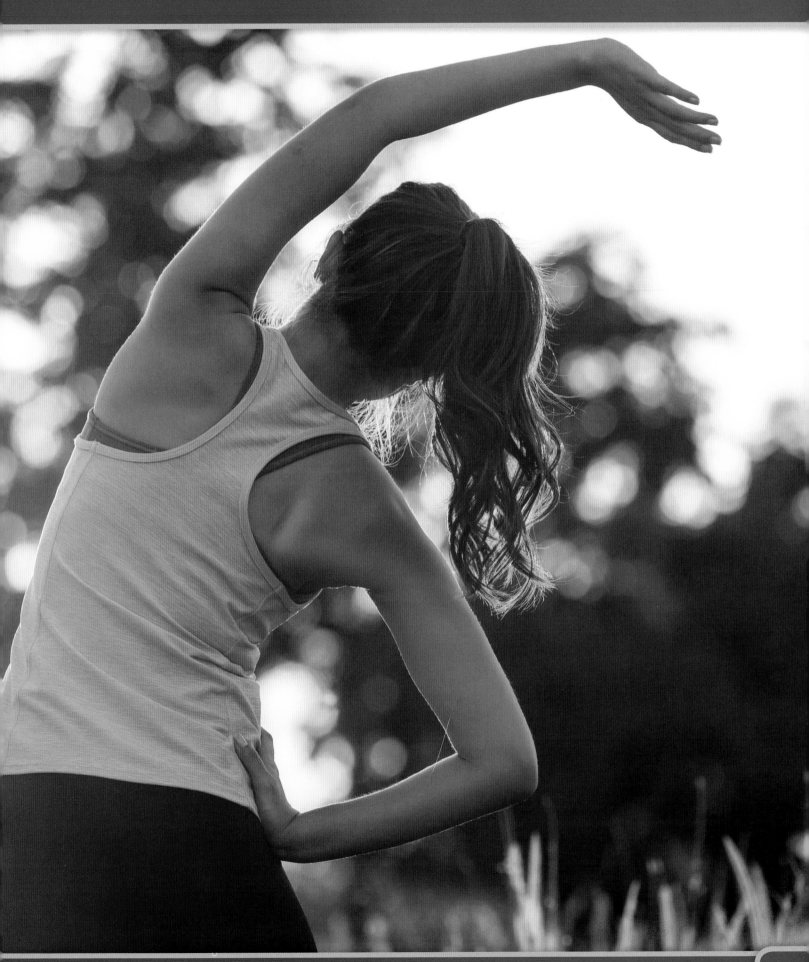

When to Avoid Stretching

Although the benefits of stretching are many, at times the physical risks of stretching may outweigh the rewards. If you have recently suffered a muscular injury, sprain, or broken bone, it is best to consult a physician or a physical therapist about which stretches would be most suitable for your recovery and when would be most appropriate for you to begin.

ACUTE MUSCLE STRAINS: People who have suffered an acute muscle strain should avoid placing further stress on the muscle through stretching activities. The injured muscle should be given time to rest. Stretching muscle fibers in the acute period can result in further injury.

FRACTURED BONES: After breaking a bone, the fracture site needs time to heal. Stretching muscles that surround this injured area could place stress on the bone and prevent it from healing, or could further displace the break. Avoid stretching a joint that surrounds a broken bone unless you have your physician's approval.

JOINT SPRAINS: When you sprain a joint, you overstretch the ligaments that help stabilize the bones of the joint. For this reason, stretching early after a joint sprain should be avoided. As with fractures, these structures need time to heal and stretching too soon after an injury might delay the healing process.

SPEAK TO A PROFESSIONAL: Stretching regularly can help your body and joints move more freely, allowing you to enjoy full functional mobility. Check in with a physical therapist to find out which stretches are best for you.

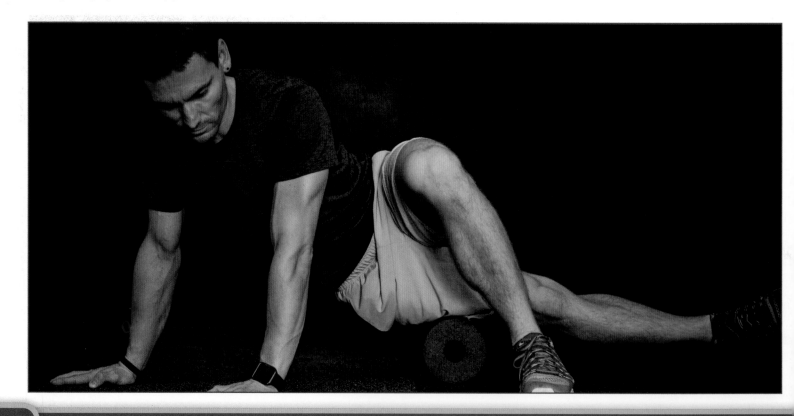

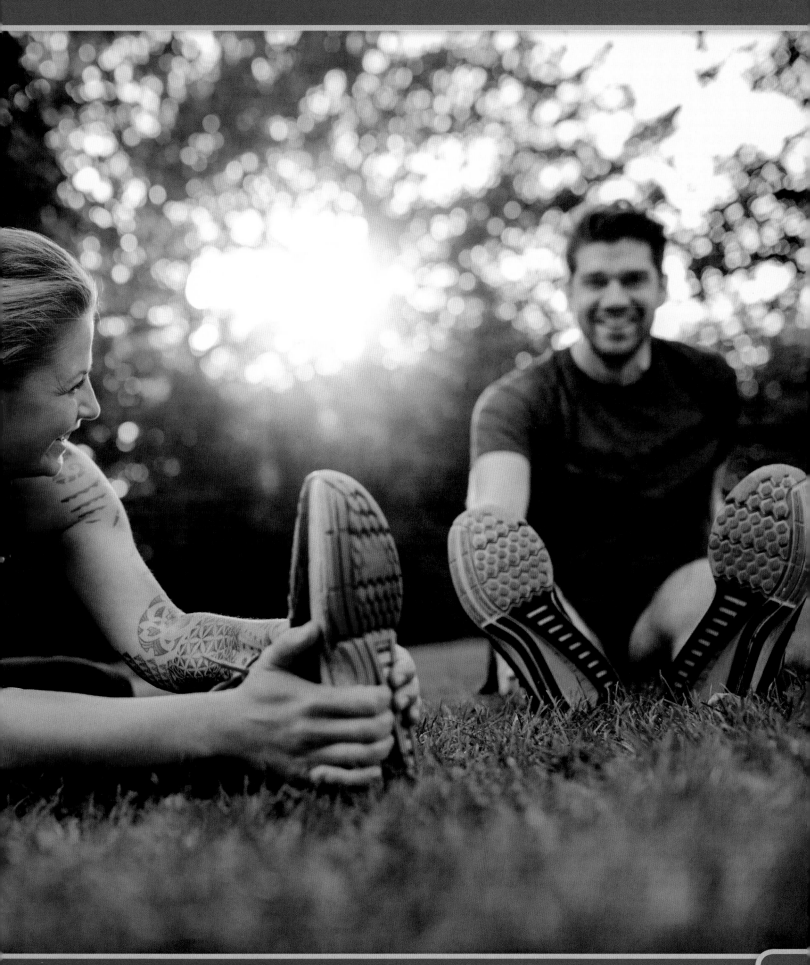

How to Use This Book

Ultimate Guide to Stretches features step-by-step instructions to 160 exercises specially selected to fit into a variety of stretching regimens.

Chapter One: Head & Neck Stretches Loosen your cervical spine and your facial and neck muscles.

Chapter Two: Arms, Shoulders, & Upper-Back Stretches Learn exercises that target these important muscle groups.

Chapter Three: Chest Stretches Home in on your pectorals and other muscles of the chest.

Chapter Four: Abdominal & Obliques Stretches Learn the best way to stretch this important group of core muscles.

Chapter Five: Lower-Back Stretches Help relieve back pain and stiffness with this group of stretches.

Chapter Six: Hips, Groin, & Glutes Stretches Open and stretch these critical muscle groups.

Chapter Seven: Leg, Ankle, & Foot Stretches Target your lower extremities with these stretches.

Chapter Eight: Stretching Routines Once you've familiarized yourself with the featured exercises, turn to this chapter to learn how to put them together in stretching routines.

KEY

KEY POSE SPREADS

❶ Category
Indicates the overall body areas targeted: your back, arms, chest, core, legs, or total body.

❷ Exercise Info
Provides the name of the exercise and some key details you need to know about it.

❸ How to Do It
Offers step-by-step instructions detailing how to perform it.

❹ Step-by-Step Photos
Shows images of the key steps to the exercise.

❺ Do It Right
Provides tips to help you perfect your form.

❻ Fact File
Lists key facts: the targeted muscles, the benefits, and any cautions that may apply.

❼ Anatomical Illustration
Indicates the key working muscles. May also include an inset showing muscles not illustrated in the main image.

❽ Modification
Shows you modifications of the pose that may be easier or harder, or variations of similar difficulty.

WORKOUT SPREADS

❶ Routine info
Gives the name of the routine and some key details you need to know about it.

❷ Exercise Info
Shows the name of the pose, the pages where you can find it, and how many breaths to hold the pose.

❸ Photo Icon
Offers a quick view of the exercise.

❹ Fact File
A quick list of key facts of the routine: the level of difficulty, its objective, the work/rest ratio, and an estimate of how long it takes to perform.

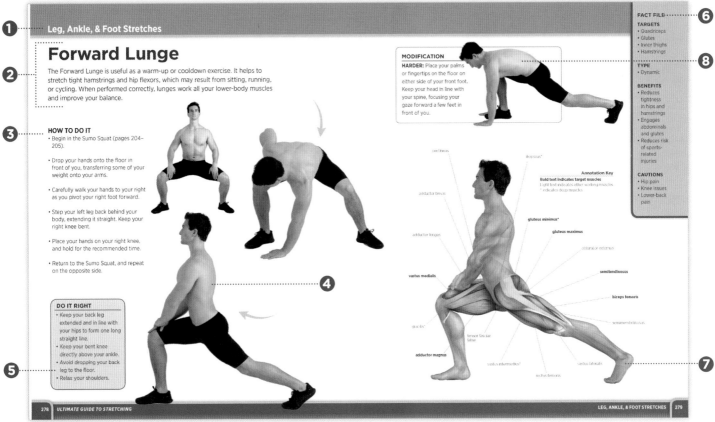

❶ Leg, Ankle, & Foot Stretches

Forward Lunge

❷ The Forward Lunge is useful as a warm-up or cooldown exercise. It helps to stretch tight hamstrings and hip flexors, which may result from sitting, running, or cycling. When performed correctly, lunges work all your lower-body muscles and improve your balance.

❸ **HOW TO DO IT**
- Begin in the Sumo Squat (pages 204–205).
- Drop your hands onto the floor in front of you, transferring some of your weight onto your arms.
- Carefully walk your hands to your right as you pivot your right foot forward.
- Step your left leg back behind your body, extending it straight. Keep your right knee bent.
- Place your hands on your right knee, and hold for the recommended time.
- Return to the Sumo Squat, and repeat on the opposite side.

DO IT RIGHT
- Keep your back leg extended and in line with your hips to form one long straight line.
- Keep your bent knee directly above your ankle.
- Avoid dropping your back leg to the floor.
- Relax your shoulders.

❺

❹

MODIFICATION
HARDER: Place your palms or fingertips on the floor on either side of your front foot. Keep your head in line with your spine, focusing your gaze forward a few feet in front of you.

❽

Annotation Key
Bold text indicates target muscles
Light text indicates other working muscles
* indicates deep muscles

pectineus*
iliopsoas*
adductor brevis
gluteus minimus*
adductor longus
gluteus maximus
obturator externus
vastus medialis
semitendinosus
biceps femoris
gracilis*
semimembranosus
tensor fasciae latae
adductor magnus
vastus intermedius*
vastus lateralis
rectus femoris

❼

❻ FACT FILE
TARGETS
- Quadriceps
- Glutes
- Inner thighs
- Hamstrings

TYPE
- Dynamic

BENEFITS
- Reduces tightness in hips and hamstrings
- Engages abdominals and glutes
- Reduces risk of sports-related injuries

CAUTIONS
- Hip pain
- Knee issues
- Lower-back pain

278 *ULTIMATE GUIDE TO STRETCHING*   LEG, ANKLE, & FOOT STRETCHES 279

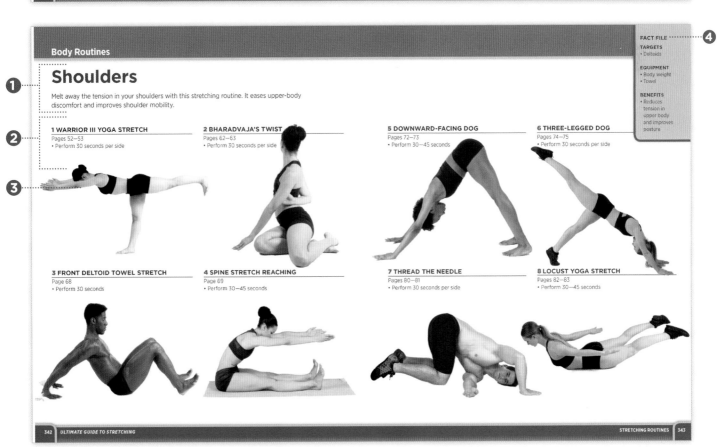

❶ Body Routines

Shoulders

Melt away the tension in your shoulders with this stretching routine. It eases upper-body discomfort and improves shoulder mobility.

❷

❸

1 WARRIOR III YOGA STRETCH
Pages 52–53
- Perform 30 seconds per side

2 BHARADVAJA'S TWIST
Pages 62–63
- Perform 30 seconds per side

5 DOWNWARD-FACING DOG
Pages 72–73
- Perform 30–45 seconds

6 THREE-LEGGED DOG
Pages 74–75
- Perform 30 seconds per side

3 FRONT DELTOID TOWEL STRETCH
Page 68
- Perform 30 seconds

4 SPINE STRETCH REACHING
Page 69
- Perform 30–45 seconds

7 THREAD THE NEEDLE
Pages 80–81
- Perform 30 seconds per side

8 LOCUST YOGA STRETCH
Pages 82–83
- Perform 30–45 seconds

❹ FACT FILE
TARGETS
- Deltoids

EQUIPMENT
- Body weight
- Towel

BENEFITS
- Reduces tension in upper body and improves posture

342 *ULTIMATE GUIDE TO STRETCHING*   STRETCHING ROUTINES 343

Full-Body Anatomy

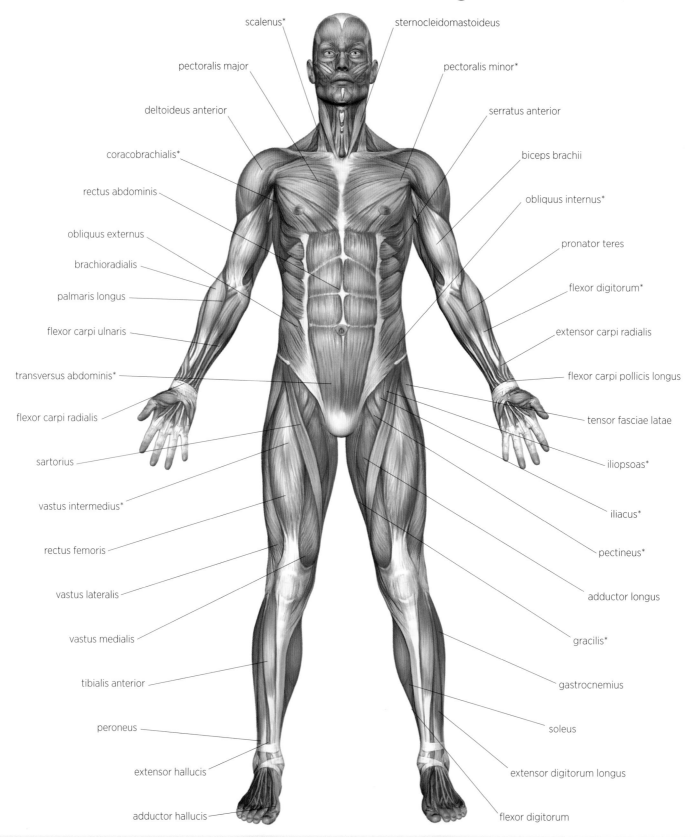

scalenus*

sternocleidomastoideus

pectoralis major

pectoralis minor*

deltoideus anterior

serratus anterior

coracobrachialis*

biceps brachii

rectus abdominis

obliquus internus*

obliquus externus

pronator teres

brachioradialis

flexor digitorum*

palmaris longus

extensor carpi radialis

flexor carpi ulnaris

flexor carpi pollicis longus

transversus abdominis*

tensor fasciae latae

flexor carpi radialis

iliopsoas*

sartorius

iliacus*

vastus intermedius*

pectineus*

rectus femoris

adductor longus

vastus lateralis

gracilis*

vastus medialis

gastrocnemius

tibialis anterior

soleus

peroneus

extensor hallucis

extensor digitorum longus

adductor hallucis

flexor digitorum

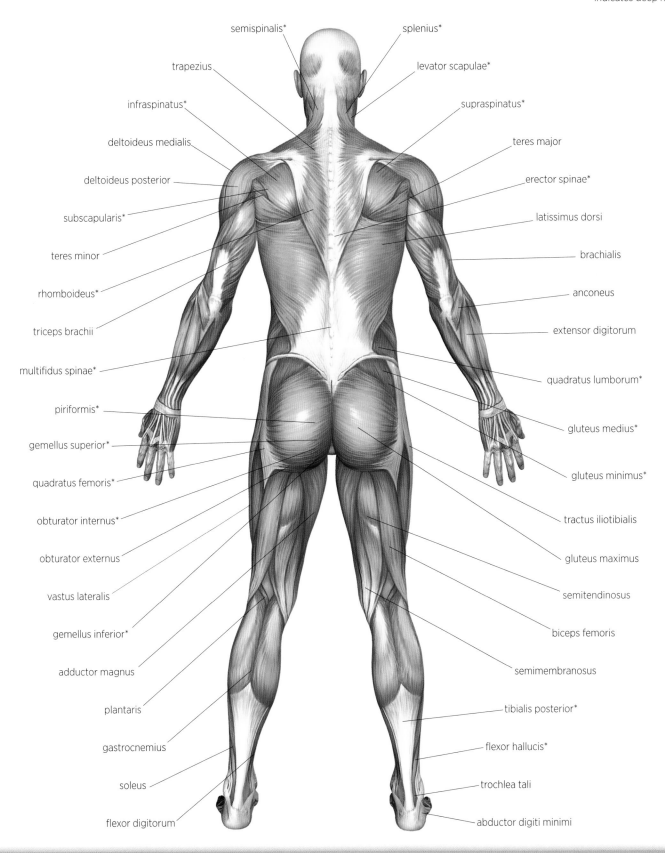

semispinalis*

splenius*

trapezius

levator scapulae*

infraspinatus*

supraspinatus*

deltoideus medialis

teres major

deltoideus posterior

erector spinae*

subscapularis*

latissimus dorsi

teres minor

brachialis

rhomboideus*

anconeus

triceps brachii

extensor digitorum

multifidus spinae*

quadratus lumborum*

piriformis*

gluteus medius*

gemellus superior*

quadratus femoris*

gluteus minimus*

obturator internus*

tractus iliotibialis

obturator externus

gluteus maximus

vastus lateralis

semitendinosus

gemellus inferior*

biceps femoris

adductor magnus

semimembranosus

plantaris

tibialis posterior*

gastrocnemius

flexor hallucis*

soleus

trochlea tali

flexor digitorum

abductor digiti minimi

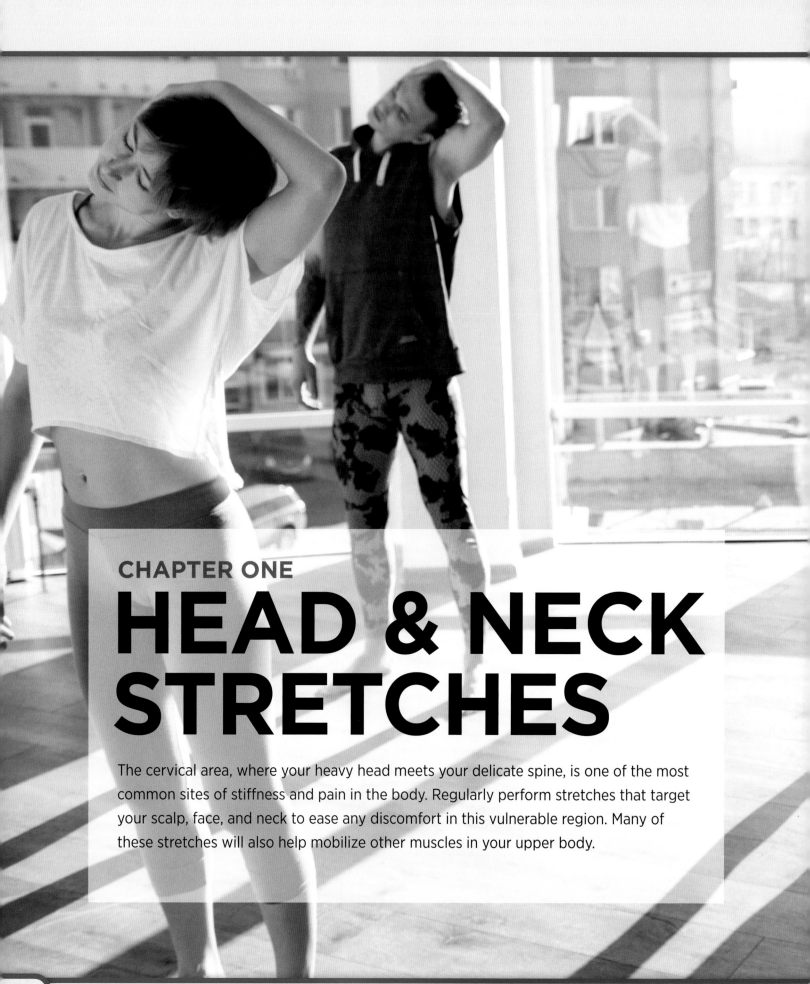

CHAPTER ONE
HEAD & NECK STRETCHES

The cervical area, where your heavy head meets your delicate spine, is one of the most common sites of stiffness and pain in the body. Regularly perform stretches that target your scalp, face, and neck to ease any discomfort in this vulnerable region. Many of these stretches will also help mobilize other muscles in your upper body.

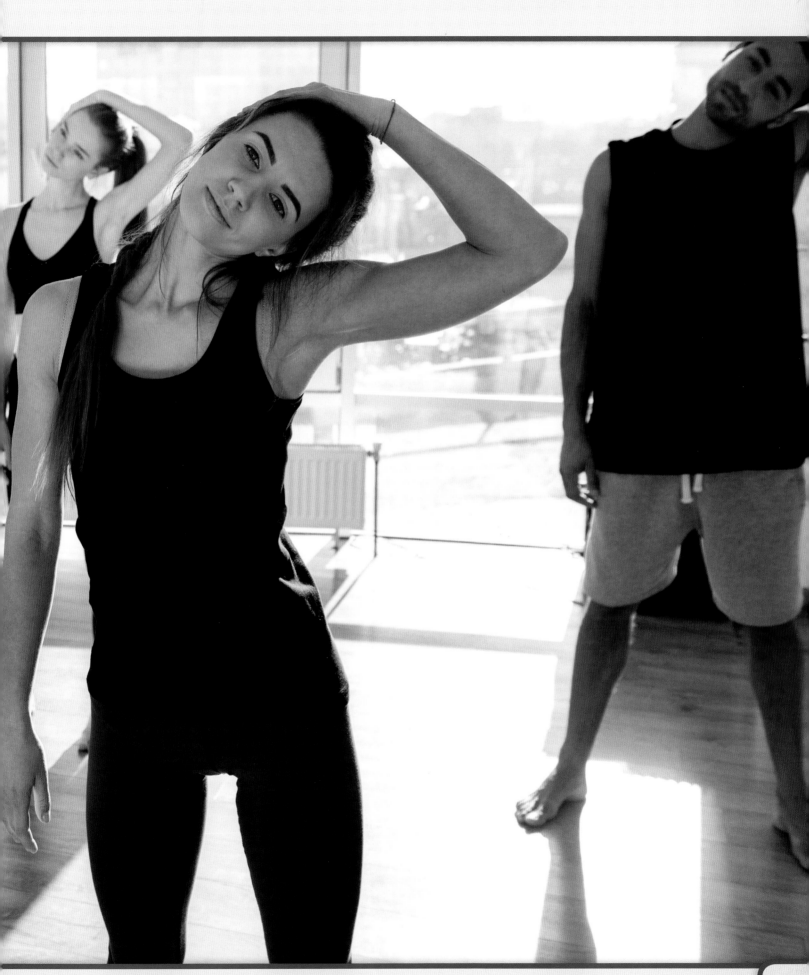

Scalp Stretch

Tightness in the scalp can arise from a variety of factors, both physical and psychological. Perform this simple stretch regularly throughout the day to alleviate some of the stress in your scalp and temples.

HOW TO DO IT

- Sit or stand, keeping your neck, shoulders, and torso in a relaxed, neutral position.

- Place your palms on your temples. Slide your fingers open and then slightly back along your scalp.

- Relying mostly on your thumbs, grasp a handful of hair on either side of your head.

- Gently pull your hair away from your head until you feel slight tension on your scalp. Hold for the recommended time, release the stretch, and then repeat for the recommended repetitions.

DO IT RIGHT

- Keep your head steady.
- Practice this stretch on various symmetrical sections of your head.

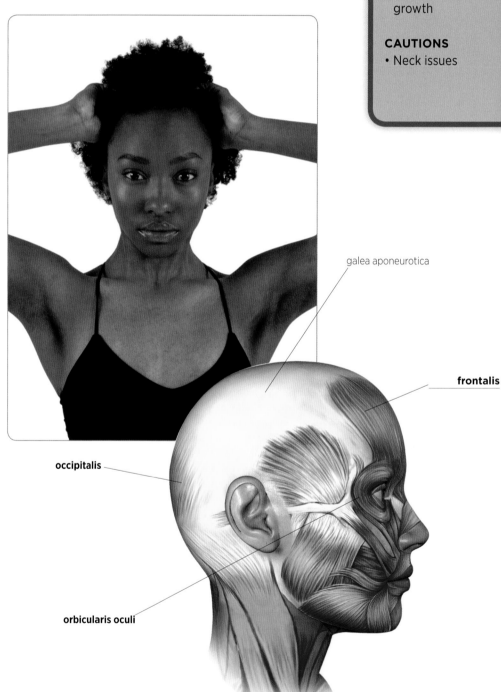

galea aponeurotica

frontalis

occipitalis

orbicularis oculi

FACT FILE

TARGETS
- Scalp
- Face

TYPE
- Static

BENEFITS
- Alleviates headaches
- Reduces tension
- Stimulates hair growth

CAUTIONS
- Neck issues

Annotation Key

Bold text indicates target muscles
Light text indicates other working muscles
* indicates deep muscles

Lion Stretch and Eye Box Stretch Combo

Spending endless hours staring at a screen can tire out your eyes and strain their supporting muscles. Revitalize these muscles and also tone your face with the Lion Stretch and Eye Box Stretch Combo. Don't worry about looking a little crazy while performing these fun exercises.

HOW TO DO IT

- Sit or stand, keeping your neck, shoulders, and torso in a relaxed, neutral position.

- To perform the Lion Stretch, raise both eyebrows as you try to lift your ears upward and backward.

- Open your mouth wide, and then place the tip of your tongue behind the back of your bottom teeth, flexing your tongue out as much as comfortably possible.

- Flare your nostrils wide. Hold this expression, and then release.

- To move into the Eye Box Stretch, look up toward the upper-right corner of your field of vision, and hold for a few seconds.

- Move your focus clockwise to the lower-right corner of your field of vision. Hold for a few seconds.

- Move your focus to the lower-left corner of your field of vision. Hold for a few seconds.

- Move your focus to the to the upper-left corner of your field of vision, hold for a few seconds, and then release the stretch.

TARGETS
- Face
- Neck
- Eyes
- Brows

TYPE
- Dynamic

BENEFITS
- Tones facial muscles
- Alleviates headaches
- Reduces facial and eye tension
- Promotes healthy skin
- Relieves tired eyes

CAUTIONS
- Neck issues

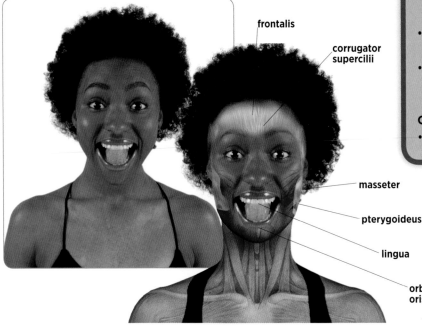

frontalis

corrugator supercilii

masseter

pterygoideus

lingua

orbicularis oris

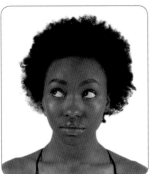
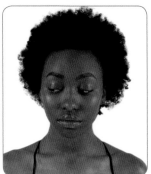
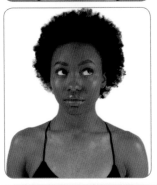
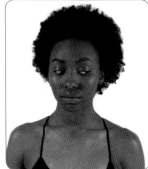

DO IT RIGHT

- Keep your head steady.
- Face forward.
- Exaggerate your facial expressions as much as possible.
- Direct your gaze as far in each direction as you can while performing the Eye Box Stretch.

Annotation Key

Bold text indicates target muscles
Light text indicates other working muscles
* indicates deep muscles

Cervical Stars

A simple but essential stretch to reduce cervical tightness and increase neck mobility. Cervical Stars effectively targets many different muscles around the neck bone.

HOW TO DO IT

• Sit or stand, keeping your neck, shoulders, and torso straight. Keeping your chin level, gaze straight ahead.

• Imagine that there is a star in front of you with a vertical line, a horizontal line, and two diagonal lines. Trace the star shape with your head and neck by following the vertical line up and down three times.

• Next, follow the horizontal line once.

• Finally, trace the two diagonal lines.

• Return to the starting position, and then repeat for the recommended repetitions.

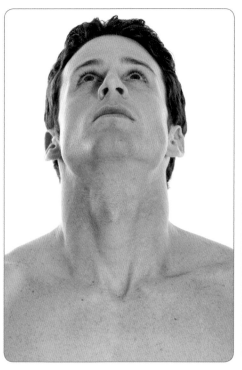
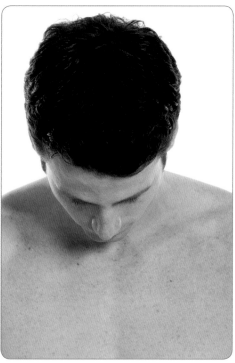
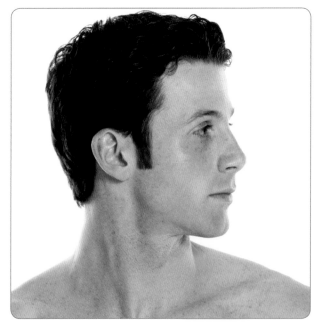
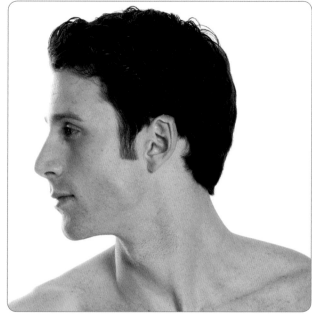

Bold text indicates target muscles
Light text indicates other working muscles
* indicates deep muscles

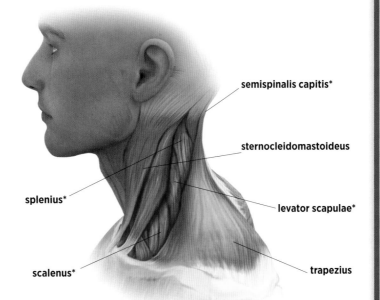

semispinalis capitis*

sternocleidomastoideus

splenius*

levator scapulae*

scalenus*

trapezius

DO IT RIGHT

- Move in a smooth, controlled manner.
- Avoid hunching or tensing your shoulders.

FACT FILE

TARGETS
- Neck rotators
- Neck flexors
- Neck extensors
- Neck lateral flexors

TYPE
- Static

BENEFITS
- Improves range of motion
- Relieves neck pain

CAUTIONS
- Numbness in arms or hands

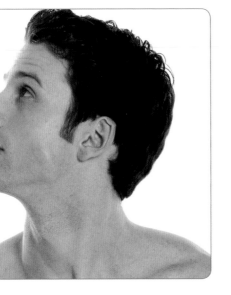

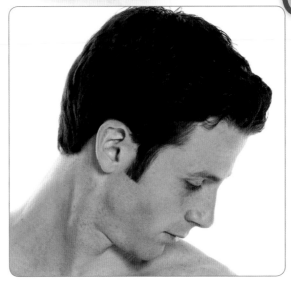

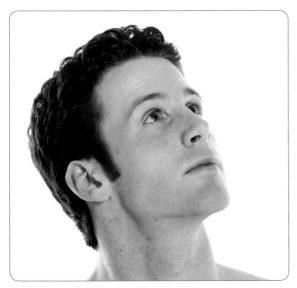

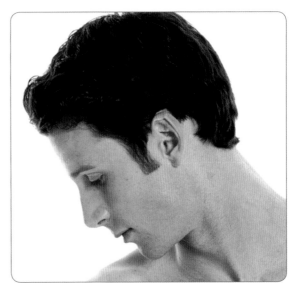

Flexion Stretch

There are two kinds of neck flexion. The first kind involves flexing the very deep muscles on the front of your neck to tuck your chin down. The second kind of flexion involves bending the whole neck forward from its base on top of the torso. Moves like the Flexion Stretch can help undo the neck stiffness that comes with a head-forward posture.

HOW TO DO IT
• Sit or stand, keeping your neck, shoulders, and torso straight. Place one or both hands behind your head.

• Slowly pull your chin toward your chest until you feel a stretch in the back of your neck.

• Hold for the recommended time, release the stretch, and then repeat for the recommended repetitions.

DO IT RIGHT
• Keep your opposite arm at your side.
• Let your gaze fall downward as you stretch.
• Move slowly and with control.
• Keep your back straight.
• Relax your shoulder muscles.
• Avoid pulling too hard with your hand.

FACT FILE
TARGETS
• Neck

TYPE
• Static

BENEFITS
• Improves range of motion
• Relieves neck pain
• Reduces tension in the shoulders and upper back

CAUTIONS
• Severe neck pain or numbness
• Spinal stenosis
• Numbness in arms or hands

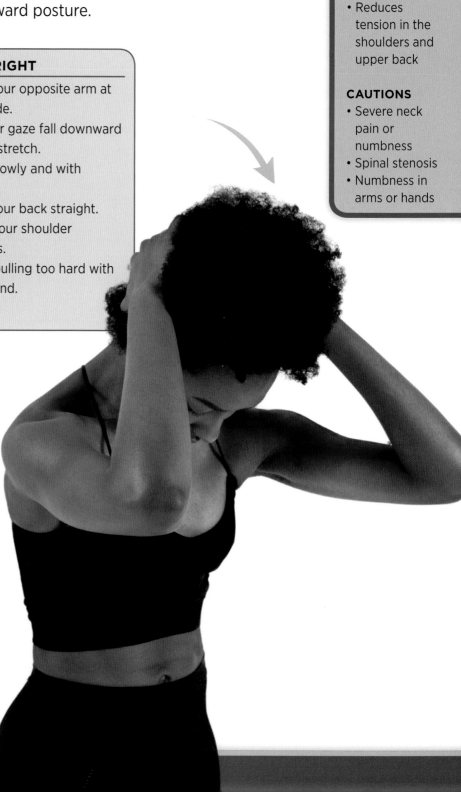

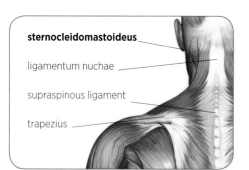

sternocleidomastoideus
ligamentum nuchae
supraspinous ligament
trapezius

Annotation Key
Bold text indicates target muscles
Light text indicates other working muscles
* indicates deep muscles

Flexion Isometric

This cervical stretch serves as a countermove to the Flexion Stretch (opposite). Isometric exercises serve to strengthen muscles without irritating ligaments, tendons, or joints.

HOW TO DO IT

- Sit or stand, keeping your neck, shoulders, and torso straight. Slightly flex your neck.

- Place your palm against your forehead, and gently push your forehead into your palm, holding the position static.

- Hold for the recommended time, release the stretch, and then repeat for the recommended repetitions.

DO IT RIGHT
- Apply only a gentle pressure.
- Avoid any movement in the neck.

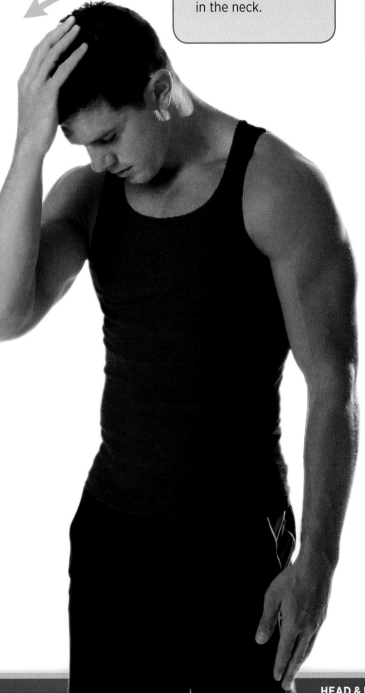

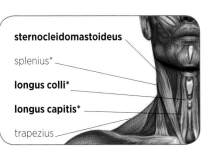

sternocleidomastoideus

splenius*

longus colli*

longus capitis*

trapezius

Annotation Key
Bold text indicates target muscles
Light text indicates other working muscles
* indicates deep muscles

Lateral Stretch

In the Lateral Stretch you move your neck from a straight position to a lateral bend in an action called lateral flexion. A group of muscles called the scalenes (or scalenus muscles) help make it happen.

HOW TO DO IT

• Sit or stand, keeping your neck, shoulders, and torso straight.

• Tilt your head down and to the side. Continue until right ear approaches your right shoulder and you feel a distinct stretch in the left side of your neck.

• Hold for the recommended time, release the stretch, and then repeat on the opposite side. Alternate sides for the recommended repetitions.

DO IT RIGHT

• Relax your shoulder muscles.
• Avoid rotating your head while tilting it.

FACT FILE

TARGETS
• Neck lateral flexors

TYPE
• Static

BENEFITS
• Improves range of motion
• Relieves neck pain

CAUTIONS
• Numbness in arms or hands

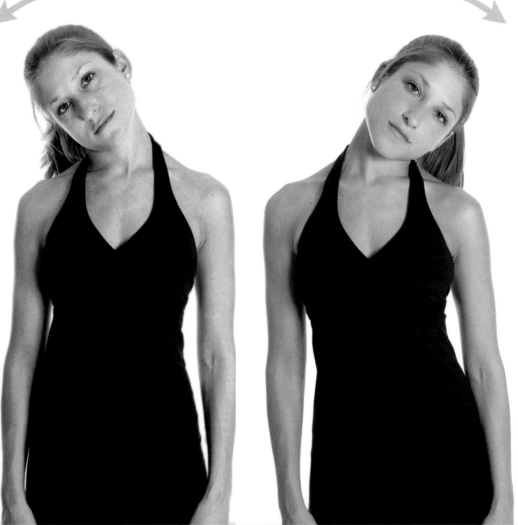

rectus capitis lateralis*

rectus capitis*

sternocleidomastoideus

scalenus*

trapezius

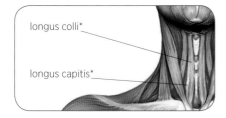

longus colli*

longus capitis*

Annotation Key
Bold text indicates target muscles
Light text indicates other working muscles
* indicates deep muscles

Lateral Isometric

This stretch helps you maintain or regain cervical mobility simply by applying pressure while you move your neck through its normal movements. Perform this stretch slowly and gently to ease and release the top of your shoulders and lower-neck muscles.

HOW TO DO IT

- Sit or stand, keeping your neck, shoulders, and torso straight. Place the palm of your right hand on the top of your head.

- Reach toward the small of your back with your left hand, bending your arm at the elbow.

- Tilt your head toward your raised elbow until you feel the stretch in the side of your neck.

- Press your head into the palm of your hand as you try to tilt your ear to your shoulder.

- Hold for the recommended time, release the stretch, and then repeat on the opposite side. Alternate sides for the recommended repetitions.

DO IT RIGHT

- Apply only a gentle pressure.
- Avoid any movement in the neck.

FACT FILE

TARGETS
- Neck lateral flexors

TYPE
- Isometric

BENEFITS
- Strengthens the lateral flexors

CAUTIONS
- Numbness in arms or hands

Annotation Key

Bold text indicates target muscles
Light text indicates other working muscles
* indicates deep muscles

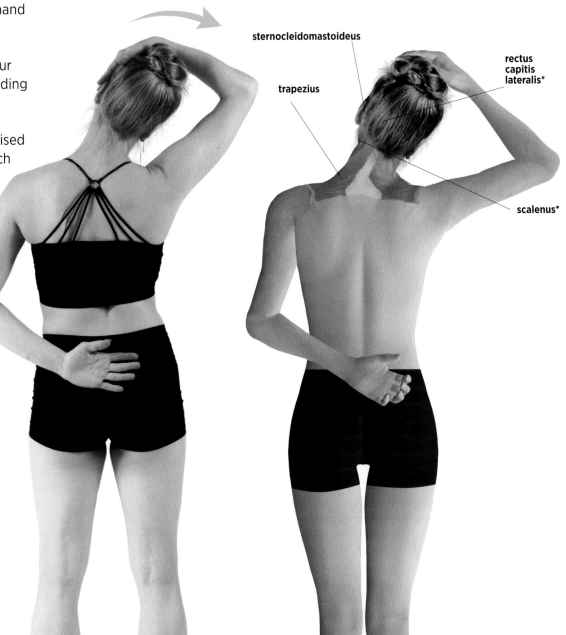

sternocleidomastoideus

trapezius

rectus capitis lateralis*

scalenus*

Rotation Stretch

The Rotation Stretch warms up the small muscles that are involved in head movement and stability. Applying very light pressure with your palm can provide a more effective stretch.

HOW TO DO IT

- Sit or stand, keeping your neck, shoulders, and torso straight.

- Place your right palm against your left temple.

- Turn your head slowly to the right, pushing gently until you feel a stretch in the left side of your neck.

- Hold for the recommended time, release the stretch, and then repeat on the opposite side. Alternate sides for the recommended repetitions.

DO IT RIGHT

- Relax your shoulder muscles.
- Keep your head in a neutral position.
- Avoid pushing too hard with your hand.

FACT FILE

TARGETS
- Neck rotators

TYPE
- Static

BENEFITS
- Improves range of motion
- Relieves neck pain

CAUTIONS
- Numbness in arms, hands, or wrists
- Severe neck or back pain

Annotation Key

Bold text indicates target muscles
Light text indicates other working muscles
* indicates deep muscles

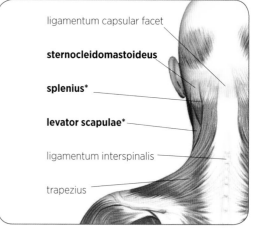

ligamentum capsular facet

sternocleidomastoideus

splenius*

levator scapulae*

ligamentum interspinalis

trapezius

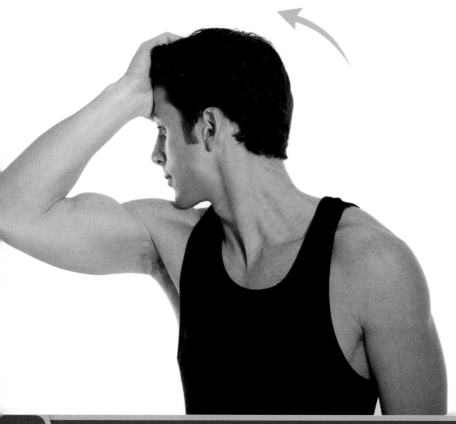

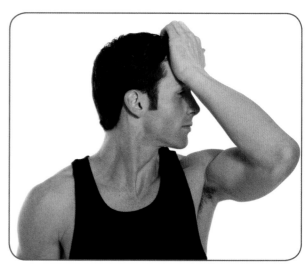

Rotation Isometric

When you engage in isometric neck exercises, such as the Rotation Isometric, you will increase the strength of the muscles of your neck, without using excessive pressure. Perform them regularly to build strength in your cervical spine, which is one of the areas most vulnerable to damage.

FACT FILE

TARGETS
• Neck rotators

TYPE
• Isometric

BENEFITS
• Strengthens the rotary muscles of the neck

CAUTIONS
• Numbness in arms, hands, or wrists
• Severe neck or back pain

HOW TO DO IT

• Sit or stand, keeping your neck, shoulders, and torso straight. Keeping your chin level, gaze straight ahead.

• Place your left palm against your left temple, and press into your palm as if you were turning your head to the left.

• Hold for the recommended time, release the stretch, and then repeat on the opposite side. Alternate sides for the recommended repetitions.

DO IT RIGHT
• Apply only a gentle pressure.
• Avoid any movement in the neck.

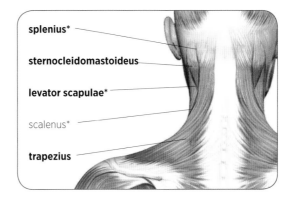

splenius*
sternocleidomastoideus
levator scapulae*
scalenus*
trapezius

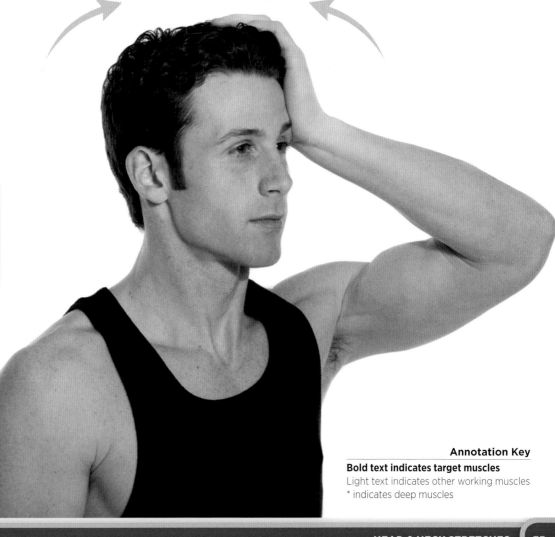

Annotation Key
Bold text indicates target muscles
Light text indicates other working muscles
* indicates deep muscles

Extension Stretch

The Extensions Stretch provides a mild stretching exercise that can help loosen postural muscles. It may also reduce neck pain without putting excessive pressure on your cervical spine.

FACT FILE

TARGETS
• Neck extensors

TYPE
• Static

BENEFITS
• Improves range of motion
• Relieves neck pain

CAUTIONS
• Numbness in arms, hands, or wrists
• Severe neck or back pain

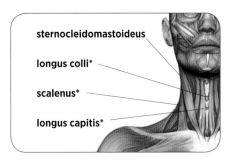

sternocleidomastoideus

longus colli*

scalenus*

longus capitis*

Annotation Key

Bold text indicates target muscles
Light text indicates other working muscles
* indicates deep muscles

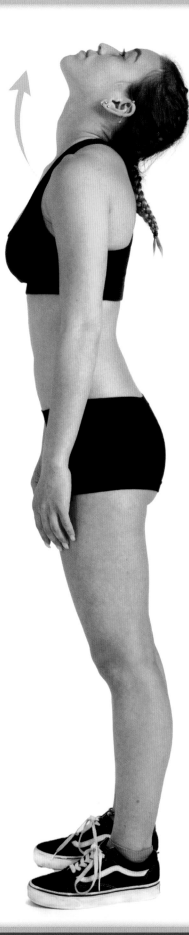

HOW TO DO IT

• Sit or stand, keeping your neck, shoulders, and torso straight. Keeping your chin level, gaze straight ahead.

• Gently bend your head backward to gaze upward toward the ceiling. Stop when you feel a stretch in the front of your neck.

• Hold for the recommended time, and then release.

DO IT RIGHT
• Relax your shoulder muscles.
• Avoid rotating your head while tilting it back.

Extension Isometric

This isometric stretch targets the hard-to-isolate muscles in the back of the neck. Pressing gently against your palm engages the muscles down the back of your neck and into the top of the cervical spine.

HOW TO DO IT

• Sit or stand, keeping your neck, shoulders, and torso straight. Keeping your chin level, gaze straight ahead.

• Clasp your hands together and place them behind your head.

• Press the back of your head into your palms.

• Hold for the recommended time, release the stretch, and then repeat for the recommended repetitions.

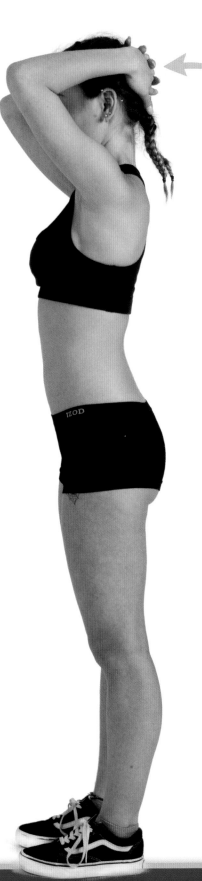

DO IT RIGHT

• Apply only a gentle pressure.
• Avoid any movement in the neck.

FACT FILE

TARGETS
• Neck extensors

TYPE
• Isometric

BENEFITS
• Strengthens the neck extensors

CAUTIONS
• Numbness in arms, hands, or wrists
• Severe neck or back pain

Upper-Trapezius Stretch

The trapezius muscles are responsible for moving and rotating your shoulder blades, stabilizing your arms, and extending your neck. To relieve tension in these muscles, you must engage your shoulder, neck, and upper back.

HOW TO DO IT

- Sit on a Swiss ball with your feet shoulder-width apart.

- Reach your left hand down the side of the ball, spreading your palm against the lower part of the ball.

- With your right hand, grasp the left side of your head. Tilt your head to the right, as if you were going to touch your right ear to your right shoulder.

- Hold for the recommended time, release the stretch, and then repeat on the opposite side. Alternate sides for the recommended repetitions.

DO IT RIGHT

- Firmly grasp the side of the ball to depress your shoulder blade.
- Avoid dropping your head forward or backward.

FACT FILE

TARGETS
- Upper trapezius

TYPE
- Static

BENEFITS
- Increases range of motion

CAUTIONS
- Neck issues

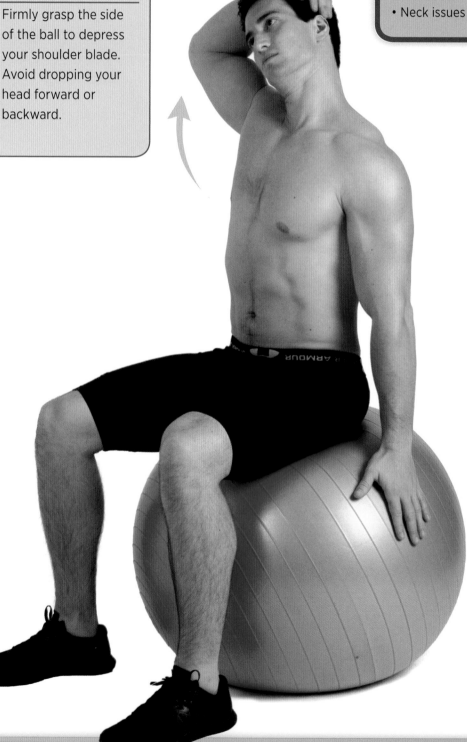

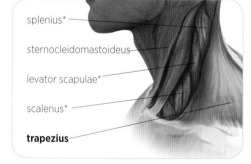

splenius*

sternocleidomastoideus

levator scapulae*

scalenus*

trapezius

Annotation Key
Bold text indicates target muscles
Light text indicates other working muscles
* indicates deep muscles

Levator Scapulae Stretch

The levator scapulae, a deep muscle, runs between the upper part of the shoulder blades and the top four cervical vertebrae. Bad posture shortens this muscle, raising the shoulder or the shoulder girdle. Lengthen this muscle by performing this ball stretch.

HOW TO DO IT

- Sit on a Swiss ball with your feet shoulder-width apart.

- Reach your right hand down the side of the ball, spreading your palm against the lower part of the ball.

- With your left hand, grasp the posterior right side of your head. Pull your chin in toward your lateral upper chest until you feel tension from the tip of your shoulder blade to the right side of your neck.

- Hold for the recommended time, release the stretch, and then repeat on the opposite side. Alternate sides for the recommended repetitions.

DO IT RIGHT
- Firmly grasp the side of the ball to depress your shoulder blade.
- Try multiple angles to find tight muscle fibers.
- Avoid excessive lateral flexion.

FACT FILE

TARGETS
- Levator scapulae

TYPE
- Static

BENEFITS
- Increases range of motion

CAUTIONS
- Neck issues

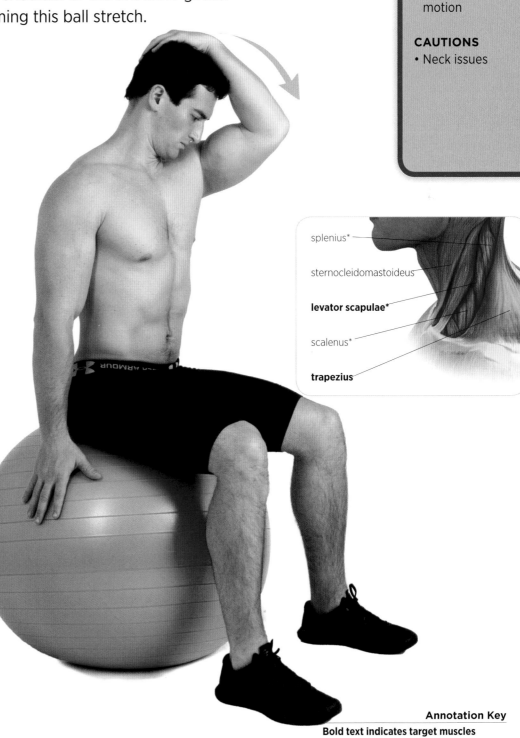

splenius*

sternocleidomastoideus

levator scapulae*

scalenus*

trapezius

Annotation Key
Bold text indicates target muscles
Light text indicates other working muscles
* indicates deep muscles

Turtle Neck

A group of muscles known as the neck flexors, which includes the sternocleidomastoid, is responsible for rotating and tilting the head to the side. The Turtle Neck stretch is an effective means of strengthening these important muscles.

HOW TO DO IT

- Sit or stand, keeping your neck, shoulders, and torso straight. Keeping your chin level, look straight ahead.

- Move your chin in as if you were a turtle drawing back into its shell until you feel a stretch in the back of your neck.

- Extend your head forward, this time as if you were a turtle coming out of its shell.

- Hold for the recommended time, release the stretch, and then repeat for the recommended repetitions.

DO IT RIGHT
- Move in a smooth, controlled manner.
- Avoid lifting your chin as you move your head back.

FACT FILE

TARGETS
- Neck flexors

TYPE
- Static

BENEFITS
- Improves range of motion
- Corrects forward head protrusion

CAUTIONS
- Numbness in arms or hands

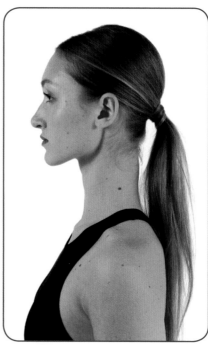
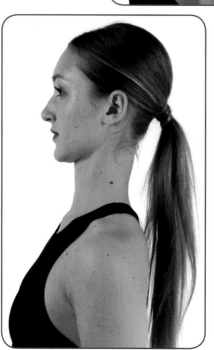
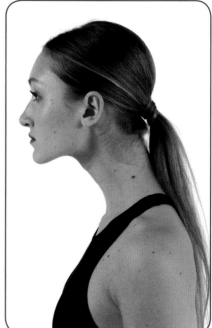
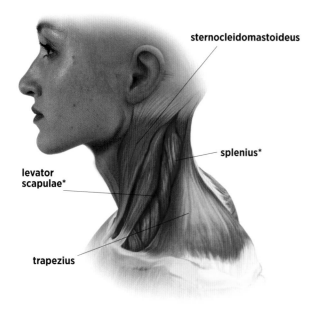

sternocleidomastoideus
splenius*
levator scapulae*
trapezius

Annotation Key
Bold text indicates target muscles
Light text indicates other working muscles
* indicates deep muscles

Shrug

It might seem like we shrug all the time, but purposefully engaging the shrug muscles can be an effective means to strengthen the neck, upper back, and shoulders.

HOW TO DO IT

- Sit on a Swiss ball or chair. Keep your back straight and your head and neck centered over the rest of your spinal column.

- With your arms at your sides, bend your elbows slightly. Hold your hands with the palms up.

- Bring your shoulders down and forward, and then lift them as high as you can.

- Return the starting position, and then repeat for the recommended repetitions.

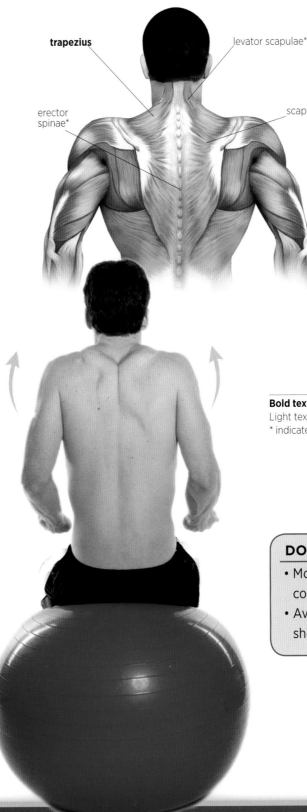

trapezius

levator scapulae*

erector spinae*

scapula

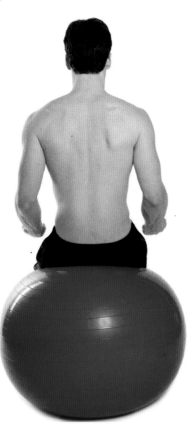

FACT FILE

TARGETS
- Neck
- Shoulders
- Scapulae

TYPE
- Dynamic

BENEFITS
- Improves range of motion.
- Relaxes tight neck, shoulder, chest, and upper-back muscles
- Stabilizes your shoulder blades

CAUTIONS
- Numbness in arms or hands
- Severe shoulder or spinal pain

Annotation Key

Bold text indicates target muscles
Light text indicates other working muscles
* indicates deep muscles

DO IT RIGHT
- Move in a smooth, controlled manner.
- Avoid rolling your shoulders.

High Plank Pike

The High Plank Pike is a challenging exercise that lengthens the spine by extending the space between each vertebrae, alleviating spinal compression. This rejuvenating inversion also improves circulation and reduces neck tension.

HOW TO DO IT

• Begin in a high plank position, with your hands planted on the floor shoulder-width apart, your arms straight, and your body lifted off the floor to form a straight line. Your feet should be parallel, with heels lifted.

• Lift your hips, forming an inverted V-position. Let your head drop, so that your gaze is out behind your legs.

• Hold for the recommended time, pushing into the stretch in your neck and upper back. Release the stretch, and slowly let your hips drop back down to a high plank position. Repeat for the recommended repetitions.

DO IT RIGHT

• Keep your spine straight.
• Engage your abdominals.
• Lengthen your hamstrings and calves.
• Control the pace of the movement, breathing rhythmically.
• Avoid tensing your shoulders.

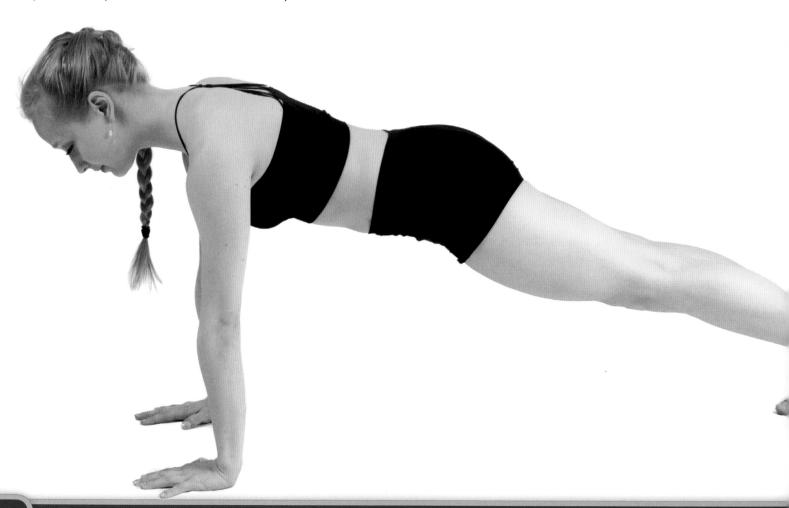

TARGETS
• Spine
• Shoulders
• Middle back

TYPE
• Static

BENEFITS
• Relaxes tight neck, shoulder, chest, and upper-back muscles
• Improves coordination and balance.
• Builds core strength
• Increases flexibility

CAUTIONS
• Back pain

Annotation Key
Bold text indicates target muscles
Light text indicates other working muscles
* indicates deep muscles

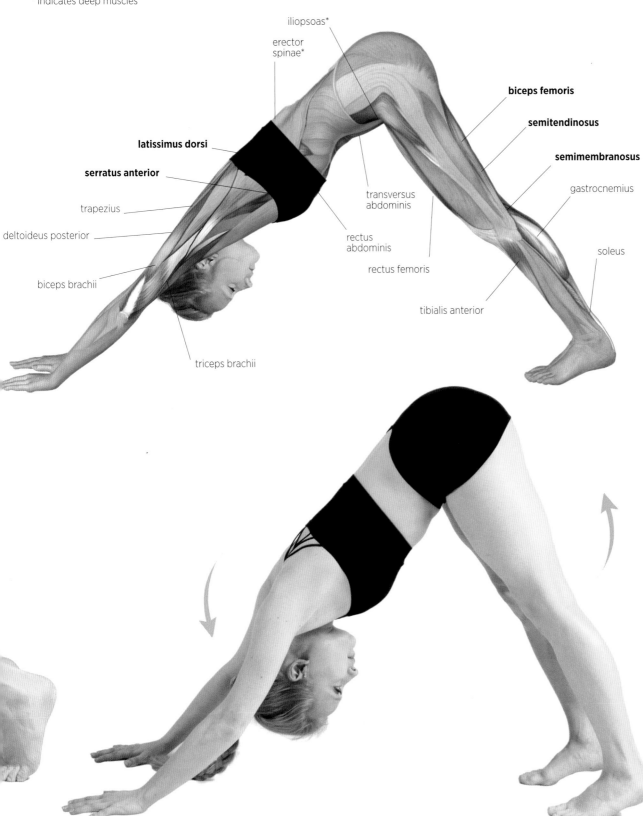

iliopsoas*

erector spinae*

biceps femoris

semitendinosus

semimembranosus

latissimus dorsi

serratus anterior

gastrocnemius

trapezius

transversus abdominis

deltoideus posterior

rectus abdominis

soleus

biceps brachii

rectus femoris

tibialis anterior

triceps brachii

CHAPTER TWO

ARMS, SHOULDERS, & UPPER-BACK STRETCHES

The muscles in your shoulders, arms, and upper back are key to mobility and posture, and are always at work, whether you are in motion or sitting still. They are also common targets for localized muscle pain, tightness, and discomfort. Regularly performing stretches that target these areas can help improve mobility throughout the whole body, as well as improve overall range-of-motion and physical health.

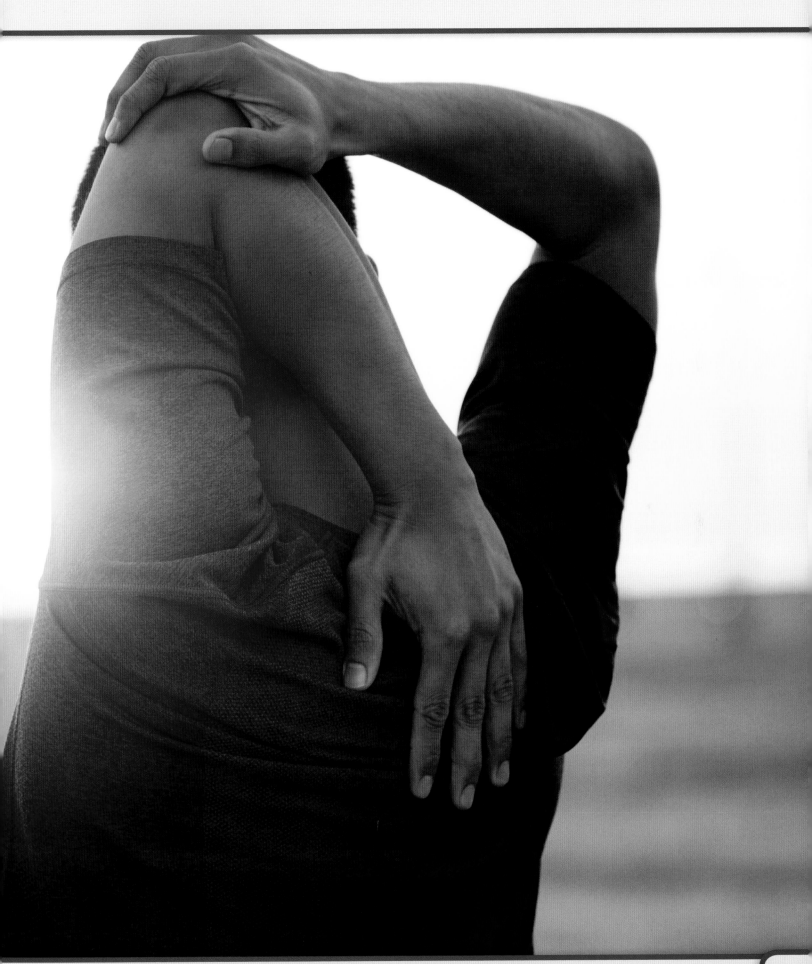

Good Morning Stretch

Perform this invigorating stretch first thing in the morning. It will engage your core and lengthen your spine while relieving any tension in your shoulders and upper back that may result from a bad night's sleep.

HOW TO DO IT

- Stand with your legs and feet parallel and shoulder-width apart. Bend your knees very slightly, and tuck your pelvis slightly forward.

- Reach your arms up toward the ceiling, keeping them long and in parallel with your body. Focus your energy on the middle of your palms, which should be facing inward, and turn your gaze upward as you stretch.

- Hold for the recommended time, release the stretch, and then repeat for the recommended repetitions.

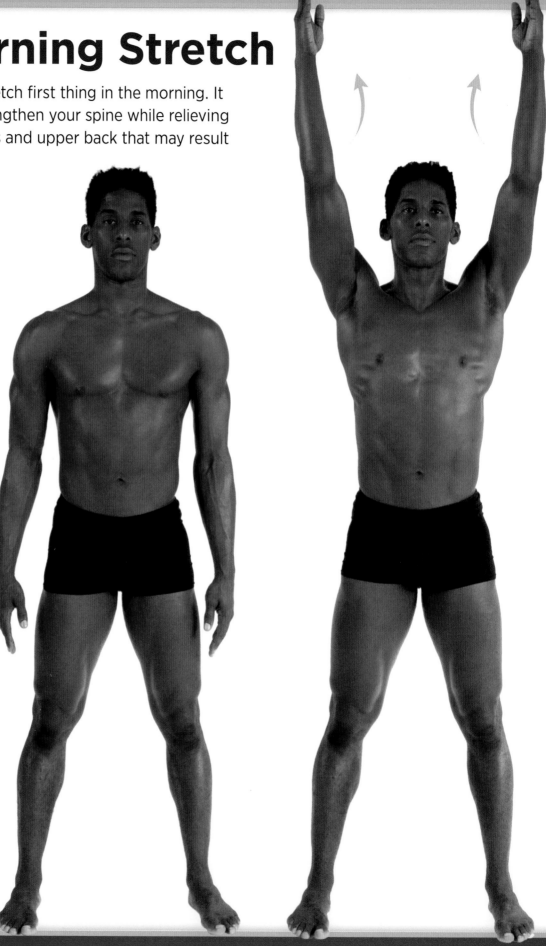

TARGETS
• Back
• Neck
• Abdominals
• Obliques
• Palms
• Forearms
• Upper arms

TYPE
• Static

BENEFITS
• Increases upper-back mobility
• Reduces shoulder tightness
• Lengthens spinal column

CAUTIONS
• Neck issues
• Shoulder issues

Annotation Key

Bold text indicates target muscles
Light text indicates other working muscles
* indicates deep muscles

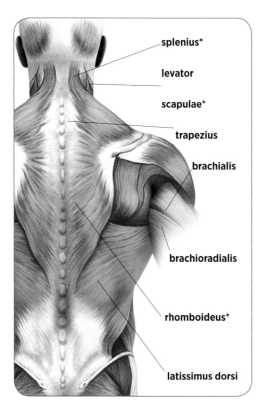

splenius*

levator

scapulae*

trapezius

brachialis

brachioradialis

rhomboideus*

latissimus dorsi

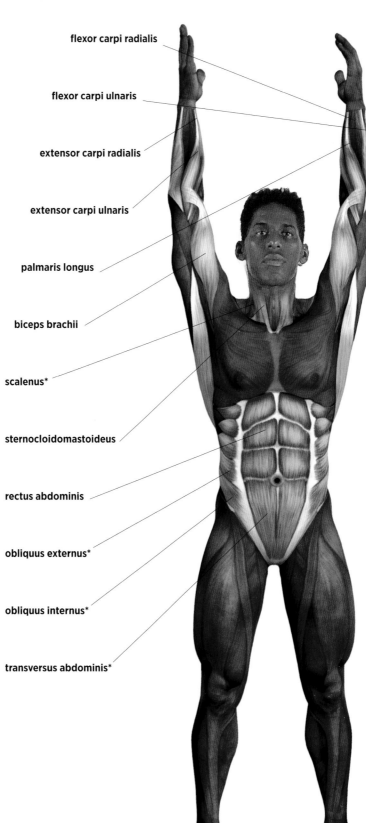

flexor carpi radialis

flexor carpi ulnaris

extensor carpi radialis

extensor carpi ulnaris

palmaris longus

biceps brachii

scalenus*

sternocloidomastoideus

rectus abdominis

obliquus externus*

obliquus internus*

transversus abdominis*

DO IT RIGHT
• Keep your elbows slightly bent.
• Tuck your pelvis.
• Avoid hyperextending either your lower back or elbows.

Chair Yoga Stretch

This stretch, known as Chair Pose in the discipline of yoga, will increase your strength, balance, and stability while activating just about every muscle in your body. It calls for you to sustain an unsupported sitting position as you extend your arms and engage the muscles in your shoulders and upper back.

HOW TO DO IT

- Stand with your feet together and arms by your sides.

- Inhale as you reach your arms out to your sides, and continue lifting until you are standing with your arms above your head. Your hands should be shoulder-width apart.

- Straighten your arms, and rotate your shoulders externally open so that the palms of your hands face each other, spreading up through your fingertips.

- Exhale, and bend your knees. Both ankles, inner thighs, and knees should be touching. Bring your weight onto your heels, shift your hips back, and draw your knees right above your ankles.

- Hold for the recommended time, release the stretch, and then repeat for the recommended repetitions.

DO IT RIGHT

- Keep your feet together.
- Keep your heels on the floor.
- Avoid overtucking your pelvis.
- Avoid overarching your lower back.
- Avoid knocking your knees inward.

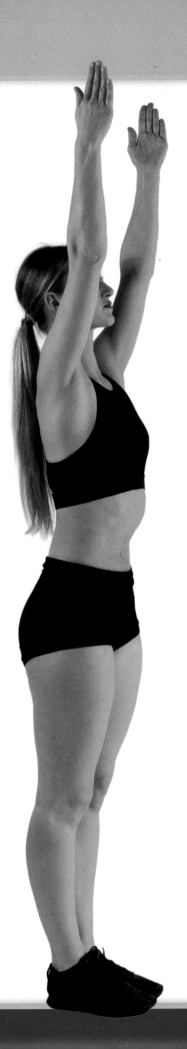

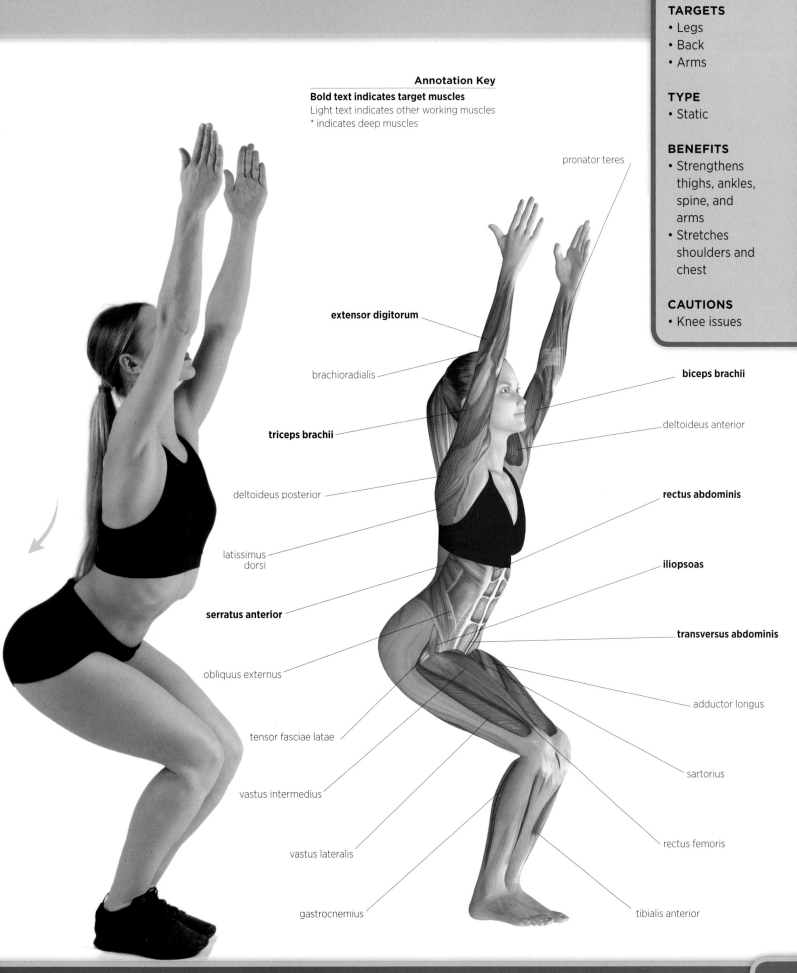

TARGETS
• Legs
• Back
• Arms

TYPE
• Static

BENEFITS
• Strengthens thighs, ankles, spine, and arms
• Stretches shoulders and chest

CAUTIONS
• Knee issues

Annotation Key

Bold text indicates target muscles
Light text indicates other working muscles
* indicates deep muscles

pronator teres

extensor digitorum

brachioradialis

biceps brachii

deltoideus anterior

triceps brachii

deltoideus posterior

rectus abdominis

latissimus dorsi

iliopsoas

serratus anterior

transversus abdominis

obliquus externus

adductor longus

tensor fasciae latae

sartorius

vastus intermedius

vastus lateralis

rectus femoris

gastrocnemius

tibialis anterior

Twisting Chair Stretch

This stretch takes the Chair Yoga Stretch a step further, challenging your sense of balance while stretching your spine, shoulders, and chest. The Twisting Chair Stretch uses just about every muscle in your body, but particularly works to strengthen your thighs, glutes, and hips.

HOW TO DO IT

- Begin in the Chair Yoga Stretch (pages 48–49), with your arms parallel to each other above your head and your knees bent deeply.

- Inhale as you lengthen your spine, and join your hands in a prayer position in front of your heart.

- Keep your hips square as you exhale and twist to the right, bringing your left elbow to the outside of your right thigh. Press your left elbow into your right knee and your knee into your elbow.

- Inhale to lengthen your spine, letting your belly move outward, and then exhale to twist as your navel draws strongly back toward your spine.

- Hold for the recommended time, and then inhale as you return to the center, reaching your arms upward. Repeat on the other side.

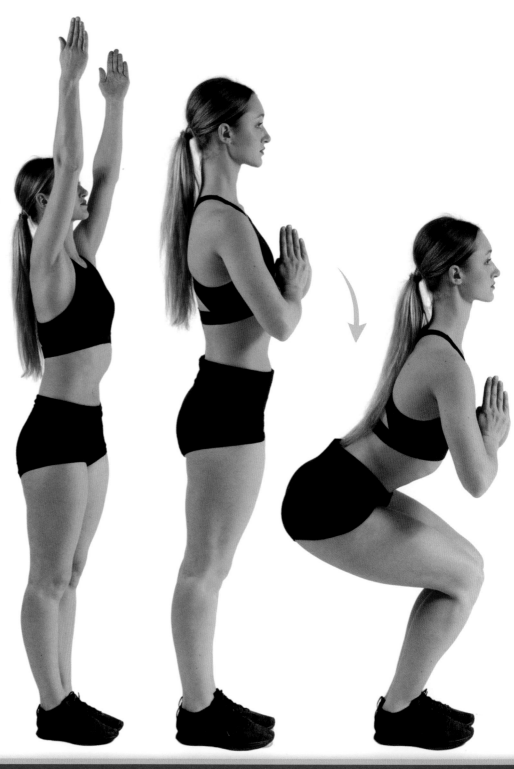

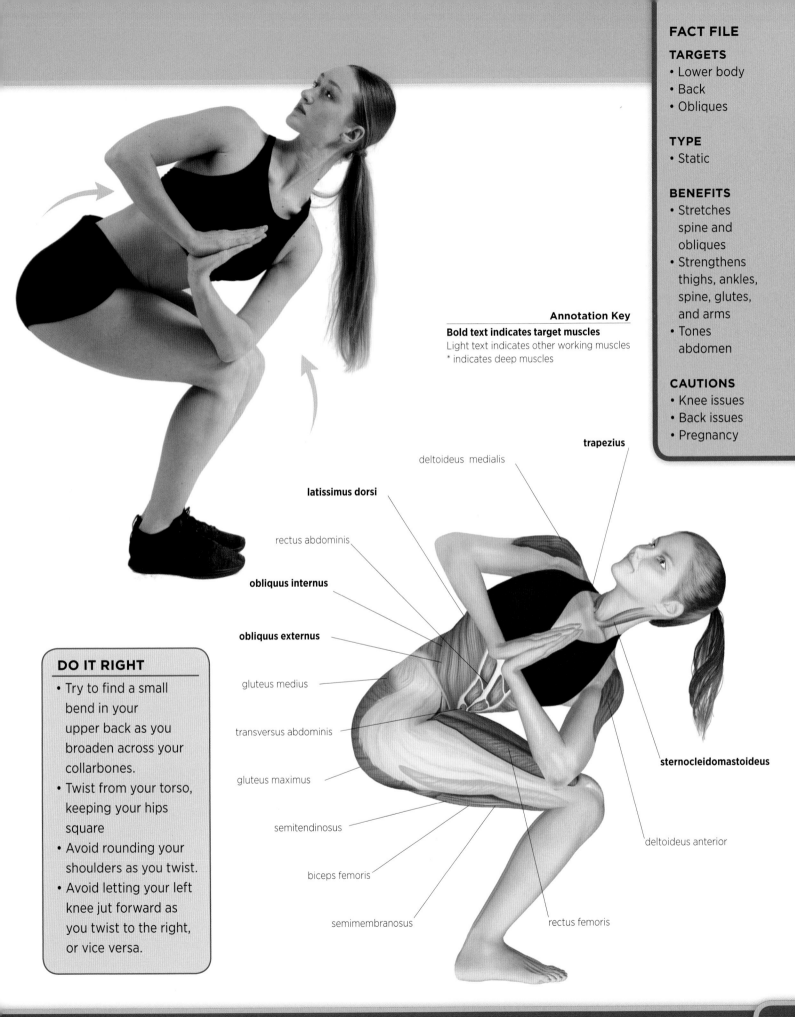

TARGETS
• Lower body
• Back
• Obliques

TYPE
• Static

BENEFITS
• Stretches spine and obliques
• Strengthens thighs, ankles, spine, glutes, and arms
• Tones abdomen

CAUTIONS
• Knee issues
• Back issues
• Pregnancy

Annotation Key
Bold text indicates target muscles
Light text indicates other working muscles
* indicates deep muscles

trapezius

deltoideus medialis

latissimus dorsi

rectus abdominis

obliquus internus

obliquus externus

gluteus medius

transversus abdominis

gluteus maximus

semitendinosus

biceps femoris

semimembranosus

sternocleidomastoideus

deltoideus anterior

rectus femoris

DO IT RIGHT
• Try to find a small bend in your upper back as you broaden across your collarbones.
• Twist from your torso, keeping your hips square
• Avoid rounding your shoulders as you twist.
• Avoid letting your left knee jut forward as you twist to the right, or vice versa.

Warrior III Yoga Stretch

Warrior III is a standing yoga pose that provides an effective arm, shoulder, and upper-back stretch. It also tones your abdominals and creates stability throughout your entire body by engaging muscles in your core, arms, and legs.

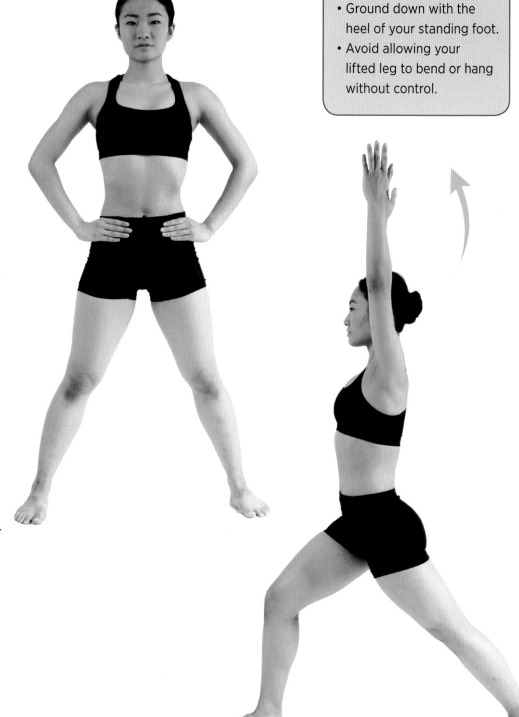

DO IT RIGHT

- Keep your hips squared.
- Keep length in your spine as you extend from your fingertips to your lifted heel.
- Energize your lifted leg to help you find balance.
- Ground down with the heel of your standing foot.
- Avoid allowing your lifted leg to bend or hang without control.

HOW TO DO IT

- Stand in the middle of a mat with your feet together and arms at your sides. Step your right foot forward about 12 inches.

- Extend your arms over your head, keeping them parallel to each other. Lift your left heel upward, shifting your weight onto the ball of your right foot.

- Square your hips to the front of the mat, drawing your right hip back and your left hip forward. Keeping your arms extended over your head, hinge your torso forward over your right thigh.

- Continue to shift your weight onto your right leg as you lift your left leg to hip height, foot flexed. Your arms and left leg should be parallel to the floor.

- Hold for the recommended time, release the stretch, and then repeat for the recommended repetitions.

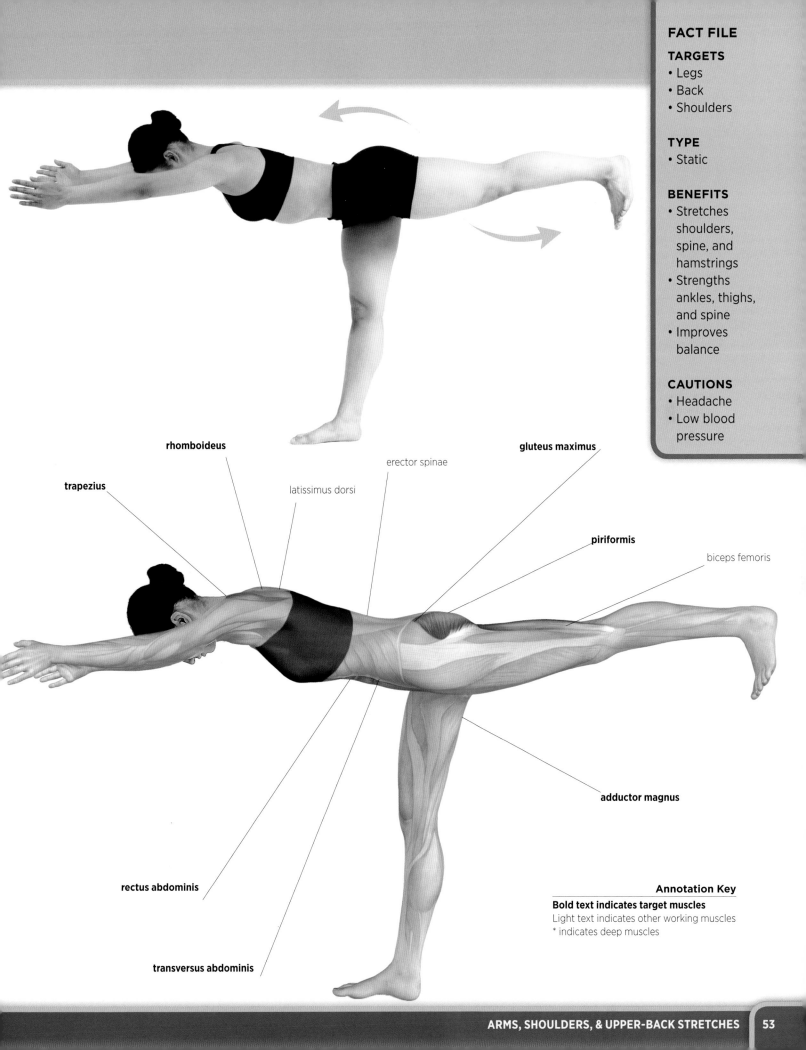

FACT FILE

TARGETS
• Legs
• Back
• Shoulders

TYPE
• Static

BENEFITS
• Stretches shoulders, spine, and hamstrings
• Strengths ankles, thighs, and spine
• Improves balance

CAUTIONS
• Headache
• Low blood pressure

rhomboideus

gluteus maximus

erector spinae

trapezius

latissimus dorsi

piriformis

biceps femoris

rectus abdominis

adductor magnus

Annotation Key
Bold text indicates target muscles
Light text indicates other working muscles
* indicates deep muscles

transversus abdominis

Upward Salute

This seemingly simple exercise targets your shoulders and upper back and, to a lesser degree, your chest, neck, biceps, forearms, triceps, middle back, and lower back. It is an effective stretch that pulls along the length of your body, from your heels to your fingertips.

HOW TO DO IT

• Stand tall with your arms at your sides and your spine straight.

• Inhale as you reach your arms out to your sides, and continue lifting them until you are standing with your arms above your head. Your hands should be shoulder-width apart.

• Straighten your arms, and rotate your shoulders externally open so that the palms of your hands face each other, spreading up through your fingertips. Gaze forward.

• Hold for the recommended time, release the stretch, and then repeat for the recommended repetitions.

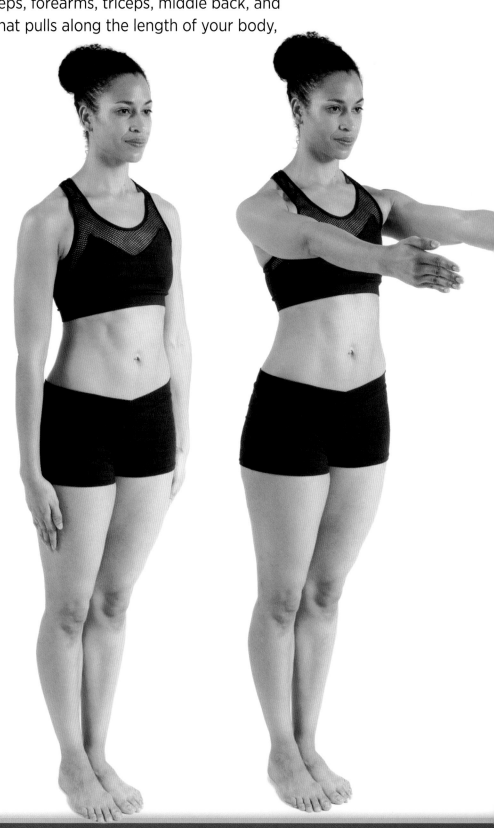

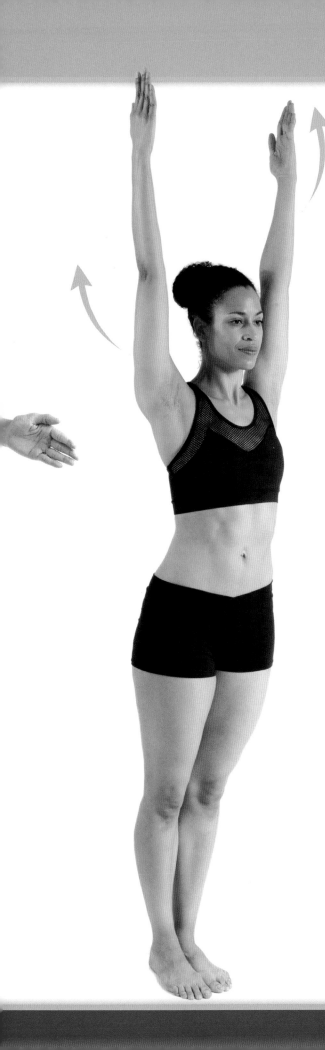

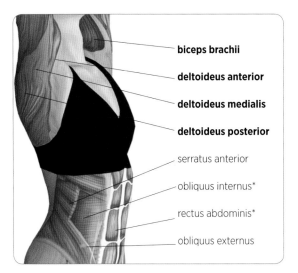

biceps brachii

deltoideus anterior

deltoideus medialis

deltoideus posterior

serratus anterior

obliquus internus*

rectus abdominis*

obliquus externus

Annotation Key
Bold text indicates target muscles
Light text indicates other working muscles
* indicates deep muscles

TARGETS
• Entire body

TYPE
• Static

BENEFITS
• Offers a full-body stretch, especially the arms, shoulders, and belly
• Alleviates backache
• Improves posture

CAUTIONS
• Shoulder issues
• Back issues
• Neck issues

DO IT RIGHT

• Stretch your arms completely straight from your elbows.
• Soften any tension in your shoulders.
• Avoid tensing your shoulders up toward your ears.

Standing Back Roll

The Standing Back Roll is a great stretch to include in your flexibility workouts, providing an easy, flowing movement from a standing forward bend to an upright posture. On its own, it is a dynamic upper-back stretch that effectively reduces tightness and tension in the rhomboid muscles.

HOW TO DO IT

- Stand with your legs and feet parallel and shoulder-width apart. Bend your knees very slightly.

- Slowly round your spine downward, from your neck through your lower back, and lower your arms down the sides of your legs. Continue bending at the waist, letting the weight of your body draw your head toward the floor as you stretch.

- Slowly roll up halfway to the point at which you feel your gluteal muscles above your hips and thighs.

- Cross your forearms to place your hands on the opposite thighs, and round your shoulders forward. Feel the heaviness of your head as you stretch your upper back between the shoulder blades.

- Slowly rise to the starting position, and then repeat for the recommended repetitions.

DO IT RIGHT

- Keep your knees slightly bent.
- Tuck your pelvis forward slightly, allowing your upper body to contract.
- Avoid allowing your knees to turn inward.

FACT FILE

TARGETS
- Upper back
- Middle back

TYPE
- Dynamic

BENEFITS
- Increases upper-back mobility
- Reduces shoulder tightness
- Lengthens spinal column

CAUTIONS
- Spinal injury
- Shoulder issues
- Hip issues

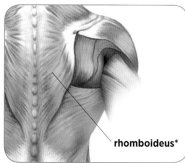

rhomboideus*

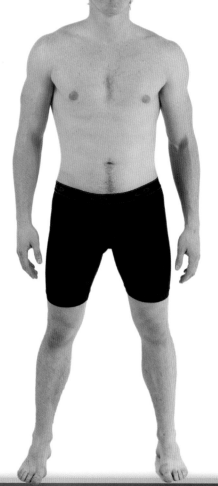

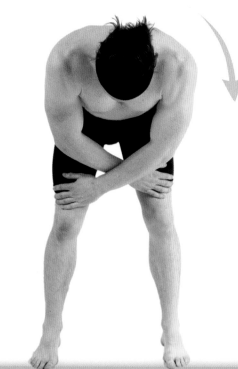

Annotation Key
Bold text indicates target muscles
Light text indicates other working muscles
* indicates deep muscles

Scoop Rhomboids

Located in the middle of the back, the rhomboid muscles retract your shoulder blades. These deep muscles are phasic, meaning they weaken with disuse. This upper-back and shoulder stretch will reduce tension in the shoulder blades, while keeping the rhomboids healthy and engaged.

HOW TO DO IT

- Sit up tall with your legs extended in front of you. Bend your knees slightly, keeping your heels on the floor, and then grasp your legs behind your knees.

- Keeping your chin down, round your upper back down as you lean back toward the floor.

- Hold for the recommended time, and then slowly roll back up to the starting position. Repeat for the recommended repetitions.

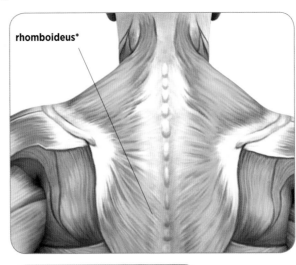

rhomboideus*

DO IT RIGHT

- Exhale as you round your upper back and lean backward.
- Avoid holding your breath.

FACT FILE

TARGETS
- Upper Back

TYPE
- Static

BENEFITS
- Increases upper-back mobility
- Reduces shoulder tightness
- Lengthens spinal column

CAUTIONS
- Shoulder issues
- Back issues

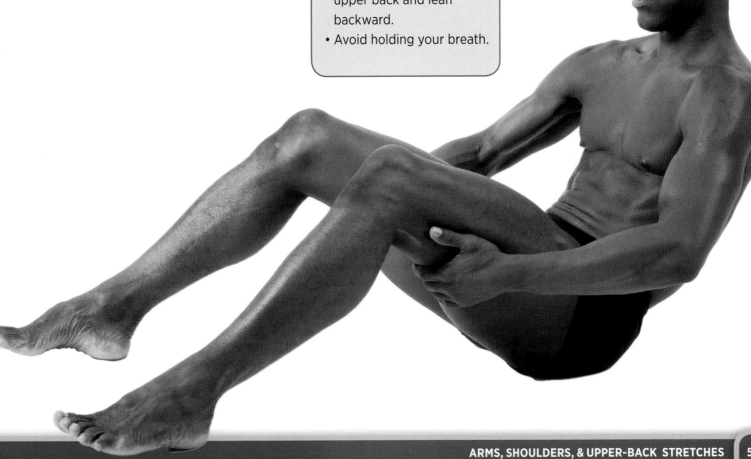

Cow Face Yoga Stretch

In yoga, Cow Face is a seated pose that targets both your hips and shoulders. It is a multipurpose stretch that engages the back of your arms, rotator cuffs, upper back, glutes, hip rotators, and chest muscles. Even without incorporating the leg position, it is still a highly effective shoulder and upper-back stretch.

HOW TO DO IT

• Sit up tall with your legs together and extended in front of you. Bend your left knee, and then cross your left leg over your right, positioning your legs so that they cross at the inner thighs.

• Bend your right leg to stack your thighs one on top of the other. Draw your shins and heels slightly forward.

• Reach your right arm out to the right, parallel to the floor. Turn your hand to face the ceiling, externally rotate your arm, and reach up by your ear. Bend your elbow so that it points toward the ceiling as your fingers point down your spine.

• Reach your left arm out to the left, parallel to the floor, internally rotating it and allowing your hand to face behind you with your thumb pointing downward. Bend your arm, pointing your elbow toward the floor, and bring your hand behind your back, palm away from your body and fingers pointing up the spine.

• Bring your hands toward each other, clasp them together, and hold for the recommended time. Release the stretch, and repeat on the other side.

DO IT RIGHT

• Position your feet so that both are the same distance from your hips.
• If your hips are uneven when you are sitting on the floor, sit on top of a block or a blanket.
• If your hands don't reach each other right away, try using a strap or band.
• Draw your elbows in opposite directions as you hold the stretch.
• Keep your head straight and gaze forward.

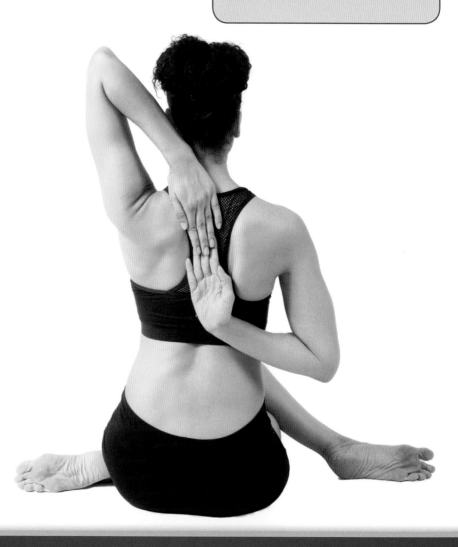

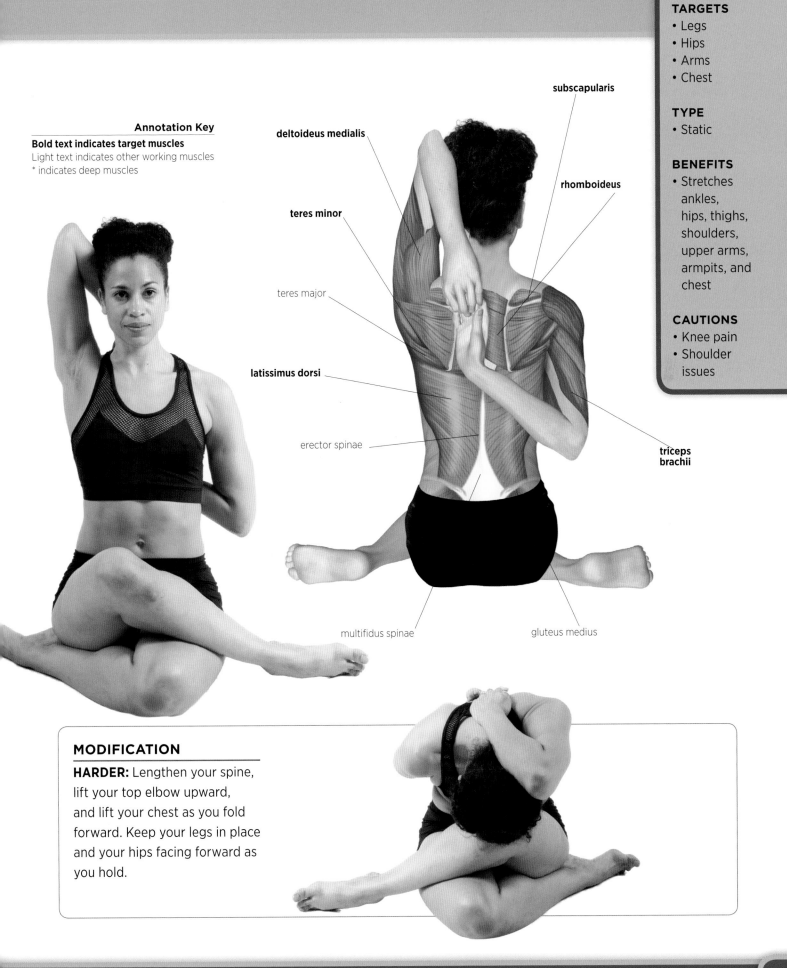

FACT FILE

TARGETS
- Legs
- Hips
- Arms
- Chest

TYPE
- Static

BENEFITS
- Stretches ankles, hips, thighs, shoulders, upper arms, armpits, and chest

CAUTIONS
- Knee pain
- Shoulder issues

subscapularis

deltoideus medialis

rhomboideus

teres minor

teres major

latissimus dorsi

erector spinae

triceps brachii

multifidus spinae

gluteus medius

Annotation Key

Bold text indicates target muscles
Light text indicates other working muscles
* indicates deep muscles

MODIFICATION

HARDER: Lengthen your spine, lift your top elbow upward, and lift your chest as you fold forward. Keep your legs in place and your hips facing forward as you hold.

Marichi's Yoga Stretch

This yoga pose helps to strengthen your back and tone your abdominals. It is a great stretch for increasing the flexibility and functioning of your spinal column.

HOW TO DO IT

- Sit up tall, with your legs together and extended in front of you. Bend your right knee, pulling your heel toward your groin. Keep your left leg extended with your toes pointed upward, and focus on keeping your leg grounded. Place your hands on the floor by your sides.

- Pushing your right foot and left leg into the floor, inhale, and lift up through your spine and chest. Keep both sit bones on the floor, and relax your shoulders.

- Exhale, and begin twisting toward your right knee. Wrap your left hand around the outside of your right thigh, pulling your knee in toward your abdominals. Press the fingertips of your right hand into the floor behind your hips.

- Turn your head to the right, and place your left elbow on the outside of your right knee. Lean back slightly, leading with your upper torso to help twist your entire spine.

- Hold for the recommended time, and then gently untwist as you exhale. Repeat on the other side.

Annotation Key
Bold text indicates target muscles
Light text indicates other working muscles
* indicates deep muscles

DO IT RIGHT
- Keep both sit bones on the floor.
- Twist from the bottom up—rotate from your lower spine, through your torso, and up through your chest.
- Avoid tensing your shoulders up toward your ears.
- Avoid rounding your spine.
- Avoid forcing a deep twist—gently ease your body into the rotation while maintaining correct posture.

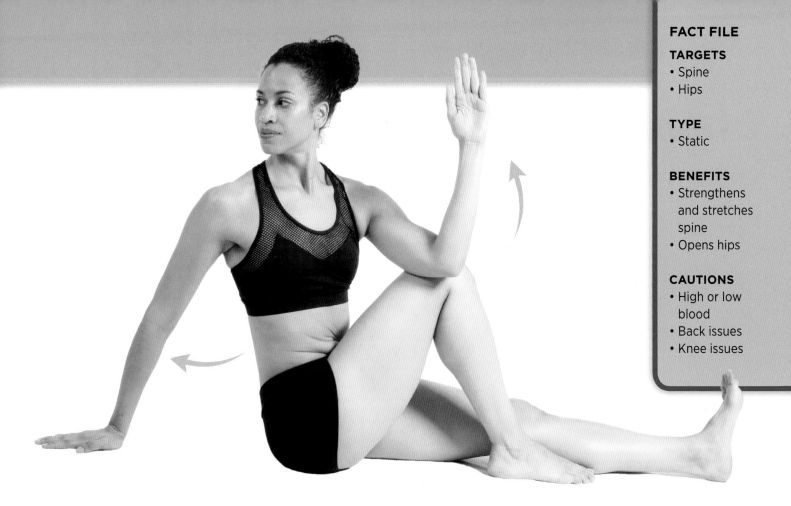

FACT FILE

TARGETS
• Spine
• Hips

TYPE
• Static

BENEFITS
• Strengthens
  and stretches
  spine
• Opens hips

CAUTIONS
• High or low
  blood
• Back issues
• Knee issues

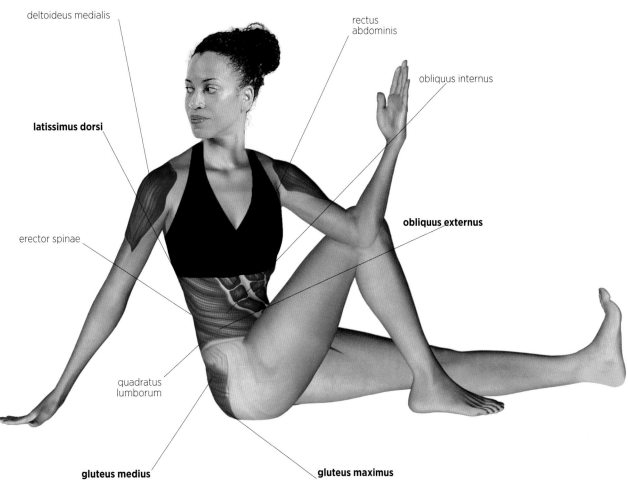

deltoideus medialis

rectus
abdominis

obliquus internus

latissimus dorsi

obliquus externus

erector spinae

quadratus
lumborum

gluteus medius

gluteus maximus

Bharadvaja's Twist

Practicing this gentle seated yoga twist will stretch your spine, oblique muscles, torso, shoulders, and hips. Bharadvaja's Twist can effectively relieve lower-back pain, neck pain, and sciatica.

HOW TO DO IT

- Sit up tall, with your legs together and extended in front of you. Shift your weight onto your right buttock, and bend your knees to the left, allowing your right thigh to rest on the floor. With your toes pointed toward your left hip, your left thigh should rest on top of your right calf, and your left ankle should sit on top of your right foot.

- Inhale, and lift up from your spine. Exhale, and twist to your right, looking over your right shoulder. Place your left hand near your right knee and your right hand on the floor beside your right hip.

- Bend your right elbow to reach across your back. Hook your right hand beneath the bend in your left elbow.

- Hold for the recommended time, and then gently untwist as you exhale, and repeat on the other side.

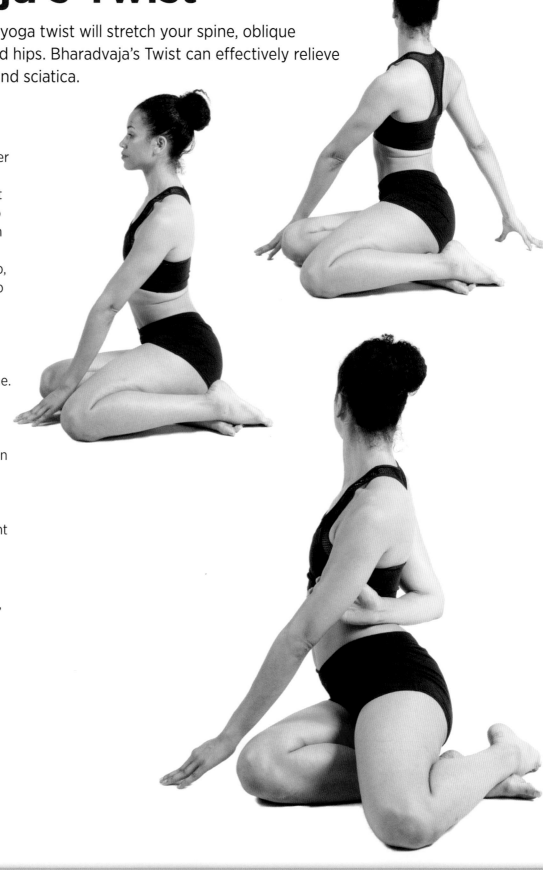

TARGETS
• Spine
• Shoulders
• Hips

TYPE
• Static

BENEFITS
• Stretches spine, shoulders, and hips
• Relieves lower-back pain, neck pain, and sciatica

CAUTIONS
• High or low blood pressure
• Knee issues
• Shoulder issues

trapezius

splenius

rhomboideus

infraspinatus

deltoideus posterior

deltoideus medialis

latissimus dorsi

teres minor

erector spinae

teres major

multifidus spinae

obliquus externus

obliquus internus

transversus abdominis

iliopsoas

Annotation Key

Bold text indicates target muscles
Light text indicates other working muscles
* indicates deep muscles

DO IT RIGHT
• Press both sit bones into the floor while twisting.
• Avoid popping your rib cage out.
• Avoid dropping your head.

Spine Twist

Stretching and strengthening the back, the Spine Twist is an excellent exercise for increasing range of motion in your torso and spine. This can help prevent future injury.

HOW TO DO IT

• Sit up tall with your legs extended in front of you slightly more than one hip-width apart.

• Keeping your back straight, raise your arms out to your sides at shoulder height, parallel to the floor.

• Pull in your lower abdominals, and twist your waist to the right taking your entire upper body with it.

• Gently untwist as you exhale, and then repeat on the opposite side. Alternate sides for the recommended repetitions.

DO IT RIGHT

• Keep your hips facing forward.
• Avoid raising your hips off the floor.
• Keep your arms parallel to the floor.

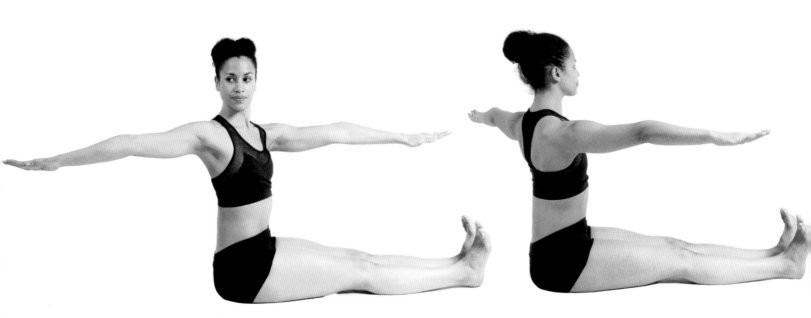

Annotation Key

Bold text indicates target muscles
Light text indicates other working muscles
* indicates deep muscles

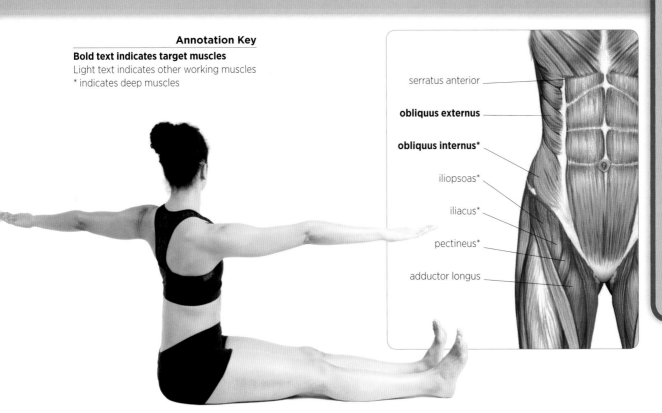

serratus anterior

obliquus externus

obliquus internus*

iliopsoas*

iliacus*

pectineus*

adductor longus

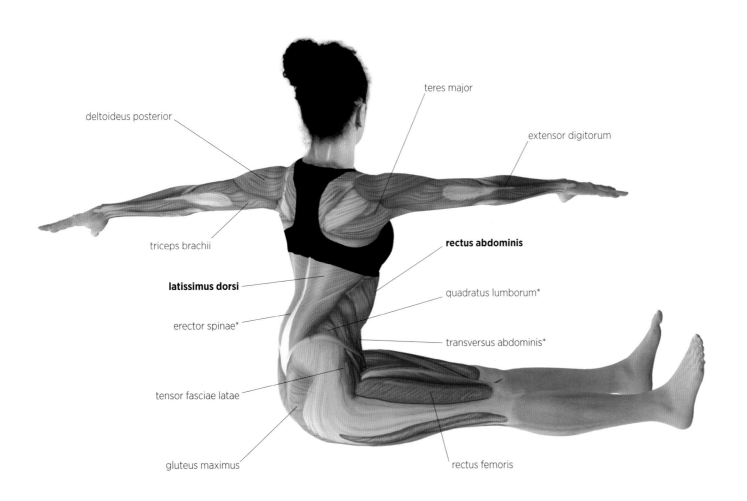

deltoideus posterior

teres major

extensor digitorum

triceps brachii

rectus abdominis

latissimus dorsi

quadratus lumborum*

erector spinae*

transversus abdominis*

tensor fasciae latae

gluteus maximus

rectus femoris

Spine Stretch Forward

The Spine Stretch Forward is a great beginner exercise that improves flexibility along your spine and in your hamstrings. As you perform this simple stretch, focus on articulating your spine as you slowly curl your body forward.

HOW TO DO IT

• Sit up tall with your legs extended in front of you slightly more than one hip-width apart.

• Flex your feet, place your palms on the floor by your hips, and inhale.

• Exhale as you curl forward, beginning with your head, neck, and upper back.

• Reach your arms forward, with palms facing up, and try to touch your feet.

• Hold for the recommended time, slowly roll back to an upright position to release the stretch, and then repeat for the recommended repetitions.

DO IT RIGHT

• Create a C-curve along your spine, from head to tailbone.

• Feel your ribcage expand outward as you inhale.

• Avoid shifting your pelvis or rolling your knees inward.

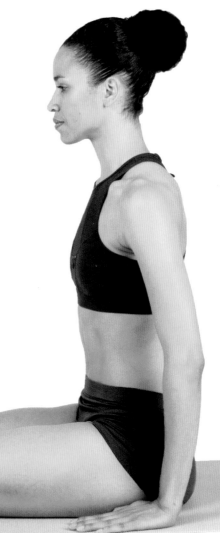

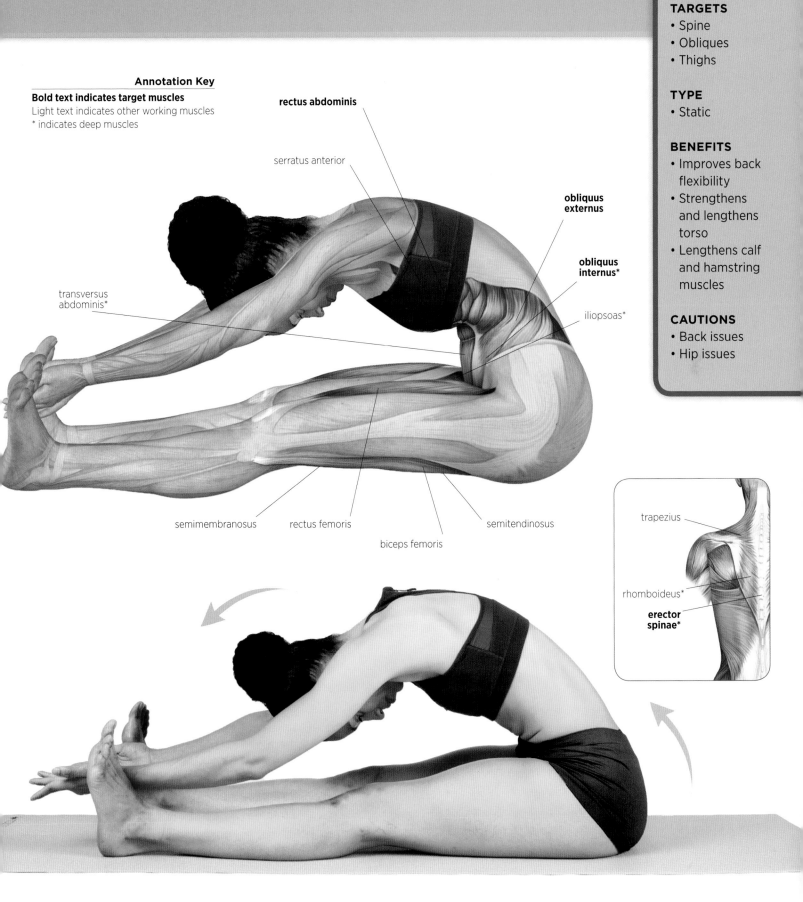

TARGETS
• Spine
• Obliques
• Thighs

TYPE
• Static

BENEFITS
• Improves back flexibility
• Strengthens and lengthens torso
• Lengthens calf and hamstring muscles

CAUTIONS
• Back issues
• Hip issues

Annotation Key

Bold text indicates target muscles
Light text indicates other working muscles
* indicates deep muscles

rectus abdominis

serratus anterior

obliquus externus

obliquus internus*

iliopsoas*

transversus abdominis*

semimembranosus

rectus femoris

biceps femoris

semitendinosus

trapezius

rhomboideus*

erector spinae*

Front Deltoid Towel Stretch

This stretch improves mobility in people who regularly perform repetitive shoulder and arm motions. Gripping the end of a short towel with either hand is a great way to target these specific shoulder muscles.

HOW TO DO IT

- Sit up tall with your legs extended in front of you. Bend your knees slightly, keeping your heels on the floor.

- Grip either end of a small towel behind your back, with your palms facing behind you.

- Gently slide your buttocks forward along the floor until you feel a comfortable stretch in your front deltoids.

- Hold for the recommended time, and then slide back up to the starting position. Repeat for the recommended repetitions.

DO IT RIGHT

- Keep your hands together while gripping the towel.
- Avoid leaning your head forward.

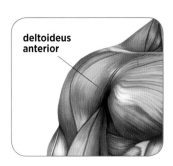

deltoideus anterior

FACT FILE

TARGETS
- Anterior deltoids

TYPE
- Static

BENEFITS
- Reduces shoulder tightness
- Increases upper-back mobility
- Expands chest

CAUTIONS
- Shoulder issues
- Back issues

Annotation Key

Bold text indicates target muscles
Light text indicates other working muscles
* indicates deep muscles

Spine Stretch Reaching

Spine Stretch Reaching eases your muscles into a full forward bend. This exercise provides a great opportunity for you to practice lengthening your shoulder blades and upper spinal column.

HOW TO DO IT

• Sit up tall with your legs extended in front of you slightly more than one hip-width apart.

• Flex your feet, place your palms on the floor by your hips, and then inhale.

• Raise your arms overhead, palms facing inward, forming a straight line with your back.

• Inhale to prepare, and then exhale as you curl forward. Reach your arms forward keeping them at shoulder height.

• Hold for the recommended time, slowly roll back to an upright position to release the stretch, and then repeat for the recommended repetitions.

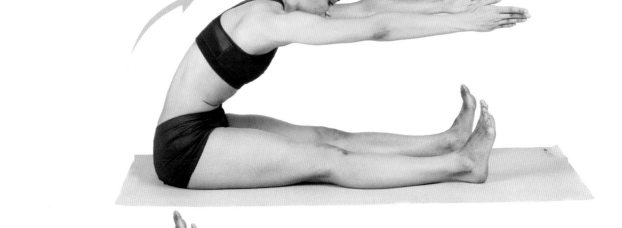

trapezius

rhomboideus*

erector spinae*

Annotation Key

Bold text indicates target muscles
Light text indicates other working muscles
* indicates deep muscles

Kneeling Lat Stretch

Your latissimus dorsi muscle is one of the widest muscles in the human body and is responsible for much of the movement of your arms from the shoulder sockets. The lats tend to be tight on most people, which can lead to forward-leaning or depressed shoulders and can limit shoulder flexion. Properly stretching the latissimus dorsi is an important part of a stretching routine.

HOW TO DO IT

• Kneel on all fours with your hands planted shoulder-width apart.

• Bring your big toes together and your knees about hip-distance apart.

• Drop your torso onto your thighs, and extend your arms on the floor above your head so that your forehead comes to rest on the floor.

• Bend your left arm so that it is perpendicular to your torso, keeping your palm flat on the floor. Lean your shoulders into this pose, feeling the stretch along the left side of your lats.

• Hold for the recommended time, and then slide back up to the starting position. Repeat for the recommended repetitions.

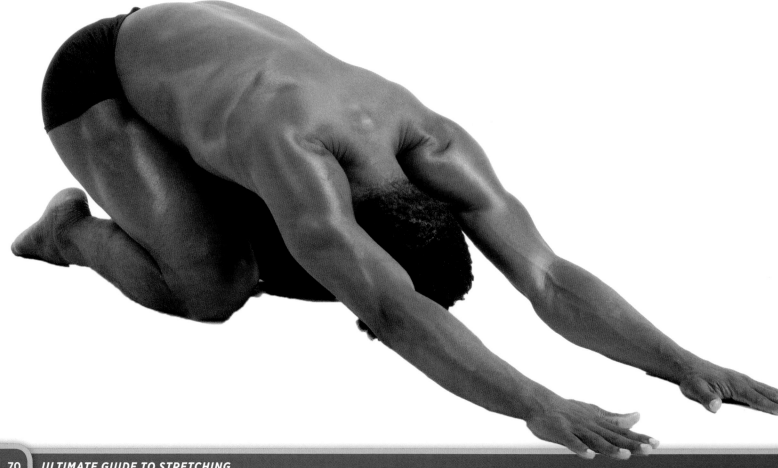

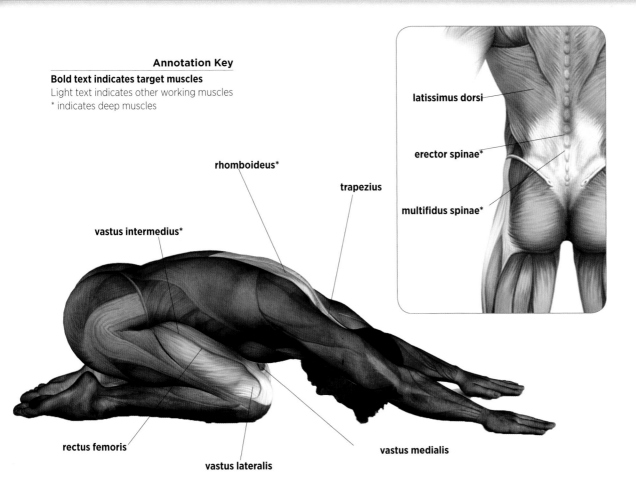

Annotation Key
Bold text indicates target muscles
Light text indicates other working muscles
* indicates deep muscles

rhomboideus*

trapezius

vastus intermedius*

latissimus dorsi

erector spinae*

multifidus spinae*

rectus femoris

vastus lateralis

vastus medialis

FACT FILE

TARGETS
• Latissimus dorsi
• Scapulae
• Rhomboids

TYPE
• Static

BENEFITS
• Improves arm mobility
• Relieves shoulder tightness

CAUTIONS
• Shoulder issues

DO IT RIGHT
• Avoid tensing your neck and shoulders.
• Breath steadily throughout this stretch.

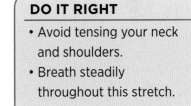

Downward-Facing Dog

Using the strength of your arms and legs to hold your body up, Downward-Facing Dog fully and evenly stretches the length of your spine. It also stretches your hips, hamstrings, and calves while strengthening your quadriceps and ankles. It opens your chest and shoulders and tones your arms and abdominals.

HOW TO DO IT

- Kneel on all fours, with your hands planted directly below your shoulders and your knees aligned beneath your hips.

- Tuck your toes under, and walk your hands forward about a palm's distance in front of your shoulders. With your hands and toes firmly planted, lift your hips as you straighten your legs and draw your heels toward the floor.

- Press your chest toward your thighs, and bring your head between your arms. Lengthen through your tailbone, and keep your thighs slightly internally rotated, finding a neutral pelvis. Gaze between your feet or toward your navel. Hold for the recommended time.

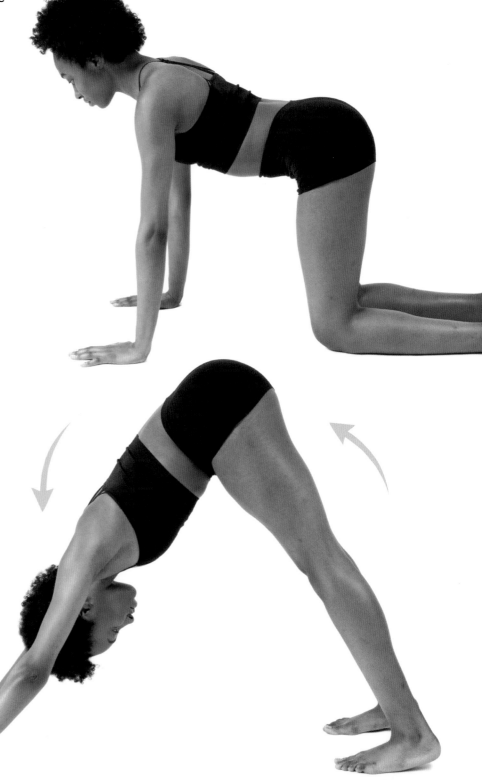

TARGETS
• Shoulders
• Arms
• Hamstrings
• Calves

TYPE
• Static

BENEFITS
• Strengthens arms and legs
• Stretches spine, hamstrings, calves, and arches

CAUTIONS
• Low blood pressure
• Shoulder issues
• Hamstring issues
• Carpal tunnel syndrome

DO IT RIGHT

• Press your hands fully into the floor at all times to avoid excess strain on your wrist joints.
• Keep your head in line with your spine.
• Keep your back flat and your chest elevated.
• Avoid holding your breath: relax your jaw slightly and breathe normally.

Annotation Key

Bold text indicates target muscles
Light text indicates other working muscles
* indicates deep muscles

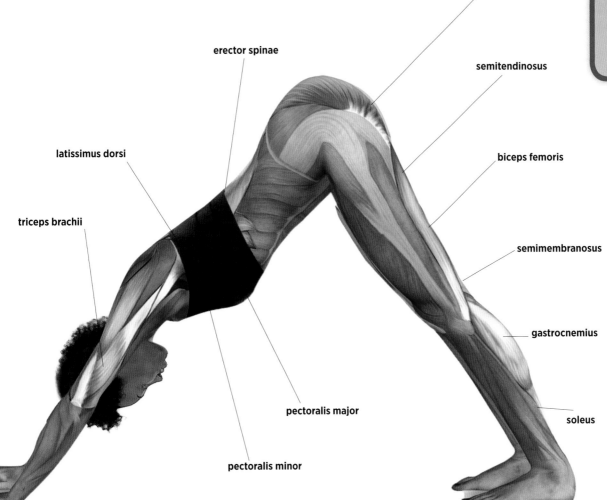

gluteus maximus

semitendinosus

erector spinae

biceps femoris

latissimus dorsi

semimembranosus

triceps brachii

gastrocnemius

pectoralis major

soleus

pectoralis minor

Three-Legged Dog

This variation of Downward-Facing Dog adds a further challenge by incorporating a backward leg extension and an asymmetrical balance. This stretching yoga pose strengthens your arm and leg muscles and also creates space in your torso for a deeper spinal and upper-back stretch.

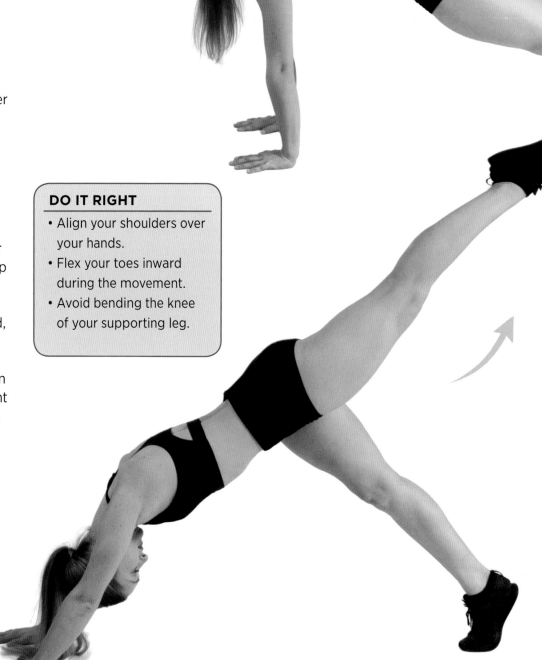

HOW TO DO IT

- Begin in a high plank position, with your shoulders directly over your hands, your torso straight, and your weight distributed evenly between your arms and legs.

- Draw your right knee into your chest, flexing your foot while rocking your body forward over your hands. You should come up on the toes of your left foot.

- Extend your left knee backward, rocking your body back and shifting your weight onto your heel. With your head in between your hands, straighten your right leg and lift it toward the ceiling.

- Release the stretch, and repeat on the opposite side. Alternate sides for the recommended repetitions.

DO IT RIGHT
- Align your shoulders over your hands.
- Flex your toes inward during the movement.
- Avoid bending the knee of your supporting leg.

FACT FILE

TARGETS
• Back
• Legs
• Shoulders
• Arms

TYPE
• Dynamic

BENEFITS
• Stabilizes core
• Stabilizes shoulders
• Stretches calves and hamstrings

CAUTIONS
• Lower-back issues
• Wrist pain
• Ankle pain

biceps femoris

semimembranosus

adductor longus

tensor fasciae latae

vastus lateralis

transversus abdominis

rectus femoris

obliquus externus

adductor magnus

latissimus dorsi

gracilis

obliquus internus

vastus medialis

teres major

sartorius

gastrocnemius

deltoideus posterior

vastus intermedius

tibialis anterior

tibialis posterior

rectus abdominis

peroneus

soleus

Annotation Key

Bold text indicates target muscles
Light text indicates other working muscles
* indicates deep muscles

Head-to-Knee Yoga Stretch

This seated, folded, forward bend is an essential exercise in many disciplines. Mastering this pose can provide a deep stretch for both your spine and hamstrings, while also opening up your hips and shoulders.

HOW TO DO IT

- Sit up tall, with your legs together and extended in front of you. Bend your right knee, and draw your heel in toward your groin, placing the sole of your foot on your left inner thigh until your right leg is at a right angle to your left shin. Draw both sit bones to the floor.

- Inhale, and lift up through your spine. As you exhale, turn your torso slightly to your left so that it aligns with your left leg. Flex your foot, and contract the muscles in your left thigh to push the back of your leg toward the floor.

- Exhale as you stretch your sternum forward to fold your torso over your left leg. Grasp the inside of your left foot with your left hand. Use your right hand to guide your torso to the left.

- Extend your right arm forward toward your left foot. You may grasp your left foot with both hands or place your hands on the floor on either side of your foot with your elbows bent. Place your forehead on your left shin. With each inhalation, lengthen your spine, and with each exhalation, deepen the stretch.

- Hold for the recommended breaths, return to the starting position, and repeat on the other side.

DO IT RIGHT

- Your abdominals should be the first part of your body to touch your thigh; your head should be the last.
- To help guide the forward bend from your hips, place a folded blanket beneath your buttocks.
- Avoid rounding your back
- Avoid allowing the foot of your bent leg to shift beneath your straight leg.

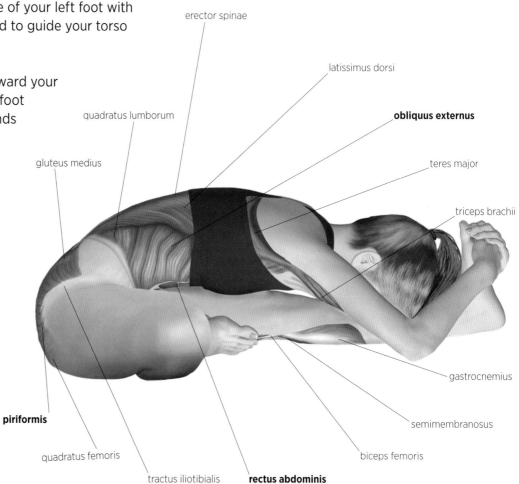

erector spinae

latissimus dorsi

obliquus externus

quadratus lumborum

teres major

gluteus medius

triceps brachii

gastrocnemius

semimembranosus

piriformis

biceps femoris

quadratus femoris

tractus iliotibialis

rectus abdominis

Annotation Key

Bold text indicates target muscles
Light text indicates other working muscles
* indicates deep muscles

TARGETS
• Hamstrings
• Groin
• Spine

TYPE
• Static

BENEFITS
• Stretches back, core, and thighs

CAUTIONS
• Knee issues
• Lower-back issues

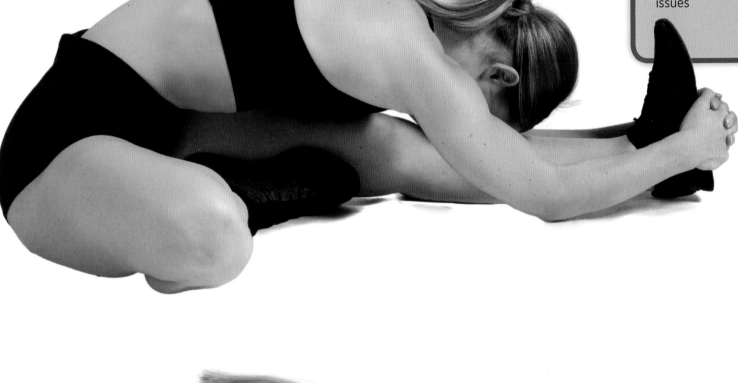

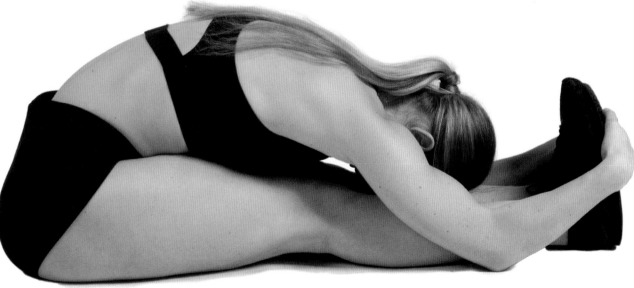

Cat-to-Cow Stretch

Cat-to-Cow alternates between two upper-back stretches to create a soothing sequence that helps keep your spine mobile. Perform it at night to release any residual tension of the day.

HOW TO DO IT

- To perform the Cat Stretch, kneel on all fours, with your hands planted directly below your shoulders and your knees aligned beneath your hips. Your hips should be in a neutral position and the tops of your feet on the floor.

- Spread your fingers wide, grounding down through your thumb and index finger. Externally rotate your arms, thinking of opening your right upper arm clockwise and your left upper arm counterclockwise.

- Drop your head as you round your upper back, and then draw your belly into your spine. Gazing down at the floor or toward your navel, hold for the recommended breaths, and then exhale to release the stretch.

- To move into the Cow Stretch, inhale, lift your sternum, and arch your upper back, raising your sit bones toward the ceiling. Hold for the recommended breaths, and then exhale to release the stretch.

- Alternate Cat-to-Cow for the recommended repetitions.

DO IT RIGHT
- Allow your shoulder blades to separate, and breathe more space into your upper spine.
- Keep your shoulders over your wrists as you round your back.
- Avoid bringing your weight back toward your knees as you round your spine.

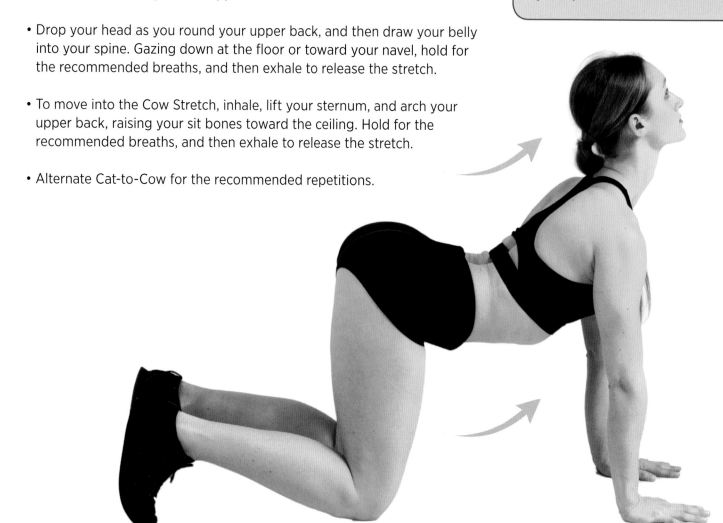

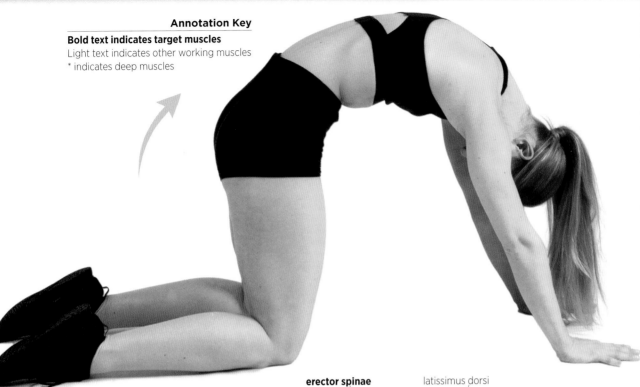

FACT FILE

TARGETS
• Spine
• Chest
• Neck

TYPE
• Static

BENEFITS
• Stretches
  upper body
  and back
• Strengthens
  hand and
  wrist muscles
• Massages
  spine
• Increases
  mobility

CAUTIONS
• Neck issues
• Wrist issues

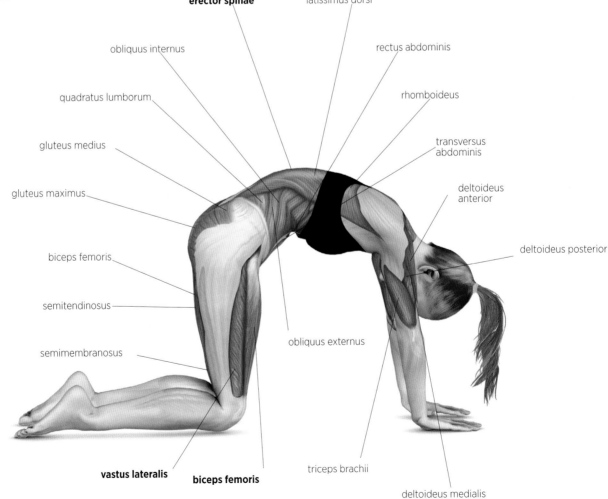

erector spinae

latissimus dorsi

obliquus internus

rectus abdominis

quadratus lumborum

rhomboideus

gluteus medius

transversus
abdominis

gluteus maximus

deltoideus
anterior

deltoideus posterior

biceps femoris

semitendinosus

obliquus externus

semimembranosus

vastus lateralis

biceps femoris

triceps brachii

deltoideus medialis

Thread the Needle

The Thread the Needle exercise stretches and opens the shoulders, chest, arms, upper back, and neck. It releases the tension that is commonly held in the upper back between the shoulder blades. This stretch incorporates a mild twist to the spine, which further reduces upper-back tension.

HOW TO DO IT

• Kneel on all fours with your back flat and hands directly below your shoulders.

• Turn your left hand over, so the back of your hand is now on the floor.

• Slide your left hand behind your right arm and out to your right side, keeping the back of your hand on the floor.

• Bend your supporting arm as you slide your left hand out farther. Continue sliding until your left shoulder rests on the floor and your supporting arm is bent perpendicular. The side of your head should be resting on the floor. Gaze to the right.

• Hold for the recommended time, and then slide back up to the starting position. Repeat on the opposite side, and the alternate sides for the recommended repetitions.

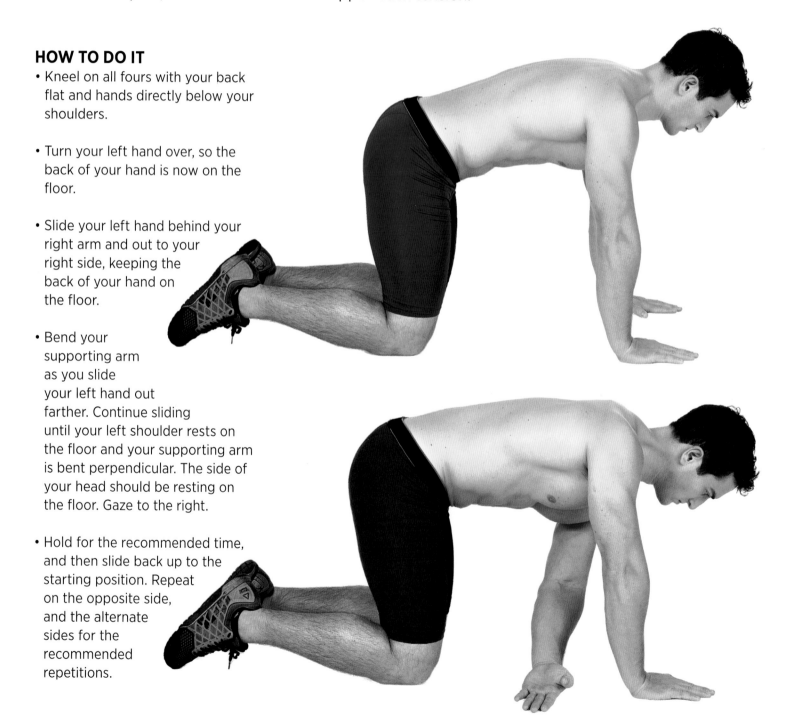

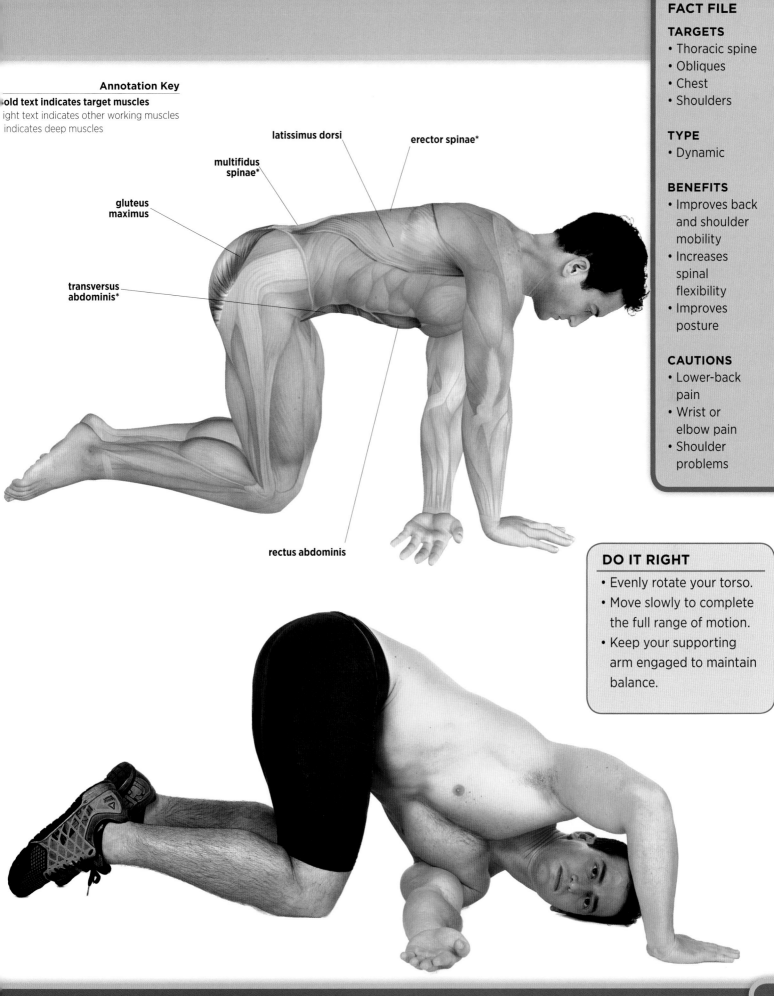

TARGETS
- Thoracic spine
- Obliques
- Chest
- Shoulders

TYPE
- Dynamic

BENEFITS
- Improves back and shoulder mobility
- Increases spinal flexibility
- Improves posture

CAUTIONS
- Lower-back pain
- Wrist or elbow pain
- Shoulder problems

Annotation Key
Bold text indicates target muscles
Light text indicates other working muscles
*indicates deep muscles

multifidus spinae*

latissimus dorsi

erector spinae*

gluteus maximus

transversus abdominis*

rectus abdominis

DO IT RIGHT
- Evenly rotate your torso.
- Move slowly to complete the full range of motion.
- Keep your supporting arm engaged to maintain balance.

Locust Yoga Stretch

The Locust, a yoga-inspired exercise, involves a mild backbend that stretches your chest, shoulders, and abdominals. It also strengthens your upper and lower back and prepares your body for deeper backbends.

HOW TO DO IT

• Lie facedown on the floor with your arms resting by your sides and the palms of your hands facing downward. Turn your legs in toward each other so that your knees point directly into the floor.

• Squeezing your buttocks, inhale, and lift up your head, chest, arms, and legs simultaneously. Extend your arms and legs behind you, with your arms parallel to the floor. Lift as high as possible, with your pelvis and lower abdominals stabilizing your body on the floor. Keep your head in a neutral position.

• Hold for the recommended time, release the stretch, and then repeat for the recommended repetitions.

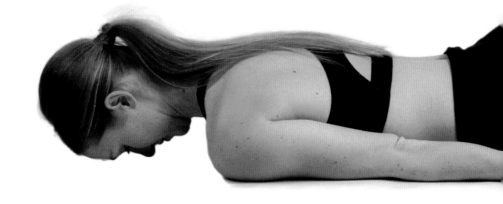

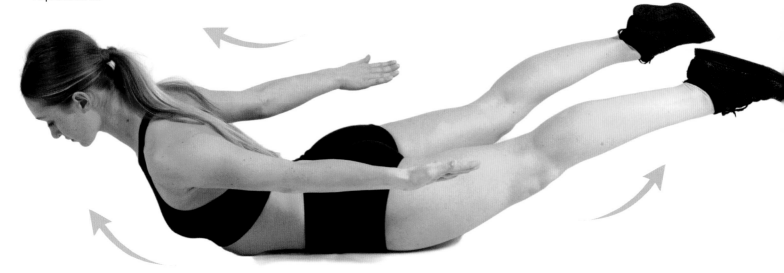

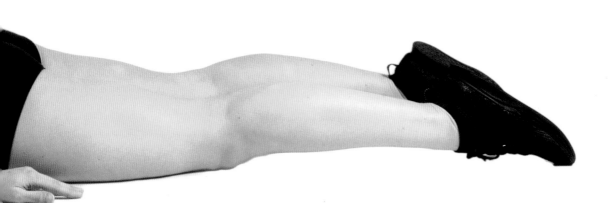

FACT FILE

TARGETS
- Chest
- Shoulders
- Abdominals
- Hips
- Spine

TYPE
- Static

BENEFITS
- Stretches hip flexors, chest, and abdominals
- Strengthens spine, glutes, arms, and legs

CAUTIONS
- Back Issues

DO IT RIGHT
- Elongate the back of your neck.
- Open your chest to extend the arch through your entire spine.
- Avoid bending your knees.
- Keep your breath even and steady.

Annotation Key

Bold text indicates target muscles
Light text indicates other working muscles
* indicates deep muscles

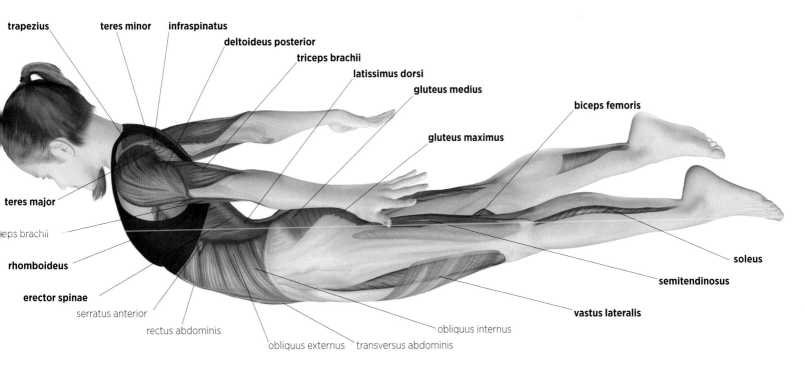

trapezius

teres minor

infraspinatus

deltoideus posterior

triceps brachii

latissimus dorsi

gluteus medius

biceps femoris

gluteus maximus

teres major

eps brachii

rhomboideus

erector spinae

serratus anterior

rectus abdominis

obliquus externus

transversus abdominis

obliquus internus

vastus lateralis

semitendinosus

soleus

Breaststroke Stretch

The Breaststroke helps to realign your spine, particularly in the upper and middle regions. This exercise strengthens the scapular muscles around the shoulder blades as you rotate your arms, and it develops the extensor muscles as you hold yourself up. If you tend to slouch, this is a great strengthening stretch.

HOW TO DO IT

- Lie facedown on a mat with your arms and legs extended and your hands shoulder-width apart.

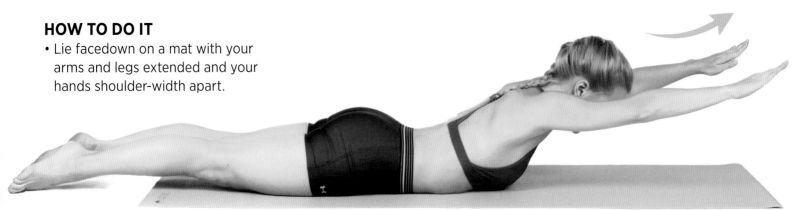

- Inhale to prepare, then exhale as you lift your arms off the mat reaching forward.

- Slowly circle your arms to the back, so that your fingers are pointed behind you.

- Bend your elbows, and return to the starting position. Repeat for the recommended repetitions.

Annotation Key

Bold text indicates target muscles
Light text indicates other working muscles
* indicates deep muscles

FACT FILE

TARGETS
• Shoulders
• Rotator cuffs
• Spine
• Upper back
• Middle back

TYPE
• Dynamic

BENEFITS
• Increases upper-back and spine mobility
• Strengthens back, spine, and core
• Engages shoulders, upper arms, hips, and glutes

CAUTIONS
• Shoulder issues
• Neck issues

DO IT RIGHT

• Keep your arms raised from the mat.
• Keep your wrists engaged.
• Keep your hip and pubic bones on the mat.
• Squeeze your legs together to engage your core.
• Align the back of your head and neck with your spine.
• Avoid lifting your torso higher than the bottom of your ribcage.

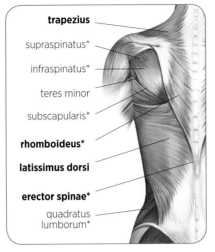

trapezius
supraspinatus*
infraspinatus*
teres minor
subscapularis*
rhomboideus*
latissimus dorsi
erector spinae*
quadratus lumborum*

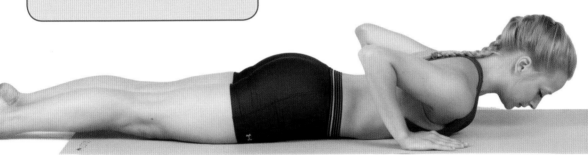

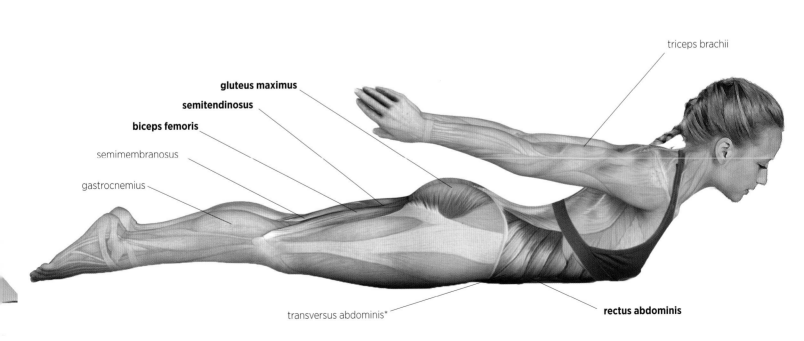

triceps brachii
gluteus maximus
semitendinosus
biceps femoris
semimembranosus
gastrocnemius
transversus abdominis*
rectus abdominis

Bridge Stretch

The Bridge is a great preparatory stretch in advance of a full-spinal lift. While preparing you for more challenging backbends, this exercise relies on the strength of your quads, glutes, and abdomen while opening your chest and stretching your spine.

HOW TO DO IT

- Lie on your back. Bend your knees, and draw you heels close to your buttocks. Place your hands flat on the floor by your sides.

- Exhale, and press down though your feet to lift your buttocks off the floor. With your feet and thighs parallel, push your arms into the floor while extending through your fingertips.

- Lengthen your neck away from your shoulders. Lift your hips higher so that your torso rises from the floor.

- Hold for the recommended time. Exhale, and release your spine onto the floor, one vertebra at a time, and then repeat for the recommended repetitions.

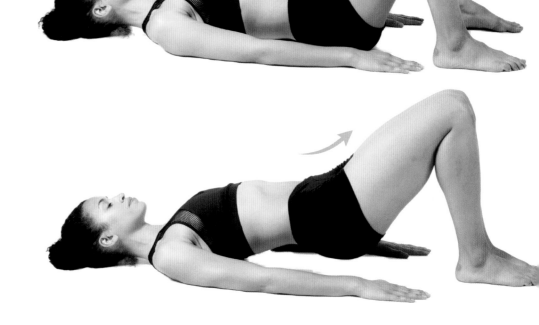

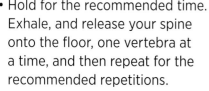

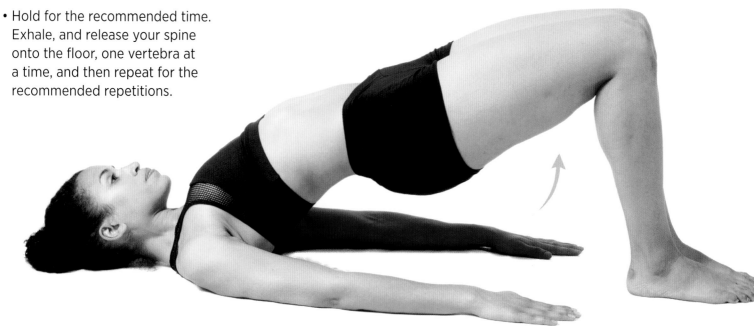

DO IT RIGHT

- Keep your knees over your heels.
- Focus on bending your upper back and chest.
- If desired, place a block beneath your sacrum to support your back.
- Contracting your hamstrings to keep your legs active.
- Avoid sticking out your stomach or ribs.
- Avoid bending from your lower back.
- Avoid clenching your buttocks.

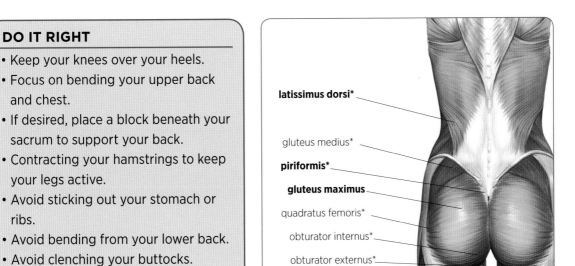

latissimus dorsi*

gluteus medius*

piriformis*

gluteus maximus

quadratus femoris*

obturator internus*

obturator externus*

FACT FILE

TARGETS
- Spine
- Chest
- Thighs
- Glutes

TYPE
- Static

BENEFITS
- Stretches chest and spine
- Strengthens thighs and glutes

CAUTIONS
- Shoulder issues
- Back issues
- Neck issues

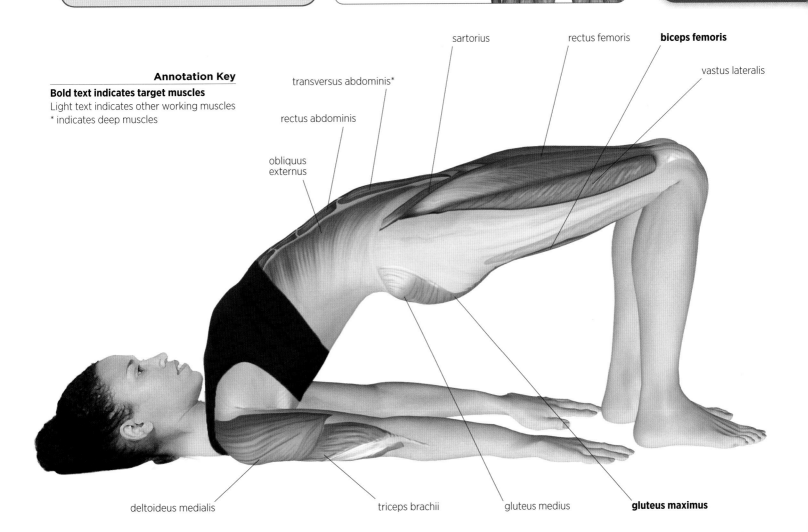

Annotation Key
Bold text indicates target muscles
Light text indicates other working muscles
* indicates deep muscles

sartorius

rectus femoris

biceps femoris

vastus lateralis

transversus abdominis*

rectus abdominis

obliquus externus

deltoideus medialis

triceps brachii

gluteus medius

gluteus maximus

Knee-to-Chest Hug

The Knee-to-Chest Hug is an easy-to-do stretch that is great for releasing tightness in the lower back and increasing range of motion along the spine. Perform it to reduce stiffness associated with spinal arthritis or spinal stenosis.

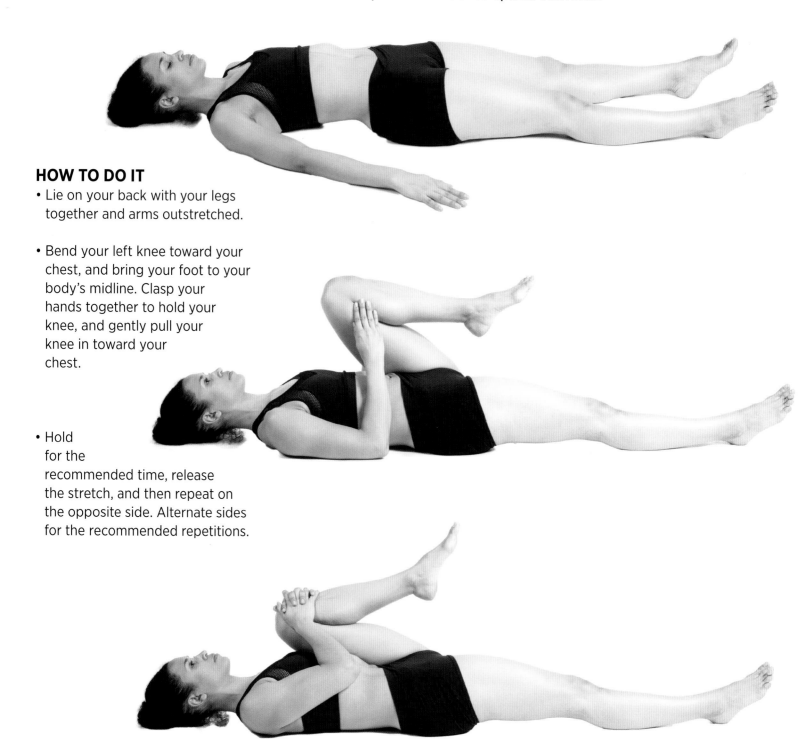

HOW TO DO IT

• Lie on your back with your legs together and arms outstretched.

• Bend your left knee toward your chest, and bring your foot to your body's midline. Clasp your hands together to hold your knee, and gently pull your knee in toward your chest.

• Hold for the recommended time, release the stretch, and then repeat on the opposite side. Alternate sides for the recommended repetitions.

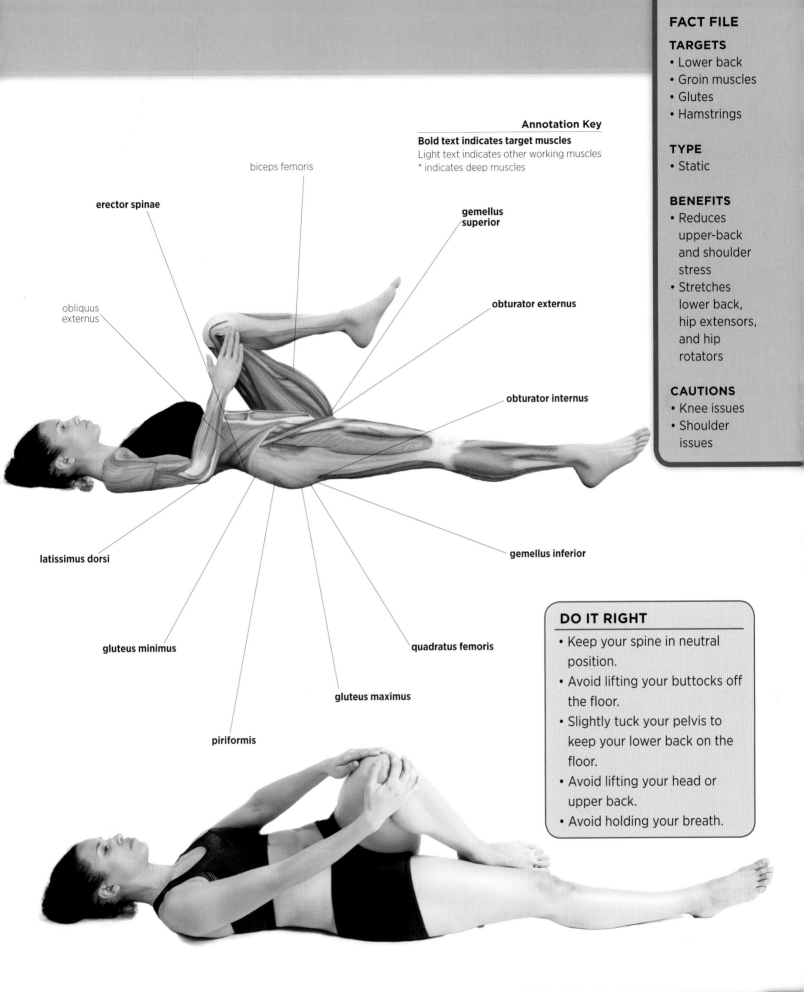

TARGETS
• Lower back
• Groin muscles
• Glutes
• Hamstrings

TYPE
• Static

BENEFITS
• Reduces upper-back and shoulder stress
• Stretches lower back, hip extensors, and hip rotators

CAUTIONS
• Knee issues
• Shoulder issues

Annotation Key

Bold text indicates target muscles
Light text indicates other working muscles
* indicates deep muscles

biceps femoris

erector spinae

gemellus superior

obliquus externus

obturator externus

obturator internus

latissimus dorsi

gemellus inferior

gluteus minimus

quadratus femoris

gluteus maximus

piriformis

DO IT RIGHT
• Keep your spine in neutral position.
• Avoid lifting your buttocks off the floor.
• Slightly tuck your pelvis to keep your lower back on the floor.
• Avoid lifting your head or upper back.
• Avoid holding your breath.

Backward Ball Stretch

An effective exercise that enhances your coordination, the Backward Ball Stretch combines an abdominal and back stretch with a core-strengthening exercise. You must fully engage your core, using steady, balanced movement to stretch your back over the Swiss ball.

HOW TO DO IT

• Sit on a Swiss ball in a well-balanced, neutral position, with your hips directly over the center of the ball.

• While maintaining good balance, begin to extend your arms behind you.

• Walk your feet forward, allowing the ball to roll up your spine.

• As your hands touch the floor, extend your legs as far forward as you comfortably can. Hold this position for about 10 seconds.

• To deepen the stretch, extend your arms, and walk your legs and hands closer to the ball. Hold this position for about 10 seconds.

• To release the stretch, bend your knees, drop your hips to the floor, lift your head off the ball, and then walk back to the starting position. Repeat for the recommended repetitions.

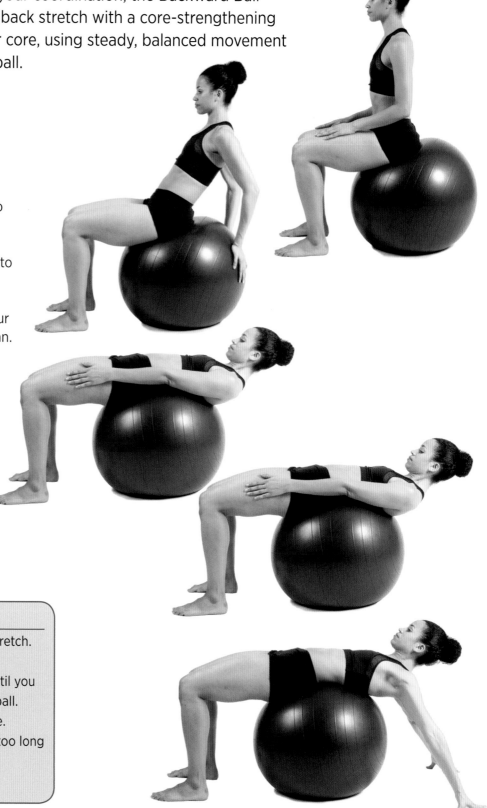

DO IT RIGHT
• Maintain good balance throughout the stretch.
• Move slowly and with control.
• Keep your head supported on the ball until you feel your torso is fully supported by the ball.
• Avoid allowing the ball to shift to the side.
• Avoid holding the extended position for too long or until you feel dizzy.

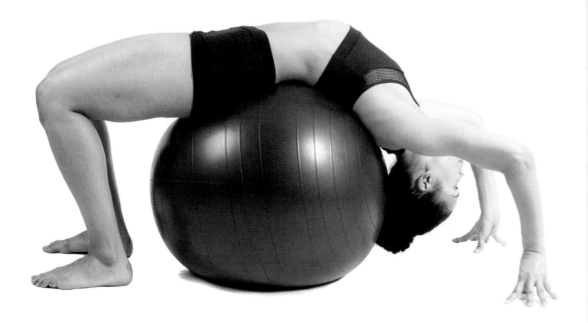

FACT FILE

TARGETS
- Thoracic spine
- Shoulders
- Middle back
- Chest

TYPE
- Static-dynamic

BENEFITS
- Stretches thoracic spine
- Increases spinal extension
- Stretches abdominals and large back muscles

CAUTIONS
- Lower-back issues
- Balancing difficulty
- Wrist issues

rectus abdominis

serratus anterior

obliquus externus

deltoideus medialis

transversus abdominis

pectoralis minor

vastus lateralis

trapezius

rectus femoris

pectoralis major

biceps femoris

biceps brachii

flexor carpi radialis

quadratus femoris

latissimus dorsi

iliopsoas

gluteus medius

ligamentum longitudinale anterius

quadratus lumborum

Annotation Key

Bold text indicates target muscles
Light text indicates other working muscles
* indicates deep muscles

Reclining Twist

This gentle supine twist stretches your glutes and spine while opening your chest. Performing this stretch regularly helps relieve lower-back pain and tension and improves shoulder mobility.

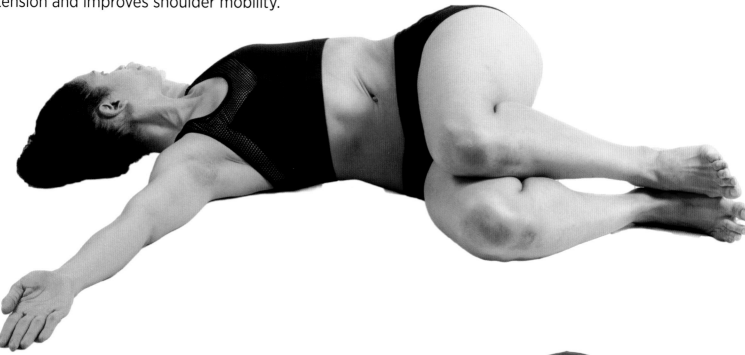

HOW TO DO IT

• Lie on your back with both legs elongated and parallel and your arms extended away from your torso, palms facing up.

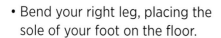

• Bend your right leg, placing the sole of your foot on the floor.

• Carefully lift your buttocks off the floor, slightly tilting your torso to your left, and cross your right leg over to your left side, with your knee bent at a right angle.

• Hold for the recommended time, release the stretch, and then repeat on the opposite side. Alternate sides for the recommended repetitions.

FACT FILE

TARGETS
• Rotator muscles
• Glutes
• Chest

TYPE
• Static

BENEFITS
• Stretches glutes
• Opens chest
• Relieves lower-back pain

CAUTIONS
• Shoulder issues

DO IT RIGHT

• Keep your elbows and wrists lower than your shoulders to protect your rotator cuffs.
• Avoid lifting your shoulders; try to keep both shoulder blades in contact with the floor throughout the stretch.

MODIFICATION

HARDER: Place the palm of your left hand on your right thigh while crossing your right leg over your left and vice versa.

Annotation Key

Bold text indicates target muscles
Light text indicates other working muscles
* indicates deep muscles

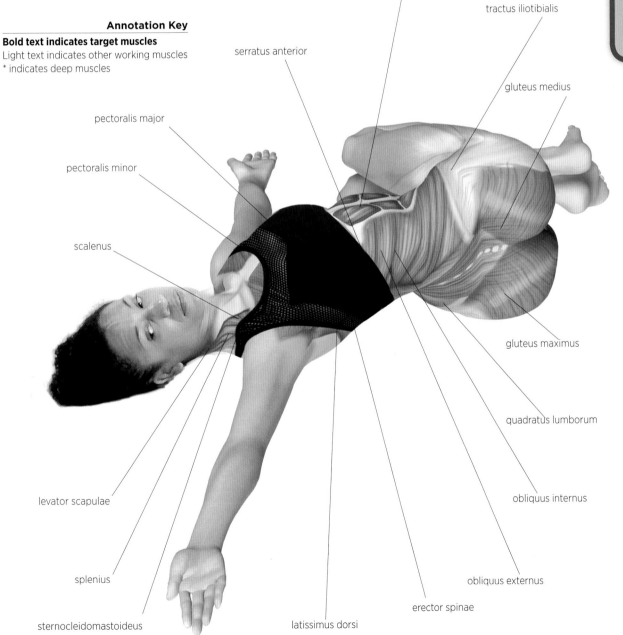

rectus abdominis

tractus iliotibialis

serratus anterior

gluteus medius

pectoralis major

pectoralis minor

scalenus

gluteus maximus

quadratus lumborum

levator scapulae

obliquus internus

splenius

obliquus externus

sternocleidomastoideus

erector spinae

latissimus dorsi

Back Roll

Foam rollers are useful tools for alleviating muscle stiffness and pain. A few minutes spent stretching and easing your back muscles with the Back Roll will reduce and relieve discomfort, especially if the exercise is performed regularly.

HOW TO DO IT

- Sit with your legs bent and feet flat on the floor in front of you. Position the foam roller behind your lower back, and then hang your arms at your sides, palms on the floor.

- Extend your legs, and begin to lean back, engaging your core muscles as you lean your lower back on the roller.

- Gradually roll forward until the roller is beneath your upper back.

- Roll back to the starting position, and then repeat the recommended repetitions.

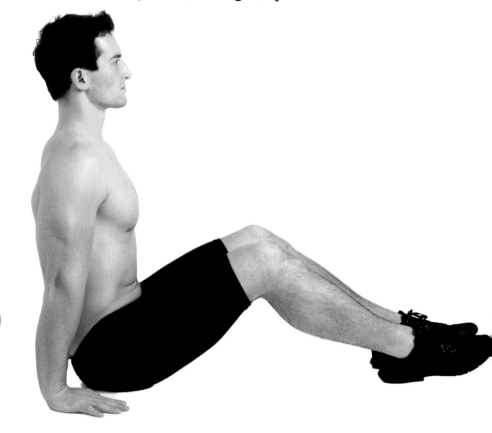

DO IT RIGHT

- Move smoothly and with control.
- Use your arms, legs, and abdominals to drive the movement.
- Keep your palms grounded on the floor.
- Press your shoulders down toward your back.
- Keep your head raised without tensing your neck.
- Avoid arching your back or hunching your shoulders

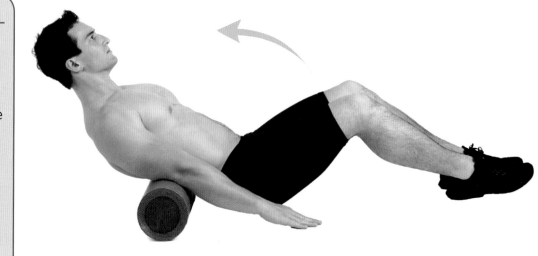

Annotation Key

Bold text indicates target muscles
Light text indicates other working muscles
* indicates deep muscles

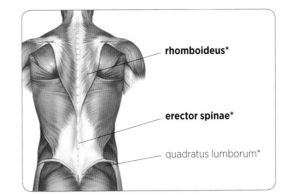

rhomboideus*

erector spinae*

quadratus lumborum*

FACT FILE

TARGETS
• Back

TYPE
• Myofascial release

BENEFITS
• Relieves back tightness or pain
• Improves range of motion

CAUTIONS
• Lower-back pain
• Shoulder issues

rectus femoris

vastus medialis

vastus lateralis

vastus intermedius*

semimembranosus

trapezius

semitendinosus

rectus abdominis

latissimus dorsi

biceps femoris

Triceps Stretch

The Triceps Stretch will quickly improve your flexibility and range of motion. After an upper-body workout, particularly one that includes pushing or pressing movements, it is important to stretch these upper-arm muscles to prevent soreness and tightening.

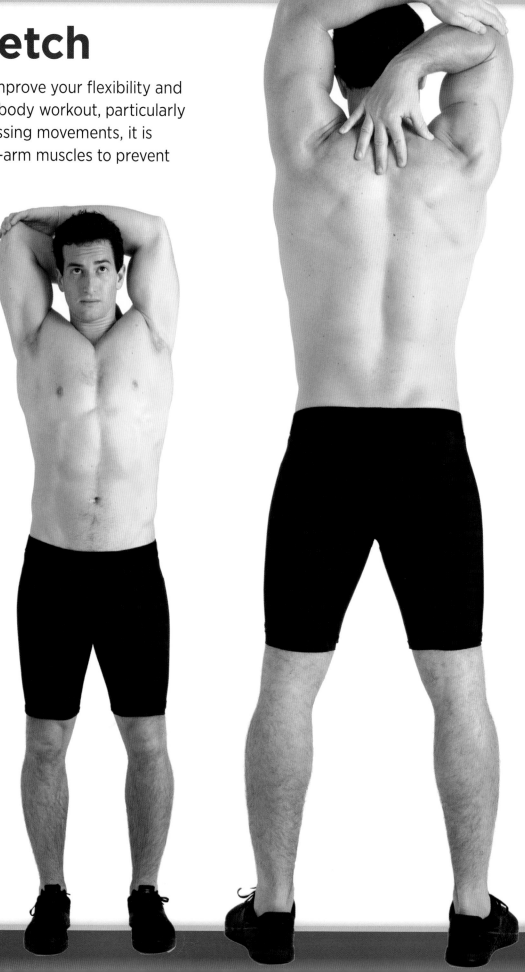

HOW TO DO IT

• Stand with your legs and feet parallel and shoulder-width apart. Bend your knees very slightly, and shift your pelvis slightly forward.

• Reach your right arm up behind your head. Bend from the elbow, aiming to bring your elbow toward the middle of the back of your head. Your right hand should fall between your shoulder blades.

• Grab your right elbow with your left hand, and gently pull down to intensify the stretch.

• Hold for the recommended time, release the stretch, and then repeat on the opposite side.

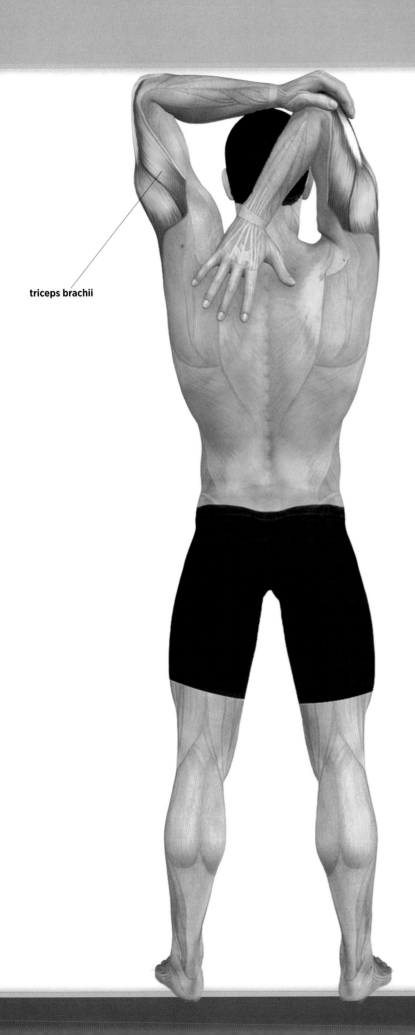

triceps brachii

TARGETS
• Triceps brachii

TYPE
• Static

BENEFITS
• Increases upper-arm mobility
• Relaxes tight shoulder joints

CAUTIONS
• Shoulder issues

Annotation Key

Bold text indicates target muscles
Light text indicates other working muscles
* indicates deep muscles

DO IT RIGHT

• Keep your shoulders pressed down and back, away from your ears.
• Maintain a firm, stable midsection, keeping your pelvis slightly tucked.
• Avoid tilting your head or neck forward.

Biceps Stretch

Your biceps are key to arm mobility. To improve their range of motion and increase muscle strength and flexibility, include the Biceps Stretch after an upper-body routine to work these muscles, as well as those in your chest and shoulders.

HOW TO DO IT

• Stand with your legs and feet parallel and shoulder-width apart. Bend your knees very slightly, and shift your pelvis slightly forward.

• Clasp your hands together behind your back with your palms together. Straighten your arms, and twist your wrists inward, pulling your palms in toward your buttocks.

• Hold for the recommended time, release the stretch, and then repeat for the recommended repetitions.

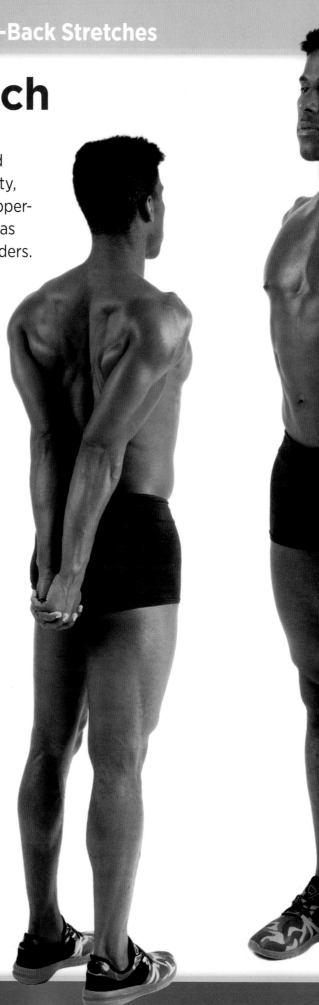
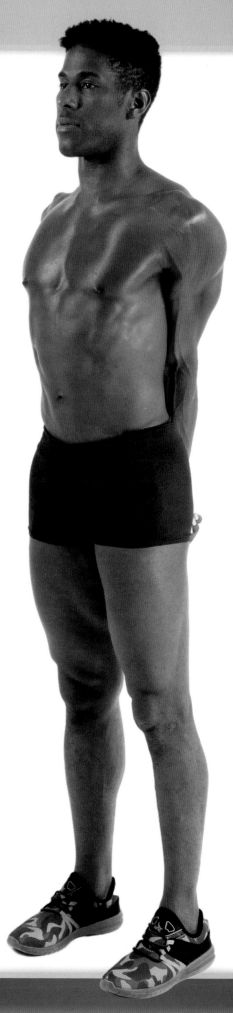

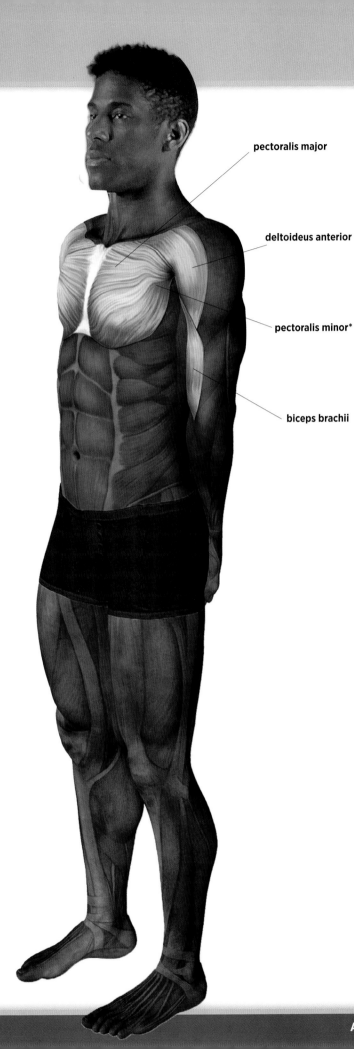

pectoralis major

deltoideus anterior

pectoralis minor*

biceps brachii

FACT FILE

TARGETS
- Biceps brachii
- Shoulders
- Chest

TYPE
- Dynamic

BENEFITS
- Stretches and strengthens arms
- Opens chest

CAUTIONS
- Shoulder issues
- Wrist issues

DO IT RIGHT
- Keep your shoulders pressed down and back, away from your ears.
- Avoid collapsing your chest forward.

Annotation Key

Bold text indicates target muscles
Light text indicates other working muscles
* indicates deep muscles

Wrist Flexion

Tension and pain can build up in the wrists and forearms from a variety of repetitive daily motions, such as typing or writing. This simple stretch uses flexion—the movement of bending the palm down toward the wrist—to alleviate stress and prevent wrist injury.

HOW TO DO IT

• Stand or sit with your arms at your sides.

• Bend your arm upward from the elbow, creating a 90-degree bend. Turn your palm downward to face the floor.

• Drop your right hand downward so that your palm faces inward.

• Place your left fingers over the back of your right hand and your left thumb on the palm of your hand, directly on the right thumb muscle.

• Gently press your left fingers into the back of your right hand, bringing your right wrist between a 60- to 90-degree bend. Push outward with your left thumb, twisting your right hand inward and creating a deeper stretch.

• Hold for the recommended time, release the stretch, and then repeat on the opposite side.

DO IT RIGHT

• Grasp the back of that hand with your other hand. Pull back so your fingers point down as you straighten your arm. Feel a stretch in your forearm and wrist.

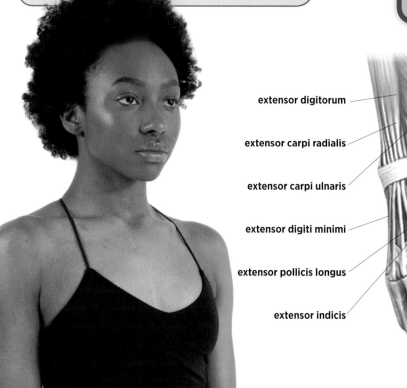

extensor digitorum

extensor carpi radialis

extensor carpi ulnaris

extensor digiti minimi

extensor pollicis longus

extensor indicis

Annotation Key
Bold text indicates target muscles
Light text indicates other working muscles
* indicates deep muscles

Wrist Extension

This stretch uses extension—the movement of raising the back of the hand—and serves as a countermove to Wrist Flexion (opposite page). Pair these moves in a simple routine at the end of your workday to loosen stiff forearm muscles.

HOW TO DO IT

• Stand or sit with your arms at your sides.

• Bend your arm upward from the elbow, creating a 90-degree bend. Turn your palm upward to face the ceiling.

• Drop your right hand downward so that your palm faces outward.

• Place your left fingers over the back of your right hand and your left thumb on the palm of your hand, directly on the right thumb muscle.

• Using your left thumb and palm, gently press your right thumb and palm in toward your body.
At the same time, use your left fingers to press on the back of your right hand, flattening your palm and creating a deeper stretch.

• Hold for the recommended time, release the stretch, and then repeat on the opposite side.

FACT FILE

TARGETS
• Wrist extensors
• Hands
• Forearms

TYPE
• Static

BENEFITS
• Relieves wrist tightness and pain
• Stretches forearm muscles

CAUTIONS
• Wrist pain

DO IT RIGHT

• Press your thumb into the meaty part of your palm, attached to the thumb, to intensify the stretch in your forearm and wrist.
• Avoid lifting or tensing your shoulders.

flexor digitorum

palmaris longus

flexor carpi ulnaris

flexor carpi radialis

flexor pollicis longus

flexor digiti minimi brevis

Annotation Key

Bold text indicates target muscles
Light text indicates other working muscles
* indicates deep muscles

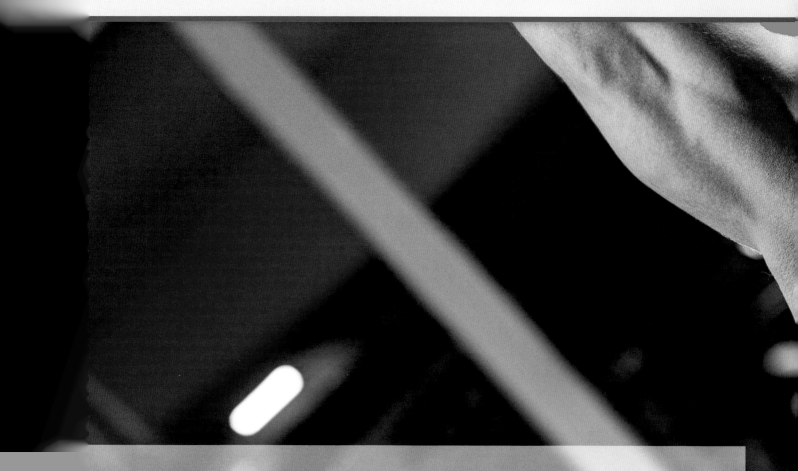

CHAPTER THREE

CHEST STRETCHES

Tightness in the chest muscles can create a variety of problems such as shoulder impingement. Incorporating chest stretches into your daily routine can help improve your body posture and function. A strong chest helps protect against chronic back pain and problems with your spine and neck. Most chest stretches target the three large muscle groups in the chest: pectoralis major, pectoralis minor, and biceps brachii. In yoga, chest stretches are often called heart openers because they increase your blood circulation and energize your body.

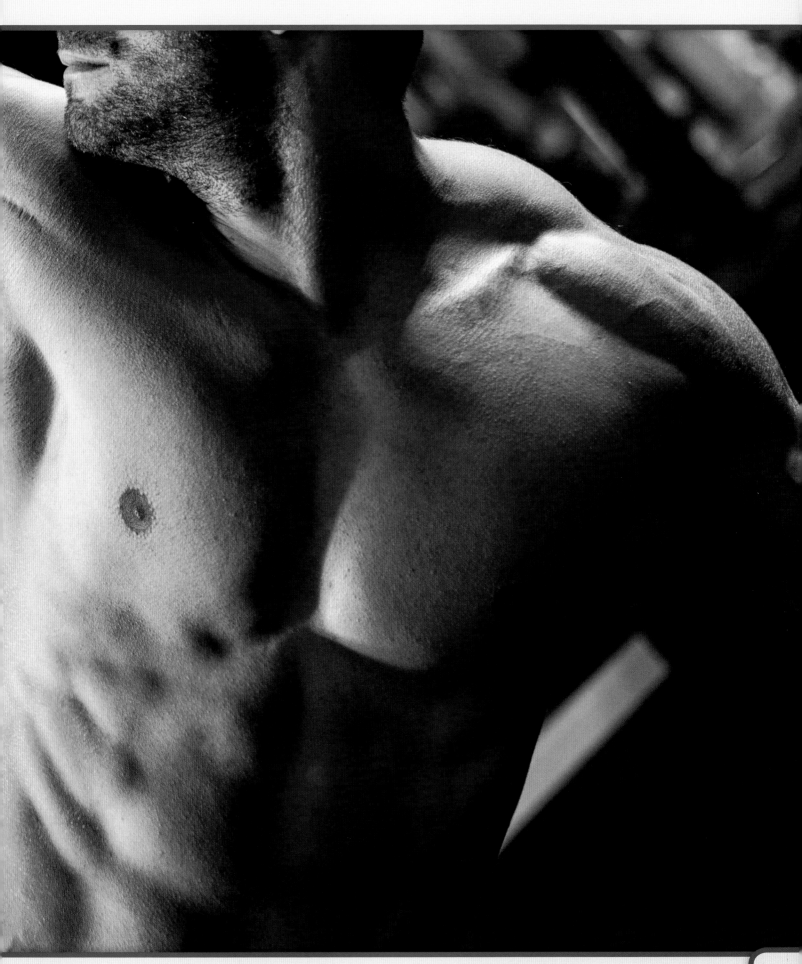

Wall-Assisted Chest Stretch

You can practice the Wall-Assisted Chest Stretch almost anywhere. This chest opener is a great exercise for relieving tension in your shoulders and pectoral muscles and for improving your posture.

HOW TO DO IT

- Stand with the left side of your body next to a wall.

- Extend your left arm toward the wall, and place your palm flat against the wall, with your fingers pointing behind you.

- Lunge forward with your left leg. Remain facing forward as you stretch.

- Place your right hand on your ribcage just below your left pectoral muscle to help keep your torso from twisting.

- Hold for the recommended time, return to the starting position, and repeat on the opposite side.

DO IT RIGHT

- Keep your shoulders pressed down and back, away from your ears.
- Position your arm at a slight downward diagonal, with your elbow slightly lower than your shoulder, to protect your rotator cuff from injury.
- Avoid rotating your chest and torso toward the wall when lunging; instead, face forward.

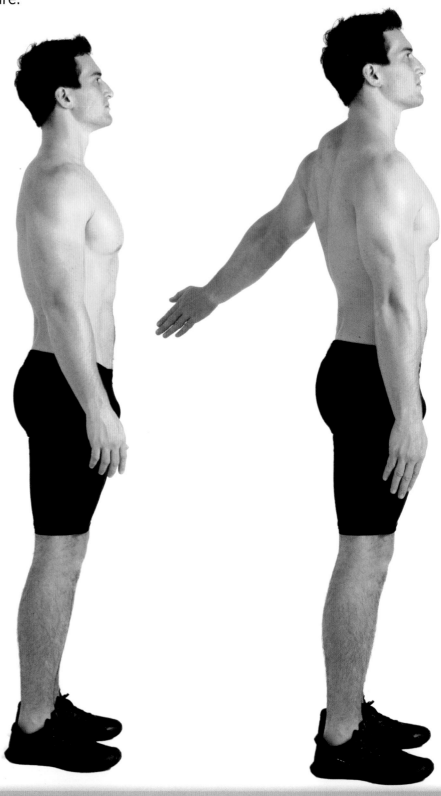

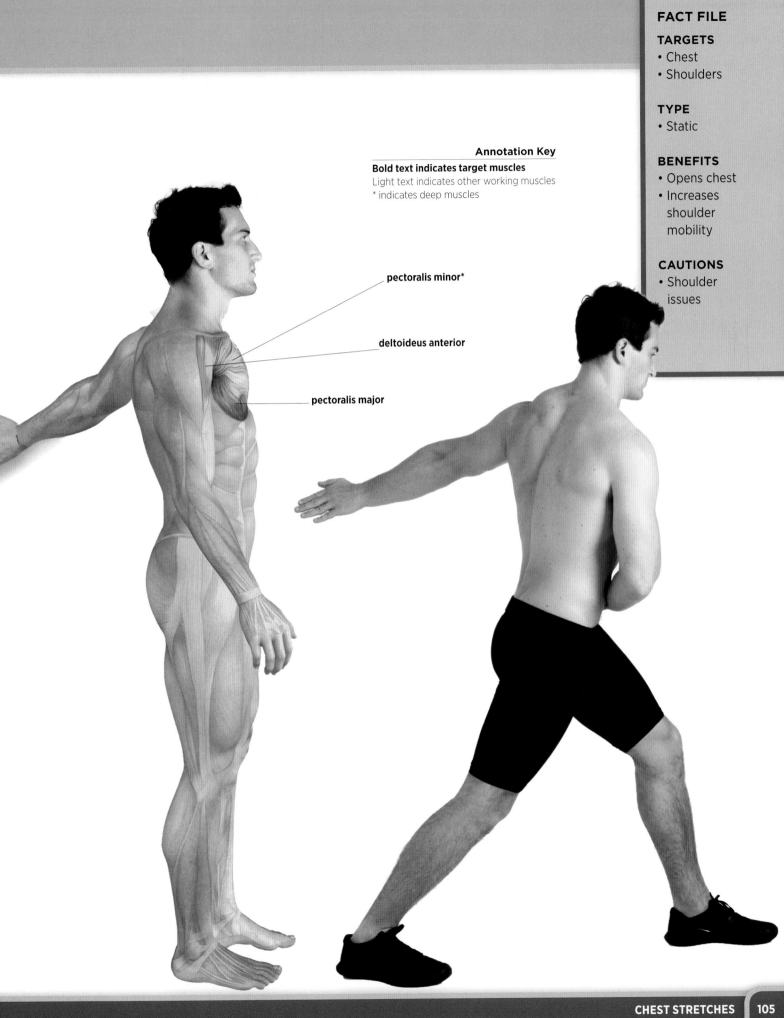

Annotation Key

Bold text indicates target muscles
Light text indicates other working muscles
* indicates deep muscles

pectoralis minor*

deltoideus anterior

pectoralis major

Camel Yoga Stretch

The yoga-inspired Camel exercise stretches nearly all the major muscles of your body, particularly your shoulders and lower back. It also tones your chest, abdomen, and thighs.

HOW TO DO IT

- Kneel on the floor, with your knees hip-width apart and your shins and feet aligned behind your knees. The tops of your feet should rest on the floor, with your toes pointing straight back.

- Bend your elbows, and bring your hands to your lower back, fingers pointing upward. Draw your elbows together, opening your chest.

- Bend from your upper back, and straighten your arms as you reach behind you to grasp your heels. Keep your hips directly above your knees; if your hips shift backward as you reach for your toes, keep your hands on your lower back instead.

- Broaden your collarbones and press your shoulder blades together to open your chest and shoulders. Allow your head to drop back. Hold for the recommended time.

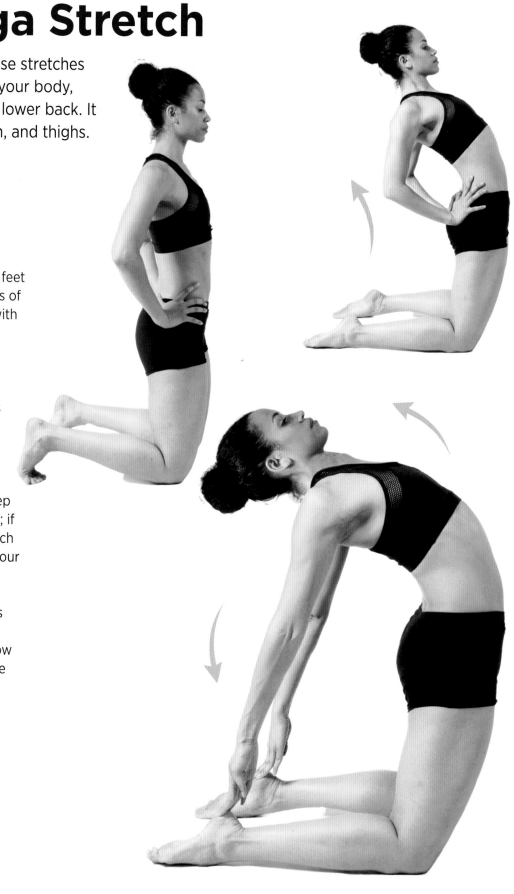

TARGETS
- Hips
- Chest
- Shoulders
- Abdominals
- Thighs

TYPE
- Static

BENEFITS
- Stretches hip flexors, thighs, and abdominals
- Opens shoulders and chest
- Improves posture

CAUTIONS
- Knee issues
- Lower-back issues
- Neck issues

Annotation Key
Bold text indicates target muscles
Light text indicates other working muscles
* indicates deep muscles

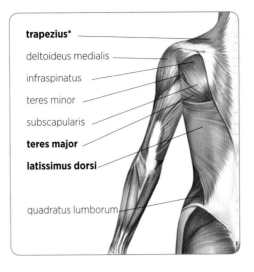

trapezius*
deltoideus medialis
infraspinatus
teres minor
subscapularis
teres major
latissimus dorsi
quadratus lumborum

scalenus*
pectoralis minor*
pectoralis major
rectus abdominis
transversus abdominis*
levator scapulae*
trapezius
gluteus medius*
gluteus maximus
deltoideus anterior
iliopsoas*
biceps femoris
rectus femoris

DO IT RIGHT
- While bending backward, keep your thighs perpendicular to the floor.
- If your neck feels strained when you drop your head backward, keep your head lifted instead and gaze forward.
- Avoid bending from your hips.
- Avoid arching your lower back.

Saw Stretch

This classic Pilates exercise uses oppositional movement to stretch your chest and upper back. The Saw improves flexibility in the spine and strengthens your abdominal obliques. This exercise helps you focus on stabilizing your pelvis during rotation.

HOW TO DO IT

- Sit upright with your legs forward. Flex your feet, and position them slightly more than hip-width apart.

- Raise your arms out to your sides, with your palms facing down. Twist your torso to your left.

- Reach your right hand over your left foot, as if "sawing" your little toe.

- Return to the starting position, and repeat on the opposite side. Perform the recommended repetitions.

DO IT RIGHT

- Keep your hips planted firmly on the floor.
- Use your legs to anchor your body.
- Lengthen your neck.
- Avoid hunching your shoulders.
- Avoid rolling your hips.

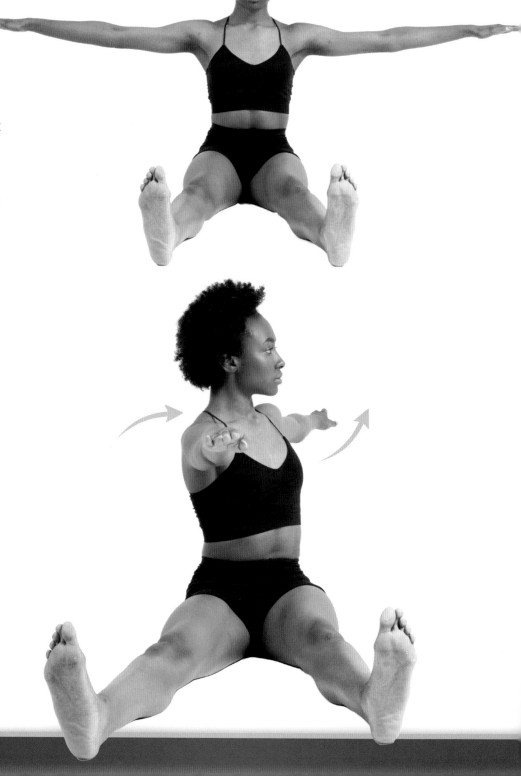

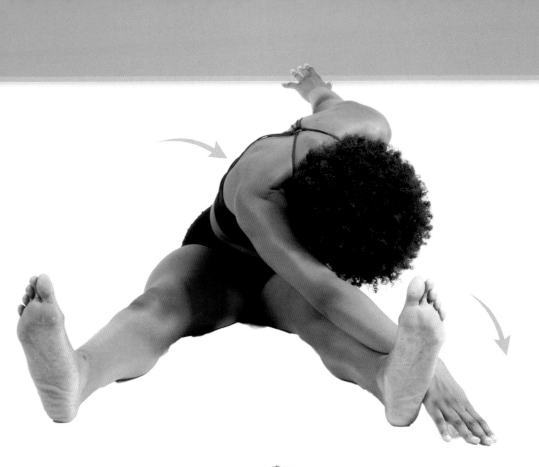

FACT FILE

TARGETS
• Chest
• Upper back
• Obliques

TYPE
• Dynamic

BENEFITS
• Stretches hip flexors, thighs, and abdominals
• Opens shoulders and chest
• Improves posture

CAUTIONS
• Knee issues
• Lower-back issues
• Neck issues

Annotation Key

Bold text indicates target muscles
Light text indicates other working muscles
* indicates deep muscles

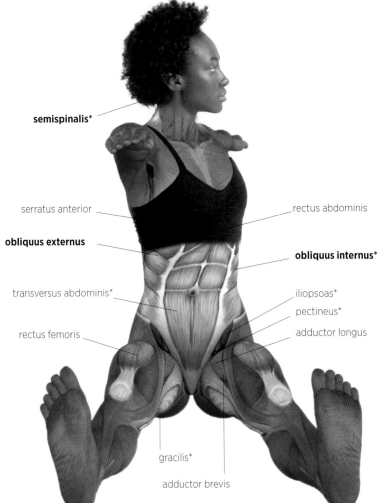

semispinalis*

serratus anterior

obliquus externus

transversus abdominis*

rectus femoris

rectus abdominis

obliquus internus*

iliopsoas*

pectineus*

adductor longus

gracilis*

adductor brevis

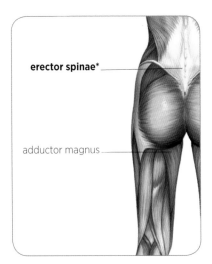

erector spinae*

adductor magnus

One-Legged Royal Pigeon Yoga Stretch

The One-Legged Royal Pigeon is an advanced stretching exercise that opens your hips, chest, and shoulders. This graceful yoga pose stretches your thighs, groin, back, glutes, and hip extensors.

HOW TO DO IT

• Begin in Downward-Facing Dog (pages 72–73). Bend your left knee, and bring it forward between your hands. Place your left leg on the floor with your knee still bent, lowering your shin and thigh to the floor. Your left heel should point toward your pubis.

• Extend your right leg behind you. Your hips should be squared forward, and your right knee should point toward the floor.

• Lift your chest, using your fingertips to bring your torso to an upright position. Press down into the floor with your hips and pubis, and lift up with your chest.

• Bend your right knee and flex your foot, drawing your heel toward your buttock. Reach your right hand behind you, and grasp your toes from the outside of your foot. You may keep your left fingertips on the floor in front of you for balance.

• Point your right elbow up toward the ceiling. Pull your sternum upward and drop your head back. Point your toes as you reach your left arm over your head and grasp your toes with your left hand. Pull your foot toward your head.

• Hold for the recommended time, return to Downward-Facing Dog, and repeat on the opposite side.

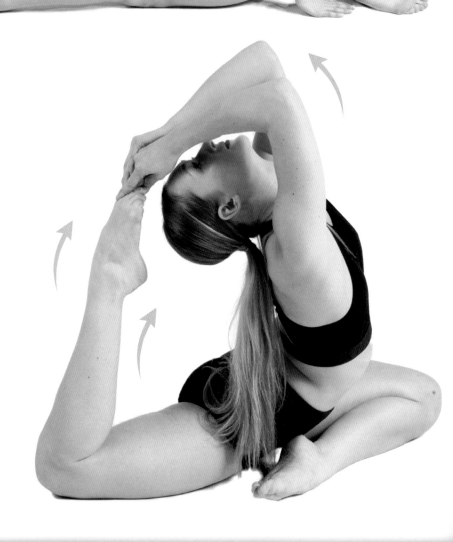

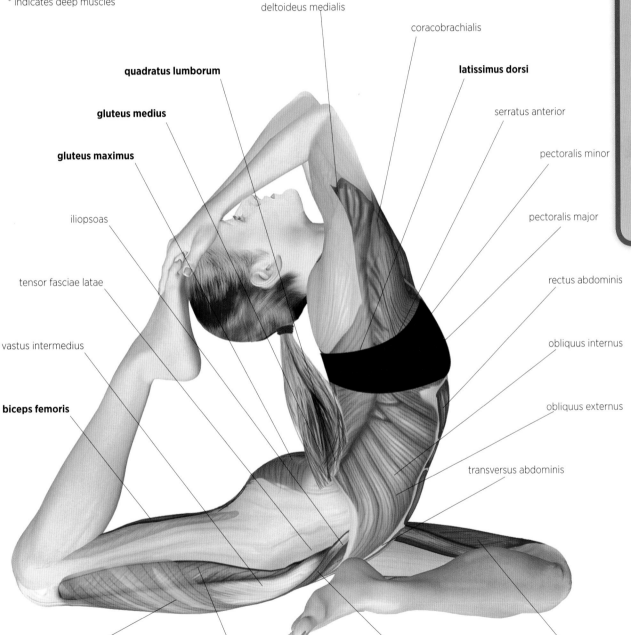

TARGETS
• Chest
• Spine
• Shoulders
• Neck
• Thighs
• Abdominals
• Hips

TYPE
• Static

BENEFITS
• Stretches hips, thighs, spine, chest, shoulders, neck, and abdominals
• Strengthens spine

CAUTIONS
• Hip issues
• Back issues
• Knee issues

DO IT RIGHT

• Keep your hips squared forward.
• Sit deeply, drawing your groin toward the floor.
• Avoid compressing your lower back to compensate for tight shoulders and chest.
• Avoid rolling your back knee to either side.

Annotation Key

Bold text indicates target muscles
Light text indicates other working muscles
* indicates deep muscles

deltoideus medialis

coracobrachialis

quadratus lumborum

latissimus dorsi

gluteus medius

serratus anterior

gluteus maximus

pectoralis minor

iliopsoas

pectoralis major

tensor fasciae latae

rectus abdominis

vastus intermedius

obliquus internus

obliquus externus

biceps femoris

transversus abdominis

vastus medialis

rectus femoris

vastus lateralis

sartorius

Upward-Facing Plank Stretch

The heart-opening Upward Plank stretches your chest and shoulders and strengthens your legs and arms. Because it stretches your pectorals and deltoids, the Upward Plank is an effective counterpose after an upper-body workout that includes push-ups.

HOW TO DO IT

• Sit with your legs extended forward. Place your palms on the floor several inches behind your hips, with your fingers facing forward.

• Draw your knees in toward your chest, placing your feet on the floor with your heels about a foot away from your buttocks. Turn your toes slightly inward towards your knees.

• Exhale, pressing down with your hands and feet and lifting your hips until your back and thighs are parallel to the floor. Your shoulders should be directly above your wrists.

• Without lowering your hips, straighten your legs one at a time.

• Lift your chest and bring your shoulder blades together. Push your hips higher, creating a slight arch in your back. Do not squeeze your buttocks to create the lift.

• Slowly and gently elongate your neck and let it drop back.

• Hold for the recommended time, release the stretch, and repeat for the recommended repetitions.

DO IT RIGHT

• Use your hamstrings and shoulders to open your hips and chest, rather than overextend your back.
• If your hamstrings are weak, keep your legs bent while holding the lift in your hips.
• Breathe steadily, using your breath to deepen the extension in your upper back.
• Avoid using your gluteal muscles to maintain the position.
• Avoid allowing your hips to sag.

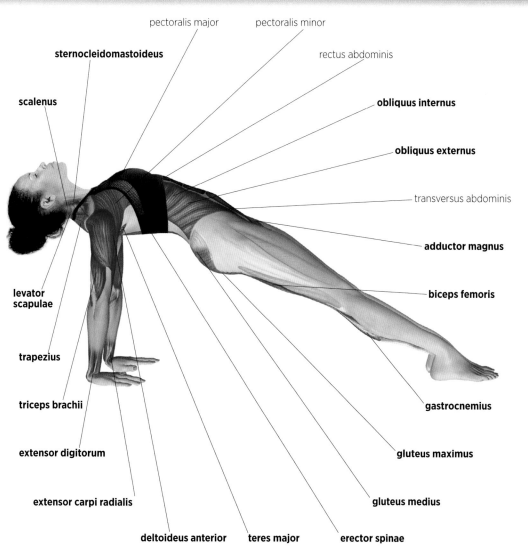

pectoralis major   pectoralis minor

sternocleidomastoideus

rectus abdominis

scalenus

obliquus internus

obliquus externus

transversus abdominis

adductor magnus

levator
scapulae

biceps femoris

trapezius

triceps brachii

gastrocnemius

extensor digitorum

gluteus maximus

extensor carpi radialis

gluteus medius

deltoideus anterior   teres major

erector spinae

FACT FILE

TARGETS
• Chest
• Shoulders
• Abdominals

TYPE
• Static

BENEFITS
• Stretches
 chest and
 shoulders
• Strengthens
 spine,
 arms, and
 hamstrings
• Extends hips
 and chest

CAUTIONS
• Neck pain
• Wrist pain

Annotation Key

Bold text indicates target muscles
Light text indicates other working muscles
* indicates deep muscles

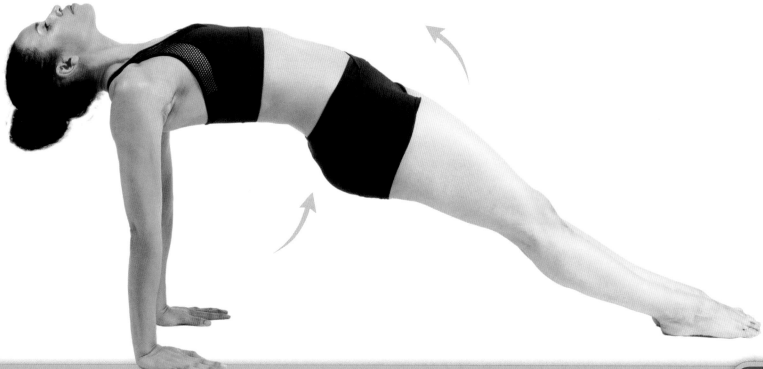

Upward-Facing Dog Yoga Stretch

The heart-opening Upward-Facing Dog Yoga Stretch stretches your chest and shoulders and strengthens your legs and arms. Because it stretches your pectorals and deltoids, the Upward Plank is an effective counterpose after an upper-body workout that includes push-ups.

HOW TO DO IT

- Sit with your legs extended forward. Place your palms on the floor several inches behind your hips, with your fingers facing forward.

- Draw your knees in toward your chest, placing your feet on the floor with your heels about a foot away from your buttocks. Turn your toes slightly inward.

- Exhale, pressing down with your hands and feet and lifting your hips until your back and thighs are parallel to the floor. Your shoulders should be directly above your wrists.

- Without lowering your hips, straighten your legs one at a time.

- Lift your chest and bring your shoulder blades together. Push your hips higher, creating a slight arch in your back. Do not squeeze your buttocks to create the lift.

- Slowly and gently elongate your neck and let it drop back.

- Hold for the recommended time, release the stretch, and repeat for the recommended repetitions.

DO IT RIGHT

- Use your hamstrings and shoulders to open your hips and chest, rather than overextend your back.
- If your hamstrings are weak, keep your legs bent while holding the lift in your hips.
- Breathe steadily, using your breath to deepen the extension in your upper back.
- Avoid using your gluteal muscles to maintain the position.
- Avoid allowing your hips to sag.

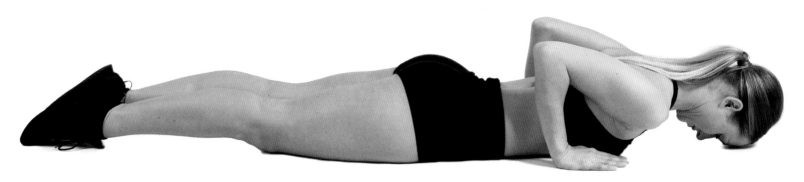

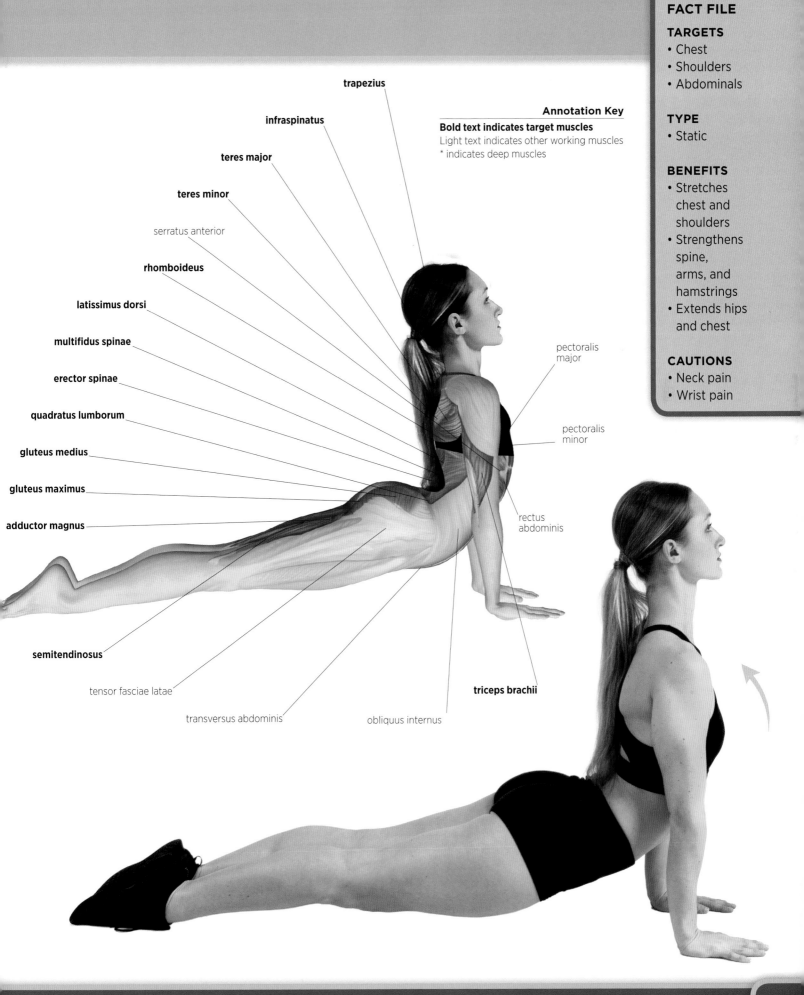

trapezius

infraspinatus

teres major

teres minor

serratus anterior

rhomboideus

latissimus dorsi

multifidus spinae

erector spinae

quadratus lumborum

gluteus medius

gluteus maximus

adductor magnus

semitendinosus

tensor fasciae latae

transversus abdominis

obliquus internus

pectoralis major

pectoralis minor

rectus abdominis

triceps brachii

Annotation Key
Bold text indicates target muscles
Light text indicates other working muscles
* indicates deep muscles

FACT FILE

TARGETS
• Chest
• Shoulders
• Abdominals

TYPE
• Static

BENEFITS
• Stretches chest and shoulders
• Strengthens spine, arms, and hamstrings
• Extends hips and chest

CAUTIONS
• Neck pain
• Wrist pain

Rising Swan Stretch

The Rising Swan is a backward extension stretch that deeply opens your chest, abdominals, and hip flexors. Perform this exercise to relax after a long day of sitting at your desk.

HOW TO DO IT

- Lie facedown on the floor with your legs and heels pressed together. Bend your arms in at your sides, and place your palms flat on the floor by your ears.

- Squeeze your inner thighs and buttocks. Inhale, and press your forearms, pubic bone, and feet into the floor. Slowly lift your torso off the floor.

- Hold for the recommended time, release the stretch, and repeat for the recommended repetitions.

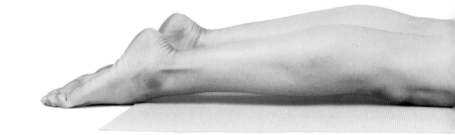

DO IT RIGHT

- Pull your chest forward and upward, while elongating your neck and spine.
- Avoid lifting your torso so high that you crunch your spine.
- Avoid using only your hands to push through the movement.

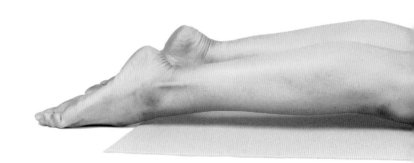

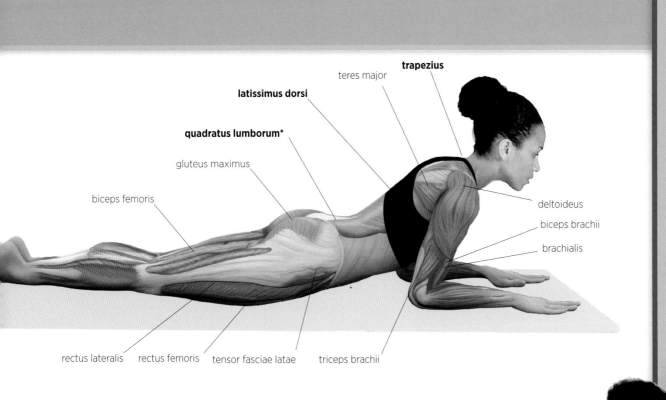

trapezius

teres major

latissimus dorsi

quadratus lumborum*

gluteus maximus

biceps femoris

deltoideus

biceps brachii

brachialis

rectus lateralis   rectus femoris   tensor fasciae latae   triceps brachii

TARGETS
• Chest
• Abdominals
• Hip flexors

TYPE
• Static

BENEFITS
• Stretches chest, abdominals, and hip flexors
• Eases upper-back tension

CAUTIONS
• Back pain
• Wrist issues

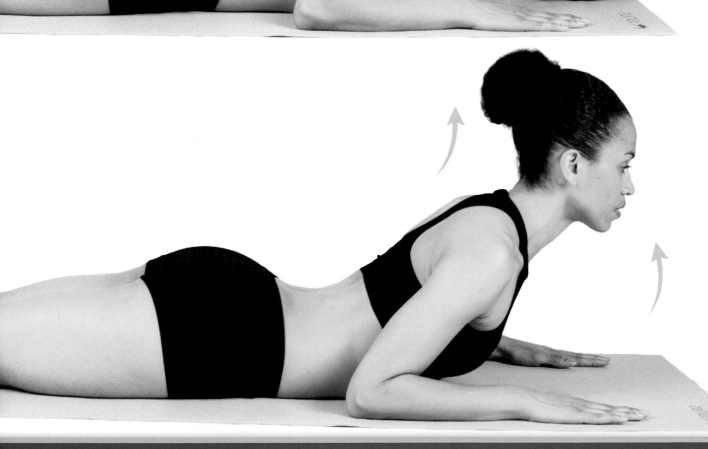

Fish Yoga Stretch

The basic Fish Yoga Stretch targets your pectoral muscles, the muscles between your ribs, and the iliopsoas muscles of your hips. As with other back-bending yoga poses, the Fish Yoga Stretch is an energizing heart opener that helps to relieve anxiety and fatigue.

HOW TO DO IT

• Lie on your back with your legs flat on the floor. Place your hands beneath your buttocks, and begin to lift your hips off the floor.

• Press your palms, elbows, and forearms into the floor. Draw your shoulder blades together, and lift your upper back, shoulders, and neck off the floor.

• Tilt your head back, so the top of your head is touching the floor. Maintain most of your weight on your forearms. Hold for the recommended time, release, and repeat for the recommended repetitions.

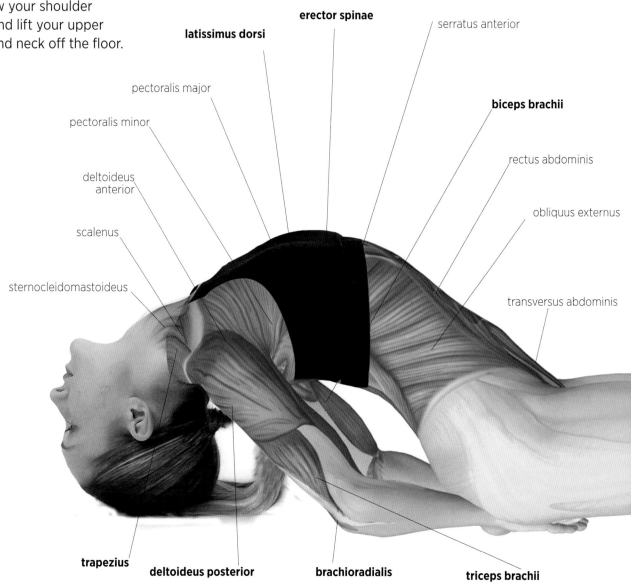

erector spinae

latissimus dorsi

serratus anterior

pectoralis major

biceps brachii

pectoralis minor

rectus abdominis

deltoideus anterior

obliquus externus

scalenus

transversus abdominis

sternocleidomastoideus

trapezius

deltoideus posterior

brachioradialis

triceps brachii

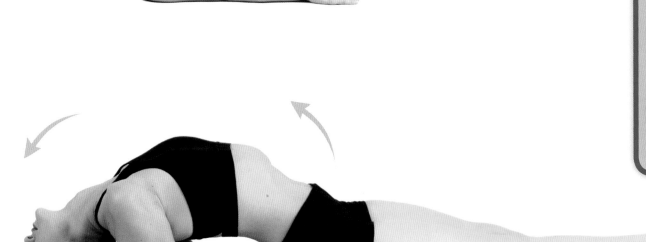

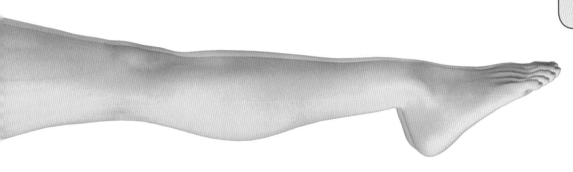

FACT FILE

TARGETS
- Chest
- Ribs
- Hips

TYPE
- Static

BENEFITS
- Opens chest
- Relieves upper-back and neck tightness
- Stretches hip flexors and intercostals
- Improves posture

CAUTIONS
- Lower-back issues
- Neck issues

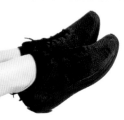

DO IT RIGHT
- Engage your stomach muscles to support your lower back.
- Avoid sinking into your lower back.

Annotation Key
Bold text indicates target muscles
Light text indicates other working muscles
* indicates deep muscles

Half-Frog Yoga Stretch

The Half Frog opens your chest and upper back. This deep stretch targets your quadriceps, abdominals, and shoulders. Be careful not to push too hard on your foot if you feel any pain in your knee.

HOW TO DO IT

- Lie facedown with your forearms and legs flat on the floor.

- Prop yourself up onto your forearms, with your elbows directly beneath your shoulders.

- Bend your left knee, bringing your heel toward your left buttock. Shift your weight onto your right hand, and reach your left hand behind you to grasp the inside of your left foot. Continue to lift your chest and push down with your right shoulder.

- Bend your left elbow up toward the ceiling, and rotate your hand so that it rests on top of your foot, with your fingers facing forward. Exhale, and press your left hand down on your foot toward your left buttock.

- Deepen the stretch by moving your left foot slightly to the outside of your left thigh, aiming the sole of your foot toward the floor.

- Hold for the recommended breaths, and repeat on the opposite side.

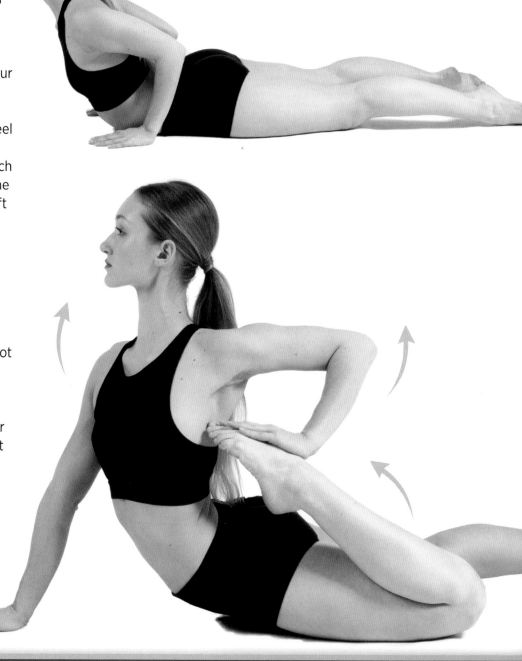

TARGETS
• Hips
• Chest
• Shoulders
• Abdominals
• Thighs
• Ankles

TYPE
• Static

BENEFITS
• Stretches shoulders, torso, neck, abdominals, thighs, hips, and ankles
• Strengthens back muscles
• Improves posture

CAUTIONS
• Lower-back issues
• Shoulder issues
• High or low blood pressure

Annotation Key

Bold text indicates target muscles
Light text indicates other working muscles
* indicates deep muscles

deltoideus medialis

latissimus dorsi

pectoralis minor

triceps brachii

pectoralis major

serratus anterior

obliquus externus

extensor hallucis

rectus abdominis

extensor digitorum longus

gluteus medius

soleus

transversus abdominis

tibialis anterior

iliopsoas

gluteus maximus

sartorius

vastus lateralis

vastus intermedius

rectus femoris

DO IT RIGHT
• Engage your abdominal muscles.
• Avoid sinking into your supporting shoulder.
• Avoid twisting your neck.

Bow Yoga Stretch

This full backward bend develops spinal strength and flexibility. The Bow is an effective counterpose to forward-bending exercises. It also strengthens your arms, legs, abdomen, and spine.

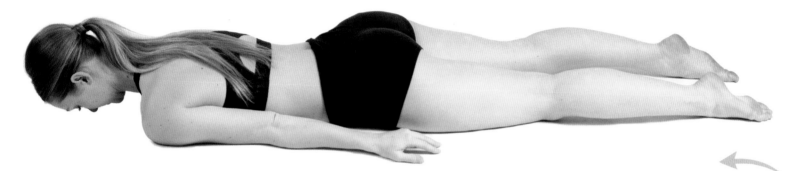

HOW TO DO IT

- Lie facedown with your forehead on the floor and your arms at your sides. Press your pelvis and lower abdomen into the floor.

- Keep your legs hip-width apart, and bend your knees so that your ankles and shins are in line above your knees.

- Inhale, and reach your arms behind you. Grab your ankles, wrapping your hands around the outside of your feet.

- Keep your arms straight, as you exhale and lift your chest and thighs from the floor. Pull your feet away from your head to help lift your chest higher.

- Rotate your thighs slightly inward. Balance on your navel to find equal extension between the lift of your chest and the lift of your legs.

- Hold for the recommended breaths, and release the stretch.

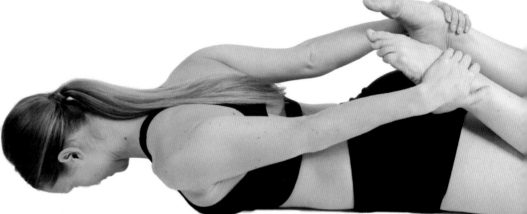

DO IT RIGHT

- Lengthen your tailbone to create space for your lower back.
- Squeeze your shoulder blades together to help lift your chest.
- Lift your chest and thighs simultaneously.
- Avoid allowing your thighs to rotate outward.

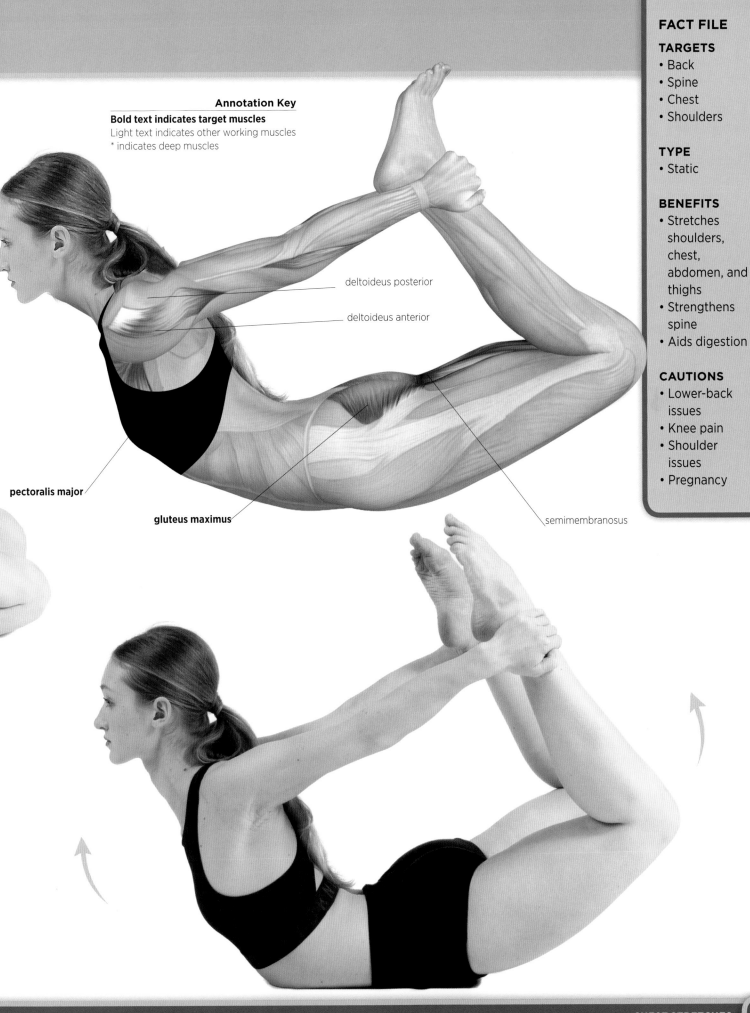

Annotation Key
Bold text indicates target muscles
Light text indicates other working muscles
* indicates deep muscles

deltoideus posterior

deltoideus anterior

pectoralis major

gluteus maximus

semimembranosus

FACT FILE

TARGETS
• Back
• Spine
• Chest
• Shoulders

TYPE
• Static

BENEFITS
• Stretches shoulders, chest, abdomen, and thighs
• Strengthens spine
• Aids digestion

CAUTIONS
• Lower-back issues
• Knee pain
• Shoulder issues
• Pregnancy

Lying-Down Pretzel Stretch

The Lying-Down Pretzel Stretch increases strength and flexibility in your hips. It can help to improve posture, alleviate lower-back pain, and stabilize your pelvis during everyday activities.

HOW TO DO IT

- Lie on your back, with both legs elongated and parallel. Extend your arms away from your torso, palms facing up. Bend your right leg and place the sole of your foot on the floor.

- Carefully lift your hip bones off the floor, shifting your torso a few inches to your left. Cross your right leg over your left leg, with your knee bent at a right angle.

- Hold for the recommended time, release the stretch, and repeat on the opposite side.

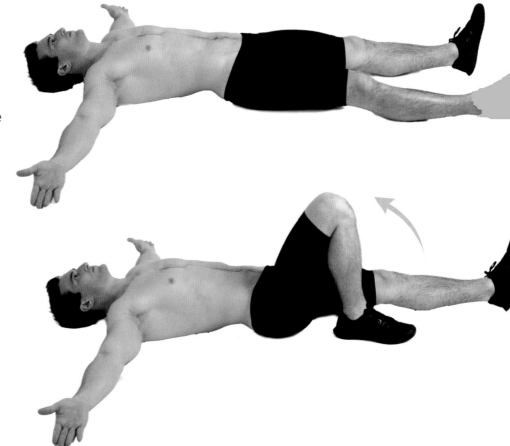

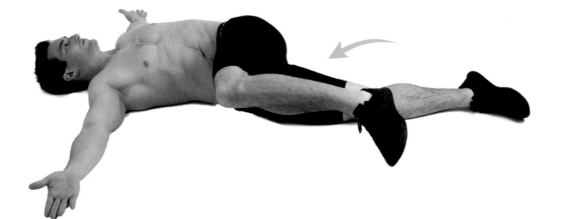

DO IT RIGHT
- Keep your elbows and wrists lower than your shoulders, protecting your rotator cuffs.
- Avoid lifting your shoulders from the floor during this stretch.

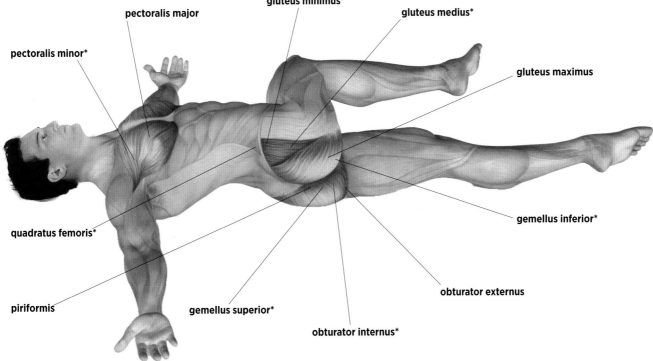

FACT FILE

TARGETS
- Chest
- Glutes

TYPE
- Static

BENEFITS
- Opens chest
- Increases hip mobility
- Stretches glutes and spine

CAUTIONS
- Lower-back pain
- Hip issues

Annotation Key

Bold text indicates target muscles
Light text indicates other working muscles
* indicates deep muscles

pectoralis minor*

pectoralis major

gluteus minimus*

gluteus medius*

gluteus maximus

quadratus femoris*

gemellus inferior*

piriformis

gemellus superior*

obturator internus*

obturator externus

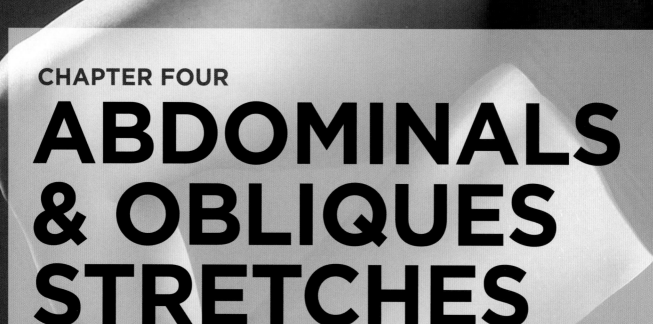

CHAPTER FOUR
ABDOMINALS & OBLIQUES STRETCHES

A limber abdominal area helps stabilize your core and prevent back injury. By stretching your abdominals regularly, you can improve your posture and take some stress off your back. Stretching your abdominal obliques increases your range of motion and your balance. Try some of these abdominal stretches before and after your exercise regimen to minimize soreness and improve overall flexibility.

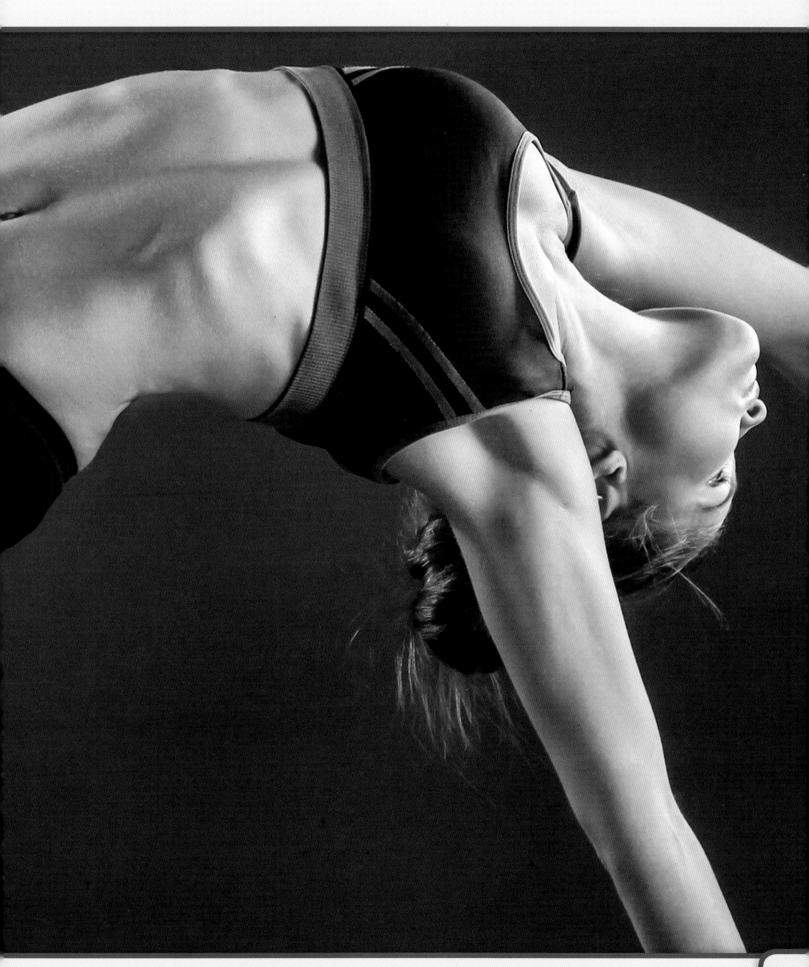

Diagonal Reach

The Diagonal Reach strengthens your abdominal muscles and stretches your obliques along the sides of your body. It also works your shoulders and arms. Move smoothly and fully extend your arms to deepen the stretch.

HOW TO DO IT

• Stand with your feet hip-width apart and your arms at your sides.

• Raise your arms diagonally upward and to your right. Follow your hands with your gaze.

• Hold for the recommended time, release the stretch, and then repeat on the opposite side. Perform the recommended repetitions.

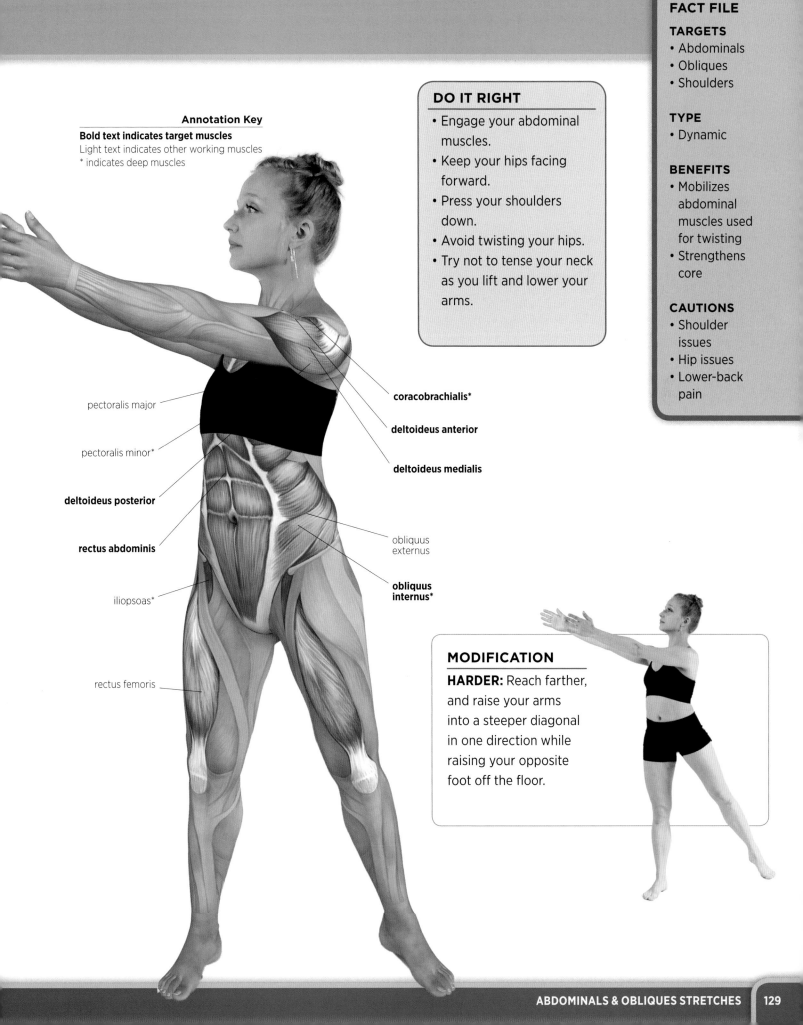

Annotation Key
Bold text indicates target muscles
Light text indicates other working muscles
* indicates deep muscles

FACT FILE
TARGETS
• Abdominals
• Obliques
• Shoulders

TYPE
• Dynamic

BENEFITS
• Mobilizes abdominal muscles used for twisting
• Strengthens core

CAUTIONS
• Shoulder issues
• Hip issues
• Lower-back pain

DO IT RIGHT
• Engage your abdominal muscles.
• Keep your hips facing forward.
• Press your shoulders down.
• Avoid twisting your hips.
• Try not to tense your neck as you lift and lower your arms.

pectoralis major

pectoralis minor*

deltoideus posterior

rectus abdominis

iliopsoas*

rectus femoris

coracobrachialis*

deltoideus anterior

deltoideus medialis

obliquus externus

obliquus internus*

MODIFICATION
HARDER: Reach farther, and raise your arms into a steeper diagonal in one direction while raising your opposite foot off the floor.

Triangle Yoga Stretch

A classic yoga pose, the Triangle stretches your torso and spine while mobilizing your hips. It also strengthens your core and helps you focus on the correct alignment of your shoulders.

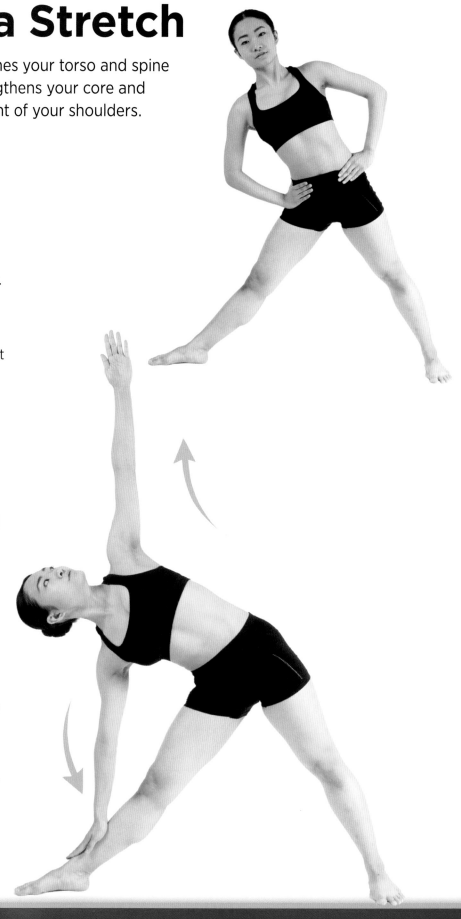

HOW TO DO IT

• Stand with your feet slightly farther than shoulder-width apart.

• Inhale, and raise both arms straight out to your sides, keeping them parallel to the floor. Your palms should be facing down.

• Exhale slowly, and without bending your knees, pivot on your heels and turn your right foot to your right and your left foot slightly toward your right, keeping your heels in line with each other.

• Lean your torso to your right side as far as is comfortable, keeping your arms parallel to the floor.

• Drop your right arm and rest your right hand on your shin or ankle. At the same time, extend your left arm straight up toward the ceiling.

• Gently twist your spine and torso counterclockwise, using your extended arms as levers, while your spinal axis remains parallel to the floor. Pull your arms away from each other in opposite directions. Turn your head to gaze at your left thumb, slightly intensifying the twist in your spine.

• Hold for the recommended time. Inhale, as you return to the standing position with your arms outstretched, strongly pressing your back heel into the floor. Reverse your foot position, and then repeat on the opposite side.

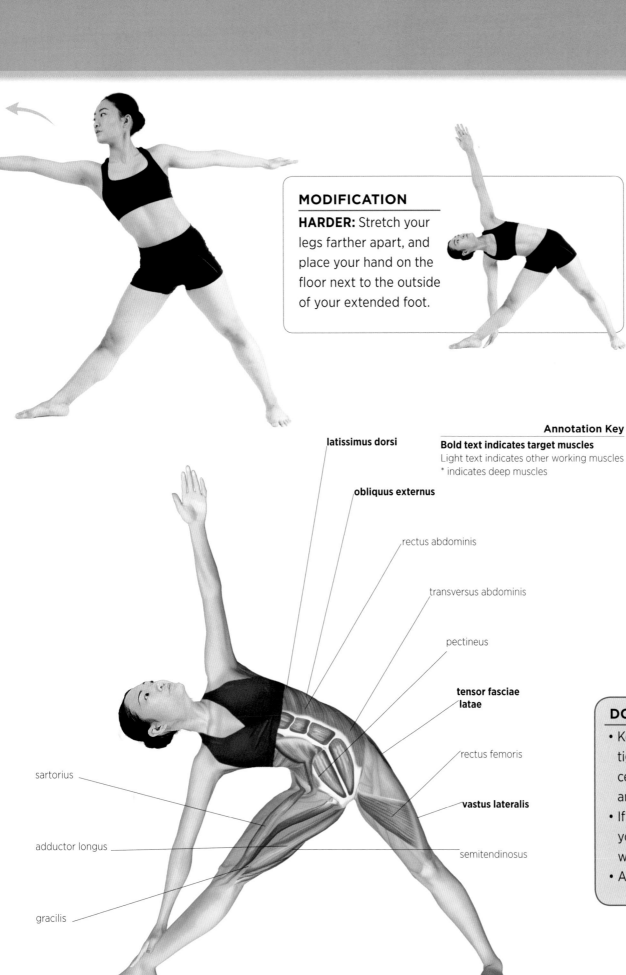

TARGETS
• Shoulders
• Chest
• Abdominals
• Spine
• Legs

TYPE
• Static

BENEFITS
• Stretches shoulders, chest, spine, and legs
• Relieves stress
• Stimulates digestion
• Relieves symptoms of menopause
• Relieves backache

CAUTIONS
• Diarrhea
• Headache
• High or low blood pressure
• Neck issues

MODIFICATION

HARDER: Stretch your legs farther apart, and place your hand on the floor next to the outside of your extended foot.

Annotation Key
Bold text indicates target muscles
Light text indicates other working muscles
* indicates deep muscles

latissimus dorsi

obliquus externus

rectus abdominis

transversus abdominis

pectineus

tensor fasciae latae

rectus femoris

vastus lateralis

sartorius

adductor longus

semitendinosus

gracilis

DO IT RIGHT
• Keep your leading knee tight and aligned with the center of your foot, shin, and thigh.
• If you feel unsteady, brace your back heel against a wall.
• Avoid twisting your hips.

Extended Side Angle Yoga Stretch

The Extended Side Angle Yoga Stretch is an excellent pose for loosening up the sides of your torso. It also strengthens your legs, core, and upper torso.

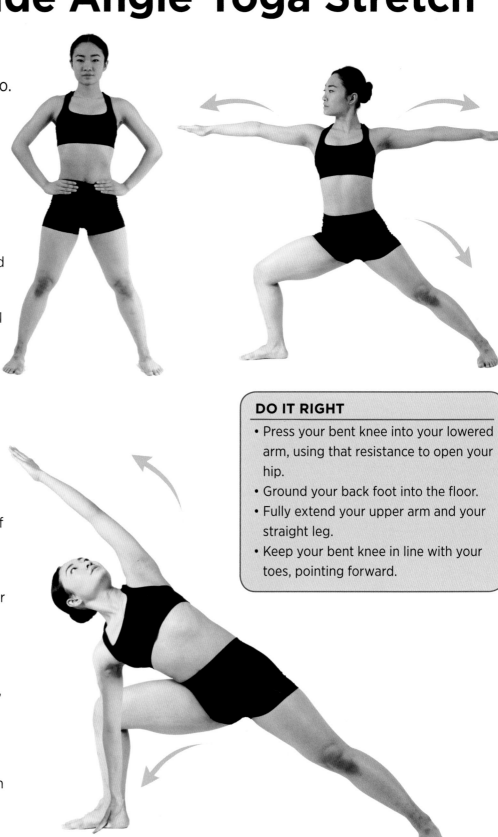

HOW TO DO IT

• Stand with your arms at your sides. Step your feet about 3 to 4 feet apart. Turn your right foot out 90 degrees and your left foot slightly inward.

• Walk your right foot to the right several inches so that your right heel aligns with the inner arch of your left foot. Extend your arms out to your sides, parallel to the floor.

• Keeping your left leg straight with the thigh slightly internally rotated, press your weight into the pinky-toe edge of your left foot. Exhale, as you extend your torso to your right, reaching your right hand to the floor on the outside of your right foot.

• Inhale, and extend your left arm straight up toward the ceiling. Turn your left hand to face the floor, externally rotating your entire arm as you exhale and reach over your left ear.

• Inhale, and lengthen your torso. Exhale, and pivot the left side of your body toward the ceiling.

• Turn your gaze upward. Hold for the recommended time, and then repeat on the opposite side.

DO IT RIGHT

• Press your bent knee into your lowered arm, using that resistance to open your hip.
• Ground your back foot into the floor.
• Fully extend your upper arm and your straight leg.
• Keep your bent knee in line with your toes, pointing forward.

FACT FILE

TARGETS
- Quadriceps
- Glutes
- Hip adductors
- Hamstrings
- Obliques
- Rib cage
- Chest
- Shoulders

TYPE
- Static

BENEFITS
- Stretches hips, groin, sides, and spine
- Strengthens and stretches thighs, knees, and ankles
- Strengthens core

CAUTIONS
- Knee issues
- Shoulder issues
- High or low blood pressure
- Neck issues

Annotation Key
Bold text indicates target muscles
Light text indicates other working muscles
* indicates deep muscles

biceps brachii

serratus anterior

obliquus internus

rectus abdominis

obliquus externus

tensor fasciae latae

transversus abdominis

pectoralis major

sartorius

triceps brachii

semitendinosus

rectus femoris

biceps femoris

gracilis

semimembranosus

MODIFICATION

EASIER : If you find it difficult to reach the floor, place the hand of your lower arm on a block. You can also rest your forearm on your thigh.

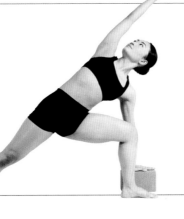

MODIFICATION

HARDER: To perform a bound version, wrap your lower arm under the thigh of your bent leg, and wrap the other arm behind your back to join your hands together.

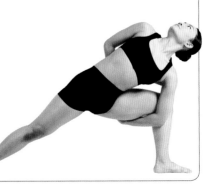

Half Moon Yoga Stretch

Half Moon opens your hips and stretches your hamstrings. It also helps you hone your balance and coordination, calling for you to balance all your weight between five fingers and one foot.

HOW TO DO IT

• Stand in Triangle Yoga Stretch (pages 130–131) with your right palm or fingertips resting on your lower shin or on the floor. Gaze down toward your right foot, and bring your left hand onto your hip.

• Bend your right knee slightly, keeping it extended over your middle toe. At the same time, shift more weight onto your left leg, and step your right foot in about 12 inches.

• Straighten your right leg, opening the thigh while lifting your left leg to hip height. Keep your left leg in a neutral position, and flex your foot.

• Once you have found your balance, extend your left arm straight up toward the ceiling, opening across the front of your chest.

• Hold for the recommended breaths, and then repeat on the opposite side.

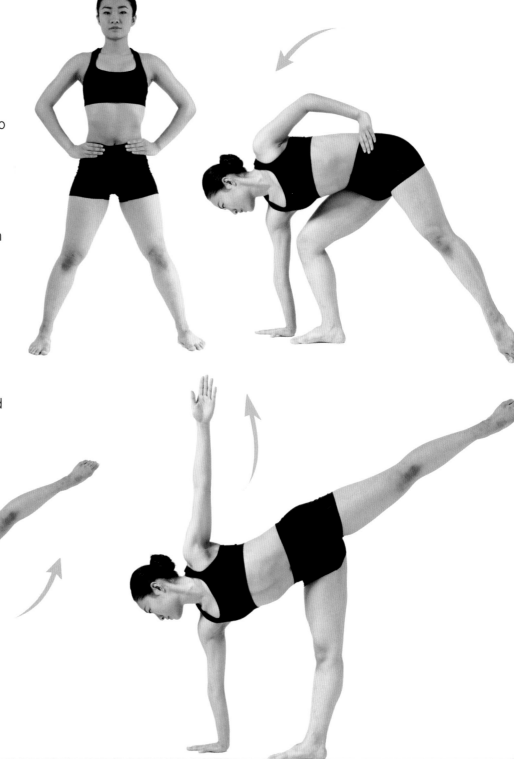

TARGETS
- Spine
- Hip adductors
- Hamstrings
- Rib cage
- Chest
- Shoulders

TYPE
- Static

BENEFITS
- Stretches hip, groin, torso, arms, and spine
- Strengthens thighs and ankles
- Stimulates digestion and elimination
- Improves balance

CAUTIONS
- Knee issues
- Shoulder issues
- High or low blood pressure
- Neck issues

Annotation Key
Bold text indicates target muscles
Light text indicates other working muscles
* indicates deep muscles

obliquus externus

obliquus internus

rectus abdominis

serratus anterior

transversus abdominis

iliopsoas

sartorius

pectineus

vastus medialis

MODIFICATION
EASIER: Use a block to steady yourself until you feel able to extend your supporting hand down to the floor.

DO IT RIGHT
- Gaze toward your raised hand.
- Imagine pressing your flexed foot into a wall behind you.
- Avoid letting your standing foot turn inward.
- Avoid allowing the knee of your standing foot to twist out of alignment.

Mermaid Stretch

Stretch out tight obliques and loosen your shoulders with the Mermaid stretch. This Pilates-inspired exercise also works the intercostals, which are the main breathing muscles around your rib cage.

HOW TO DO IT

• Sit with your knees bent and your legs tucked at your left side.

• Inhale, and place your left hand on your outer ankle. Extend your right arm upward.

• Exhale, and bend your torso to your left. Reach your right arm overhead, and gaze upward.

• Hold for the recommended time, and then repeat on the opposite side.

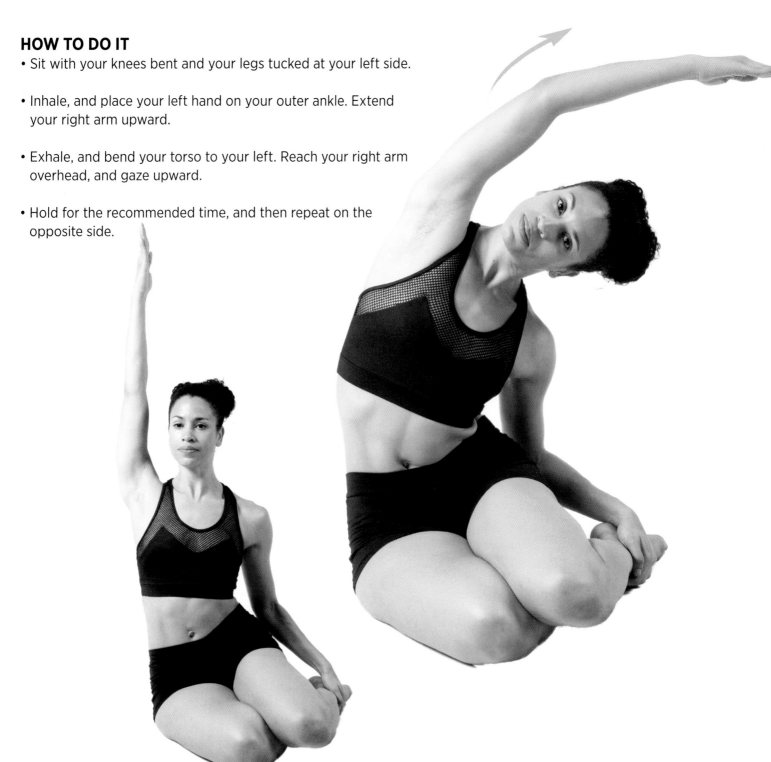

Annotation Key

Bold text indicates target muscles
Light text indicates other working muscles
* indicates deep muscles

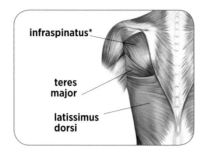

infraspinatus*

teres
major

latissimus
dorsi

FACT FILE

TARGETS
• Obliques
• Abdominals
• Middle back

TYPE
• Static

BENEFITS
• Intense side
  stretch
• Shoulder
  opener
• Reduces neck
  pain

CAUTIONS
• Spinal injury
• Shoulder
  issues

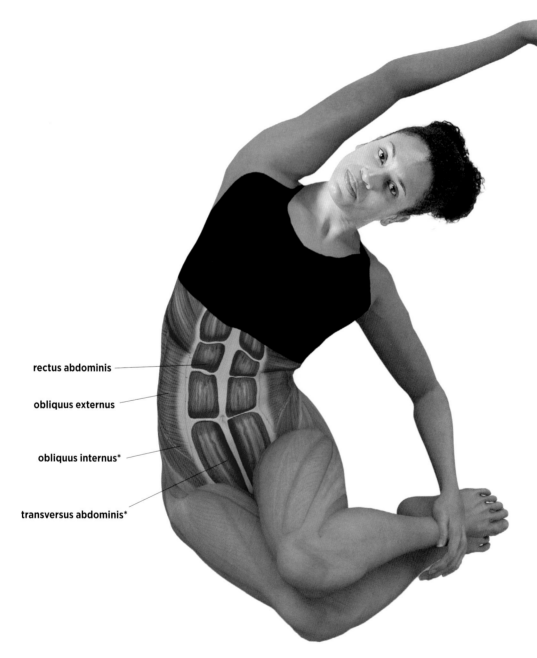

rectus abdominis

obliquus externus

obliquus internus*

transversus abdominis*

DO IT RIGHT

• Lengthen your spine and
  feel the energy release
  through your raised arm.
• Keep the lower hip
  grounded throughout.
• Avoid popping out your
  rib cage.
• Avoid arching your back.

Half Straddle Stretch

The Half Straddle Stretch benefits your lower torso and your legs, opening your hips and lengthening your obliques, thighs, quads, and calves.

HOW TO DO IT

• Sit upright with your knees bent.

• Keeping your right knee bent, lower it to the floor, and draw your right foot in toward your groin.

• Extend your left leg straight out to your left side.

• Plant your arms on the floor behind you to support your lower back as you stretch.

• Hold for the recommended time, release the stretch, and then repeat on the opposite side.

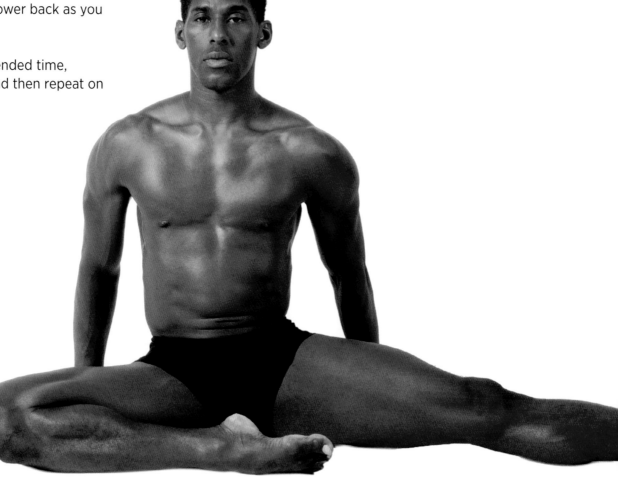

TARGETS
- Hamstrings
- Quadriceps
- Inner thighs
- Calves
- Obliques

TYPE
- Static

BENEFITS
- Stretches obliques, quads, and hamstrings
- Improves lower-body flexibility

CAUTIONS
- Groin injury
- Lower-back issues

Annotation Key

Bold text indicates target muscles
Light text indicates other working muscles
* indicates deep muscles

pectineus*

adductor magnus

adductor brevis

adductor longus

gracilis*

gastrocnemius

soleus

obturator externus

biceps femoris

semitendinosus

semimembranosus

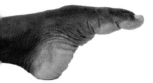

DO IT RIGHT
- Lean your back against a sofa, if necessary, to stabilize yourself and to correctly align your hip bones on the floor.
- Avoid raising your grounded thigh from the floor.

Side-Leaning Half Straddle

This Side-Leaning Half Straddle Stretch increases the benefits provided by the Half Straddle Stretch, deepening the effects on your obliques as you bend your torso to your side.

HOW TO DO IT

- Begin in the Half Straddle Stretch (pages 138–139), seated upright, with your left knee bent and resting on the floor. Extend your right leg out to your right side. Bend your right elbow, and rest your right forearm on your right thigh.

- Raise your left arm over your head, palm inward.

- Bend slightly forward at the hips, and slowly lean toward your right side until you feel a comfortable stretch along your left side.

- Hold for the recommended time, release the stretch, and then repeat on the opposite side.

DO IT RIGHT

- Lean from your hips, elongating your upper torso.
- Avoid lifting your buttocks from the floor.

MODIFICATION

HARDER: Lower your resting elbow and forearm to the floor in front of your inner thigh

FACT FILE

TARGETS
- Obliques
- Quadriceps
- Calves
- Hamstrings

TYPE
- Static

BENEFITS
- Stretches core
- Loosens tight leg muscles
- Decompresses spine
- Improves lower-body flexibility

CAUTIONS
- Groin injury
- Lower-back issues

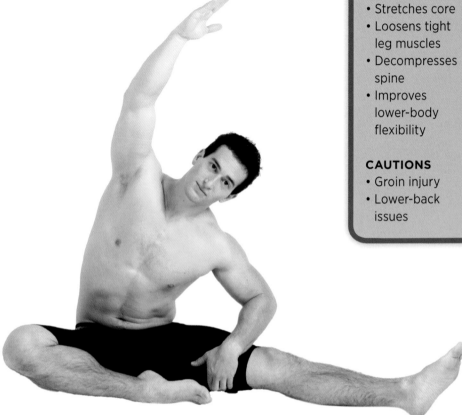

obliquus externus

obliquus internus*

Annotation Key
Bold text indicates target muscles
Light text indicates other working muscles
* indicates deep muscles

Lying-Down Arch Stretch

This basic lying-down arch exercise effectively pulls along the length of your entire body. By pushing your fingertips and toes in opposite directions, you alleviate any tightness in your abdominals, intercostal muscles, and lower back.

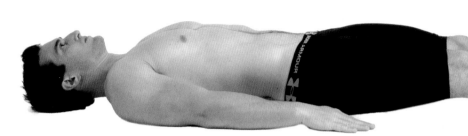

HOW TO DO IT

• Lie flat on your back with your legs extended in front of you and your toes pointed.

• Extend your arms on the floor above your head.

• Your biceps should be on either side of your ears, and your fingers should be pointed out away from you.

• Pull along the length of your entire body as you stretch, attempting to push your toes and fingertips in opposite directions.

• Release slowly and return to the starting position.

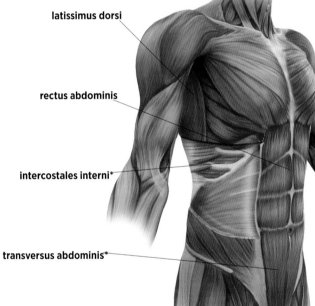

latissimus dorsi

rectus abdominis

intercostales interni*

transversus abdominis*

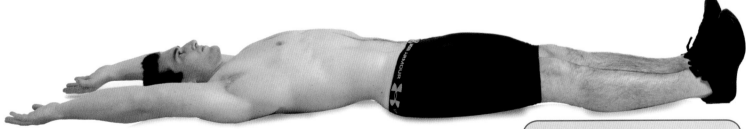

Annotation Key
Bold text indicates target muscles
Light text indicates other working muscles
* indicates deep muscles

DO IT RIGHT
• Form one long line from your fingertips to your toes.
• Avoid overarching your lower back.

Revolved Head-to-Knee Yoga Stretch

This versatile seated yoga stretch engages your obliques, shoulders, spine, and hamstrings. It also expands the intercostal muscles within your rib cage, which can help improve your lung capacity. Perform this stretch to relieve the symptoms of painful menstruation, fatigue, and headache.

HOW TO DO IT

- Sit with your legs extended in front of you and your feet flexed.

- Bend your left knee, and draw your heel in toward your groin, placing the sole of your foot on your right inner thigh. Your left shin should be at a right angle to your right thigh. Draw both sit bones to the floor.

- Inhale, and lift up through your spine. As you exhale, turn your torso slightly to your left so that it aligns with your right leg. Flex your foot, and contract the muscles in your right thigh to push the back of your leg toward the floor.

- Exhale, and stretch your sternum forward to bend your torso over your right leg. Grasp the inside of your right foot with your right hand.

- Extend your left arm overhead, arching toward your right, and rotate your torso toward the ceiling. Reach your left hand down to your right foot. Turn your face upward as you bend over your right leg. With each inhalation, lengthen your spine; with each exhalation, deepen the stretch.

- Hold for the recommended time, return to the starting position, and then repeat on the opposite side.

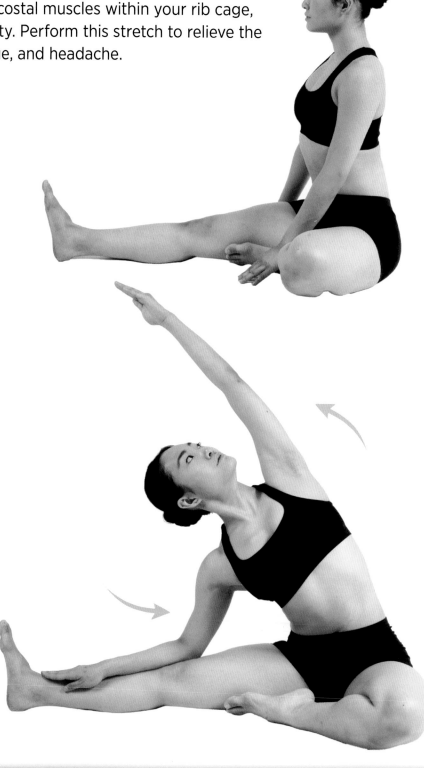

FACT FILE

TARGETS
- Hamstrings
- Groin
- Spine

TYPE
- Static

BENEFITS
- Stretches back, core, and thighs
- Stimulates digestion
- Alleviates high blood pressure
- Eases stress and mild depression

CAUTIONS
- Knee issues
- Lower-back issues
- Diarrhea

Annotation Key

Bold text indicates target muscles
Light text indicates other working muscles
* indicates deep muscles

obliquus internus

obliquus externus

rectus abdominis

iliopsoas

transversus abdominis

deltoideus anterior

tensor fasciae latae

sartorius

adductor longus

adductor magnus

deltoideus medialis

soleus

gastrocnemius

gracilis

semimembranosus

semitendinosus

biceps femoris

DO IT RIGHT
- To help guide the bend from your hips, place a folded blanket beneath your buttocks.
- Avoid rounding your back or allowing the foot of your bent leg to shift beneath your straight leg.

Side Plank

A powerful stretching exercise, the Side Plank strengthens your wrists, arms, legs, and abdominals. It will also help you build your core balance.

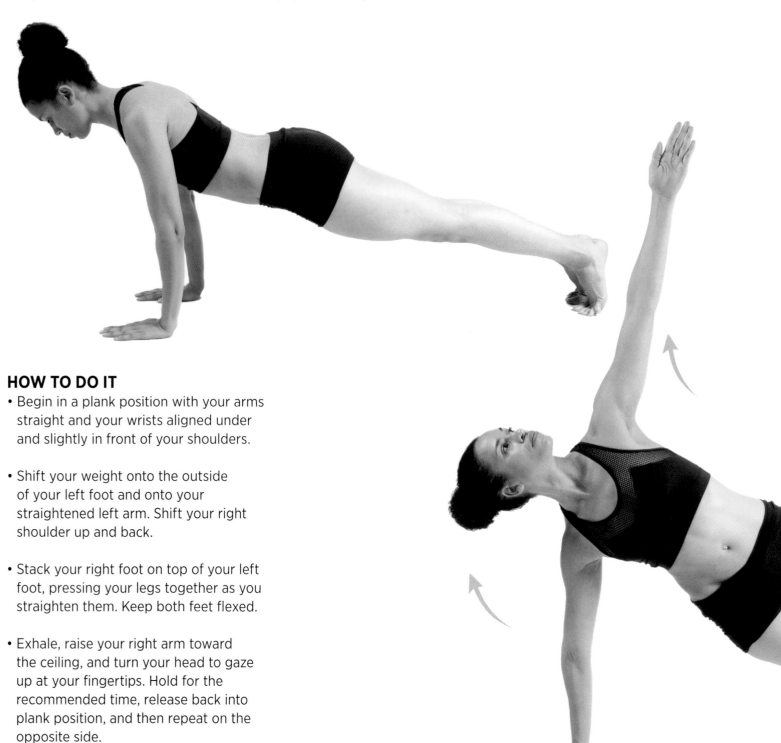

HOW TO DO IT

• Begin in a plank position with your arms straight and your wrists aligned under and slightly in front of your shoulders.

• Shift your weight onto the outside of your left foot and onto your straightened left arm. Shift your right shoulder up and back.

• Stack your right foot on top of your left foot, pressing your legs together as you straighten them. Keep both feet flexed.

• Exhale, raise your right arm toward the ceiling, and turn your head to gaze up at your fingertips. Hold for the recommended time, release back into plank position, and then repeat on the opposite side.

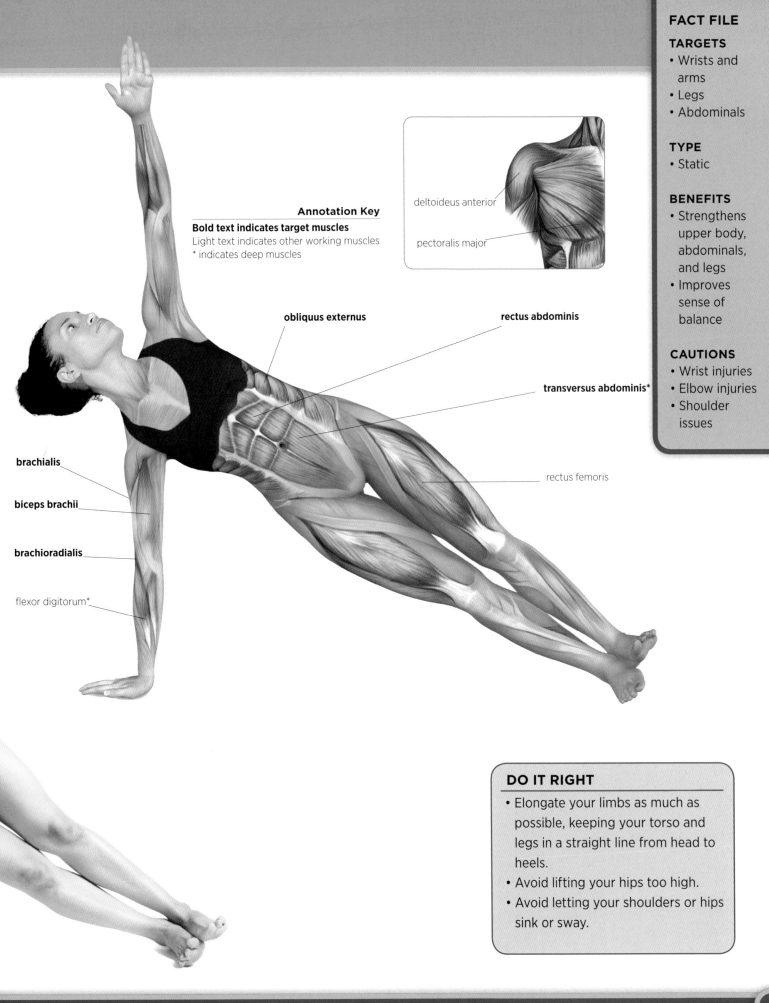

TARGETS
- Wrists and arms
- Legs
- Abdominals

TYPE
- Static

BENEFITS
- Strengthens upper body, abdominals, and legs
- Improves sense of balance

CAUTIONS
- Wrist injuries
- Elbow injuries
- Shoulder issues

deltoideus anterior

pectoralis major

Annotation Key

Bold text indicates target muscles
Light text indicates other working muscles
* indicates deep muscles

obliquus externus

rectus abdominis

transversus abdominis*

brachialis

biceps brachii

brachioradialis

flexor digitorum*

rectus femoris

DO IT RIGHT
- Elongate your limbs as much as possible, keeping your torso and legs in a straight line from head to heels.
- Avoid lifting your hips too high.
- Avoid letting your shoulders or hips sink or sway.

Side-Lying Rib Stretch

Your core helps you stay balanced and assists as you perform many of your daily activities without falling over or straining your back. Your obliques in particular are important for keeping your body stable, strong, and flexible. This Side-Lying Rib Stretch is a great way to keep your oblique muscles active.

HOW TO DO IT

• Lie on your right side with your legs extended and pressed together.

• Lift your upper body slightly off the floor and support yourself on your right forearm. Place both palms on the floor in front of your body.

• Bend your left leg, and place the sole of your foot just in front of your right thigh, your knee pointing up toward the ceiling.

• Keeping your legs in place, press down with your hands, and straighten both arms as you raise your body upward, feeling a stretch around the right side of your rib cage.

• Hold for the recommended time, release the stretch, and then repeat on the opposite side.

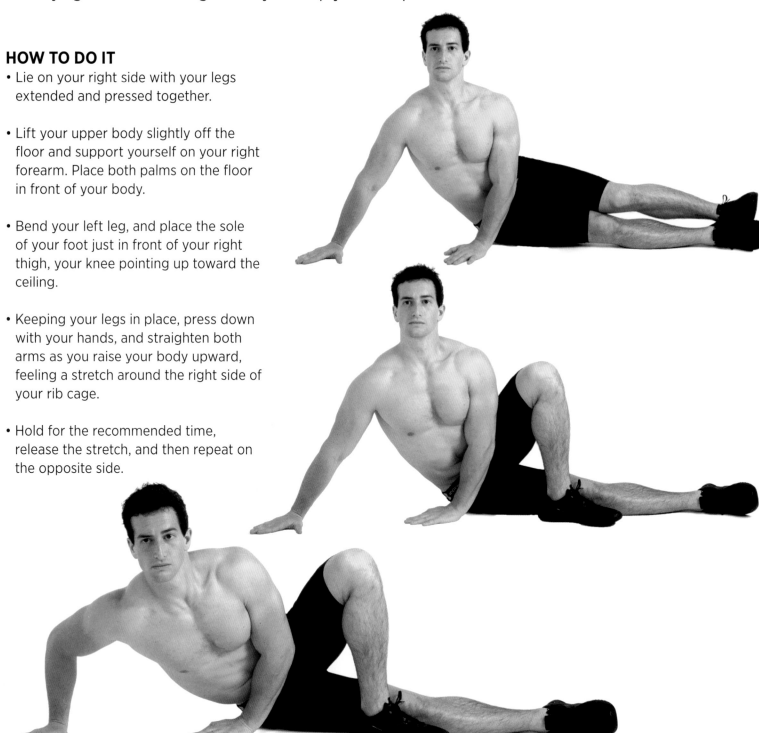

FACT FILE

TARGETS
• Obliques

TYPE
• Static

BENEFITS
• Increases lower-back mobility
• Strengthens core
• Opens hips

CAUTIONS
• Hip pain
• Lower-back pain

Annotation Key

Bold text indicates target muscles
Light text indicates other working muscles
* indicates deep muscles

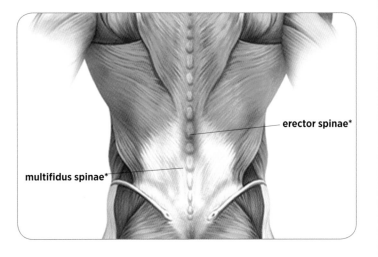

erector spinae*

multifidus spinae*

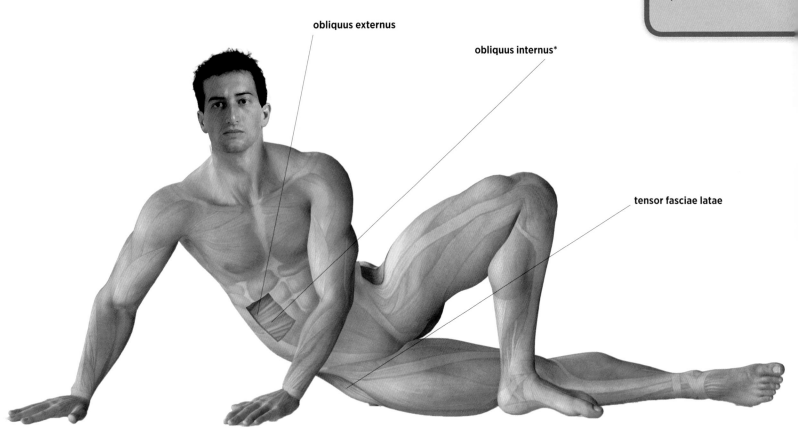

obliquus externus

obliquus internus*

tensor fasciae latae

DO IT RIGHT

• Shift your weight forward on your supporting hip.
• Place a towel under your bottom hip if it feels uncomfortable to rest directly on the floor.
• Avoid tightening your jaw, which can cause tension in your neck.

Reverse Bridge Rotation

This dynamic core exercise, performed on a Swiss ball, requires a great deal of core strength and stability. When practiced correctly, the Reverse Bridge Rotation also provides a highly effective abdominal and oblique stretch and can improve mobility throughout your midsection.

HOW TO DO IT

• Sit on a Swiss ball while holding a medicine ball in your lap. Slowly walk your feet out in front of you and lean back until your back and shoulders are flat on the Swiss ball. Place your feet hip-width apart, and bend your knees 90 degrees.

• Lift the medicine ball straight up above your chest.

• Rotate your upper body to the left, rolling your weight onto your left shoulder while balancing on the Swiss ball.

• Hold for the recommended time, and then slowly roll back to the starting position with the medicine ball above your chest. Repeat on the opposite side.

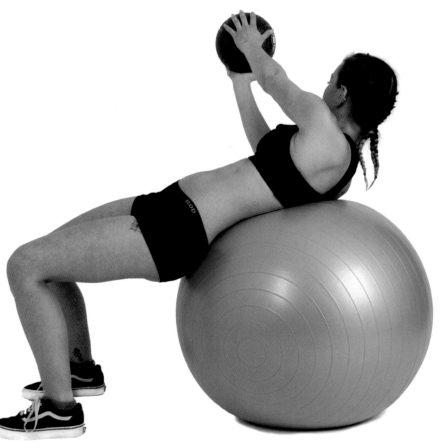

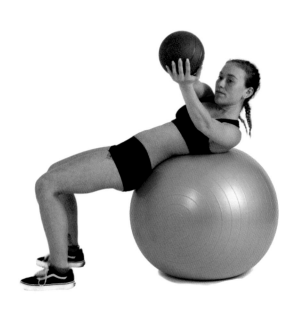

DO IT RIGHT

- Position the Swiss ball directly between your shoulder blades.
- Activate your abdominals so that you maintain neutral alignment.
- Keep your hips in line with your knees as you turn your upper body and work your spinal rotators.
- Avoid bending your arms.

FACT FILE

TARGETS
- Obliques
- Abdominals

TYPE
- Dynamic

BENEFITS
- Stabilizes core
- Strengthens obliques and abdominals

CAUTIONS
- Neck pain
- Lower-back issues

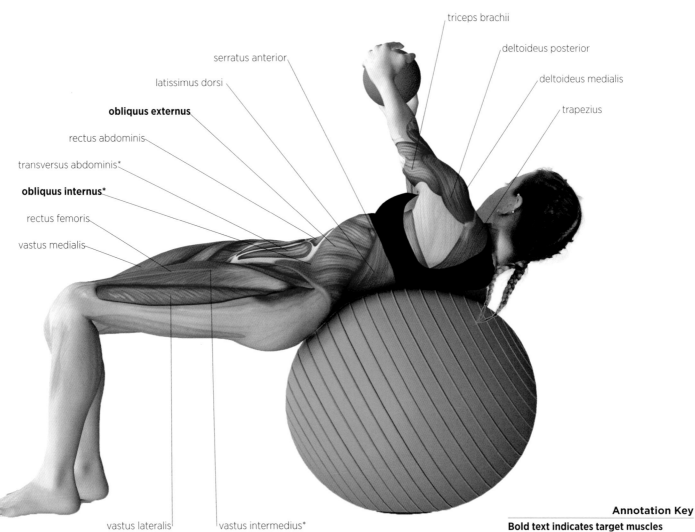

deltoideus anterior

biceps brachii

triceps brachii

serratus anterior

latissimus dorsi

obliquus externus

rectus abdominis

transversus abdominis*

obliquus internus*

rectus femoris

vastus medialis

deltoideus posterior

deltoideus medialis

trapezius

vastus lateralis

vastus intermedius*

Annotation Key

Bold text indicates target muscles
Light text indicates other working muscles
* indicates deep muscles

Reverse Bridge Ball Roll

This variation on a Reverse Bridge Stretch, which is practiced on a Swiss Ball, is a great chest opener, core strengthener, and oblique stretch. For an easier variation and greater stability, plant your feet wide apart in front of the ball.

HOW TO DO IT

• Lie supine with your lower back on a Swiss ball and your feet together. Keep your knees bent at 90 degrees and your feet planted on the floor in front of the ball. Stretch your arms out to your sides, palms facing upward.

• Move your upper body across the ball to your left, rolling across the ball so it is beneath your left shoulder.

• Hold for the recommended time, and then slowly roll back to the starting position, with the Swiss ball centered between your shoulder blades. Repeat on the opposite side, and perform the recommended repetitions.

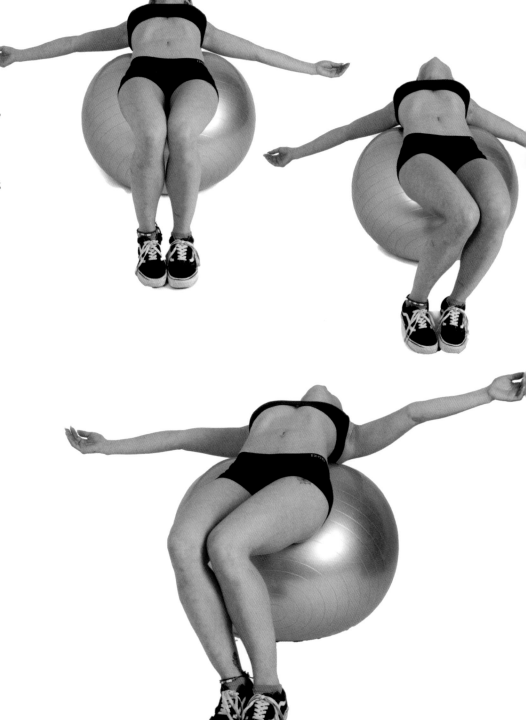

DO IT RIGHT

• Exhale as you roll to the side, and inhale as you return to the starting position.
• Hold your body stable as you roll across the ball, keeping your core engaged.
• If necessary, increase the space between your feet to maintain your balance.
• Avoid allowing your pelvis to drop—your body should form a straight line from your shoulders to your knees.

FACT FILE

TARGETS
• Obliques
• Abdominals

TYPE
• Dynamic

BENEFITS
• Stabilizes core
• Strengthens obliques and abdominals

CAUTIONS
• Neck pain
• Lower-back pain
• Spinal problems

MODIFICATION

EASIER: Rather than keeping your feet together, position them about shoulder-width apart.

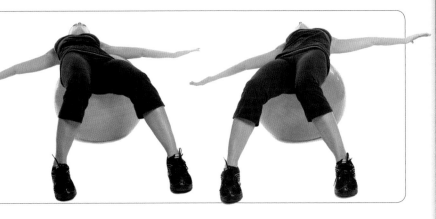

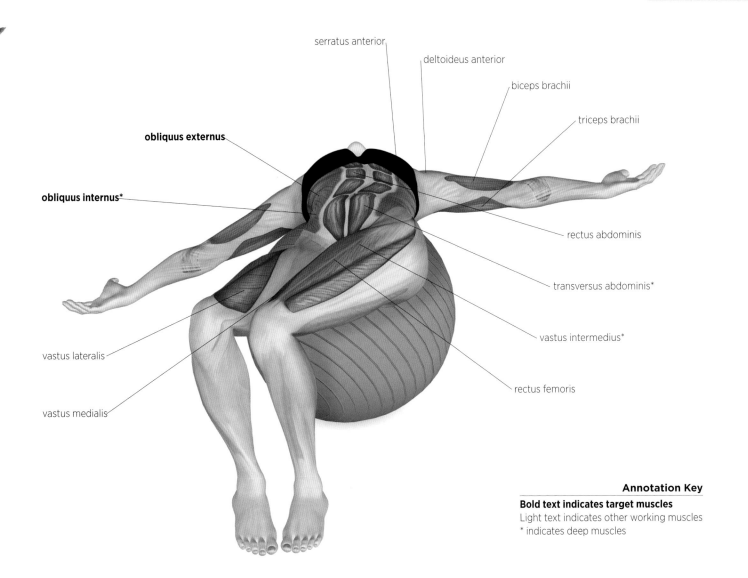

serratus anterior

deltoideus anterior

biceps brachii

triceps brachii

obliquus externus

obliquus internus*

rectus abdominis

transversus abdominis*

vastus intermedius*

vastus lateralis

rectus femoris

vastus medialis

Annotation Key
Bold text indicates target muscles
Light text indicates other working muscles
* indicates deep muscles

Wheel Yoga Stretch

Performing a full bridge is physically challenging but provides an uplifting reward once perfected. This full backbend improves spinal flexibility and stretches your abdominals, chest, and shoulders. It also helps to strengthen your arms, legs, and spine.

HOW TO DO IT

- Lie on your back, with your knees bent and your feet hip-width apart. Inhale, and raise your arms straight up toward the ceiling with your palms facing away from you.

- Bend your arms back, and place your hands on the floor next to your ears, shoulder-width apart, with your fingers facing the same direction as your toes.

- Press your hands and feet into the floor as you lift your hips.

- Lift onto the crown of your head. Pause, then press your palms into the floor, spreading your fingers wide and grounding down through every knuckle and through the base of your thumb and index finger.

- Straighten your arms, and wrap your outer, upper arms inward to find external rotation. Press down through all four corners of your feet, shifting your weight onto your heels. Let your head fall between your shoulders in a comfortable position. Hold for the recommended breaths.

- To come out of the pose, bend your arms and shift your body weight toward your shoulders as you slowly descend, landing on the back of your head and your shoulder blades.

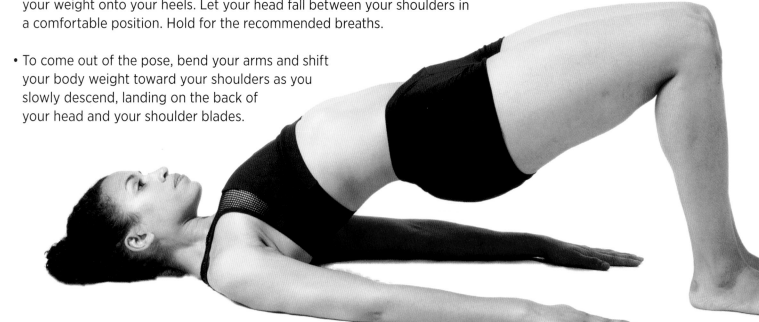

FACT FILE

TARGETS
• Abdominals
• Chest
• Shoulders

TYPE
• Static

BENEFITS
• Increases spinal flexibility
• Improves posture
• Builds stamina and strength

CAUTIONS
• Elbow issues
• Knee issues
• Lower-back issues
• Neck issues
• Wrist issues
• Pregnancy

Annotation Key

Bold text indicates target muscles
Light text indicates other working muscles
* indicates deep muscles

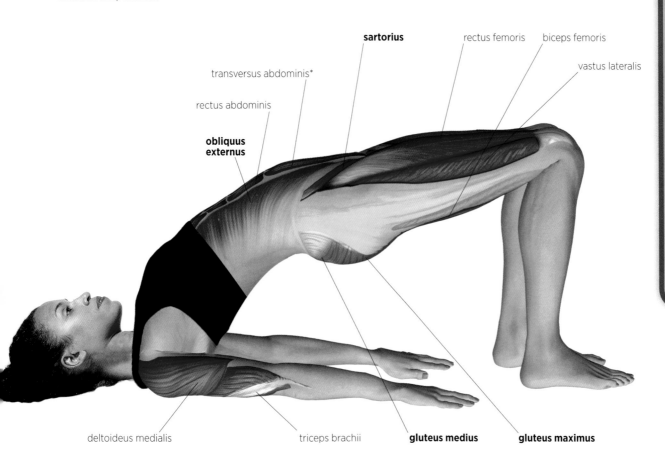

transversus abdominis*

rectus abdominis

obliquus externus

sartorius

rectus femoris

biceps femoris

vastus lateralis

deltoideus medialis

triceps brachii

gluteus medius

gluteus maximus

DO IT RIGHT

• After lifting onto the crown of your head, squeeze your elbows toward each other to keep your elbows over your wrists.
• Draw your tailbone down toward your knees and lift your frontal hip bones up toward your ribs.
• Avoid letting your thighs externally rotate, as this can cause compression in your lower back.

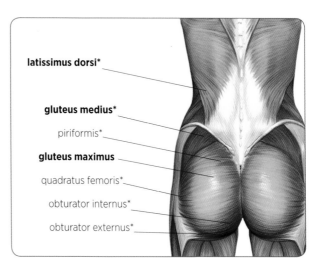

latissimus dorsi*

gluteus medius*

piriformis*

gluteus maximus*

quadratus femoris*

obturator internus*

obturator externus*

Single-Leg Stretch

The single-leg stretch can be performed as a standalone stretch, or as part of a dynamic exercise that involves rhythmic arm and leg movements. As a standalone stretch, it provides an effective abdominal stabilizer and strengthener, while also targeting the muscles in your upper legs.

HOW TO DO IT

• Lie on your back with your knees raised directly above your hips, and your legs bent at 90 degrees. Place your arms at your sides, palms down.

• Inhale, and curl your head and neck off the floor.

• Reach both hands to your left shin. Exhale, and extend your right leg out straight, keeping it raised off the floor. With both hands, pull your left leg in toward your chest, feeling the stretch.

• Release your leg, bring both legs back to the starting position, and then repeat on the opposite

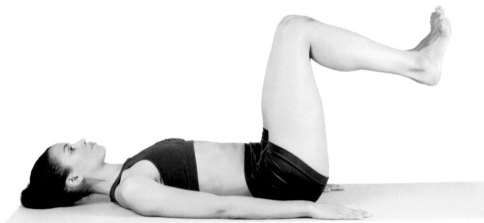

DO IT RIGHT

• Lengthen your neck.
• Engage your deep abdominals and glutes for stability.
• Don't hunch your shoulders.

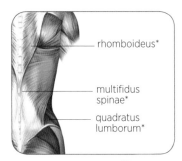

rhomboideus*

multifidus
spinae*

quadratus
lumborum*

Annotation Key

Bold text indicates target muscles
Light text indicates other working muscles
* indicates deep muscles

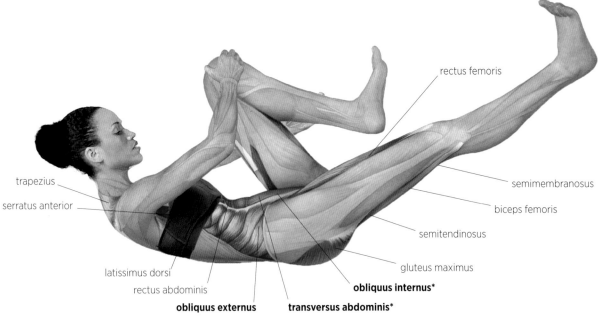

rectus femoris

trapezius

serratus anterior

semimembranosus

biceps femoris

semitendinosus

gluteus maximus

latissimus dorsi

rectus abdominis

obliquus internus*

obliquus externus

transversus abdominis*

FACT FILE

TARGETS
• Abdominals
• Obliques

TYPE
• Static

BENEFITS
• Core stabilizer
• Abdominal
  strengthener

CAUTIONS
• Hip pain
• Upper- or
  lower-back
  sensitivity

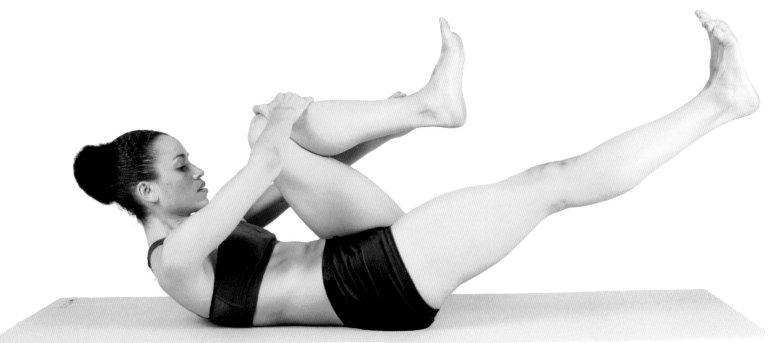

Double-Leg Stretch

The Double-Leg Stretch challenges your abdominals, especially your obliques and transverse muscles. The lower you hold your arms and legs, the harder the exercise. Begin by extending your arms and legs at a steep diagonal.

HOW TO DO IT

- Lie on your back with your legs bent and perpendicular. Flex your feet. Inhale, and curl your head and neck from the mat.

- Place your hands on the outside of your knees. Exhale and extend your arms and legs to 45 degrees, pointing your toes.

- Hold this pose for the recommended time.

- Inhale, and return your legs to the original position.

- Circle your arms out to your sides and back to your knees.

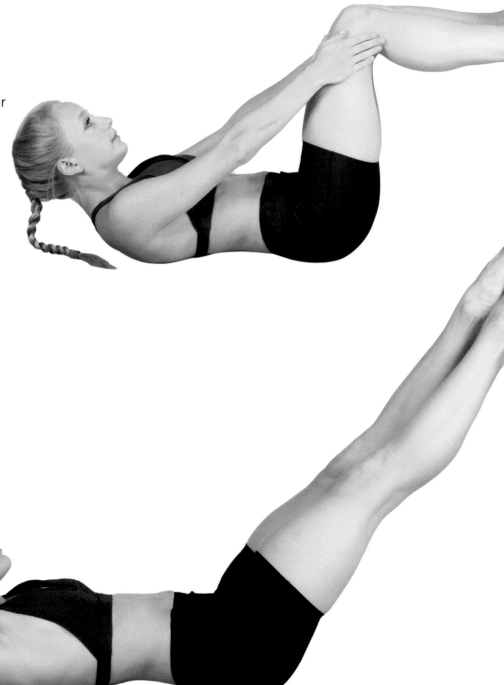

TARGETS
- Obliques
- Abdominals
- Thighs

TYPE
- Static

BENEFITS
- Abdominal strengthener
- Core stabilizer

CAUTIONS
- Shoulder pain
- Spinal problems

DO IT RIGHT

- Stabilize your torso and hips and keep your abdominals flat.
- Focus your gaze on your knees to steady your movements.
- Avoid swinging your knees into your chest.

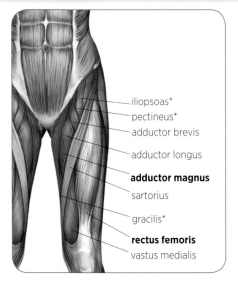

iliopsoas*
pectineus*
adductor brevis
adductor longus
adductor magnus
sartorius
gracilis*
rectus femoris
vastus medialis

Annotation Key

Bold text indicates target muscles
Light text indicates other working muscles
* indicates deep muscles

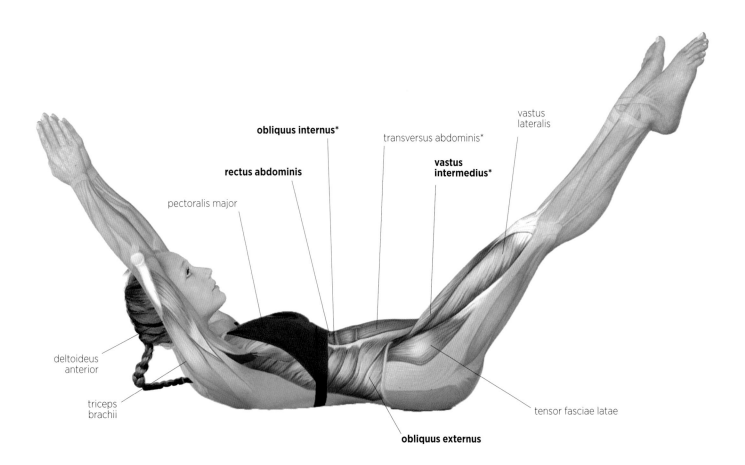

obliquus internus*
transversus abdominis*
vastus lateralis
rectus abdominis
vastus intermedius*
pectoralis major
deltoideus anterior
triceps brachii
tensor fasciae latae
obliquus externus

Reclining Hero Yoga Stretch

Reclining Hero provides an intense stretch in your thighs, hip flexors, and ankles. This exercise also deeply stretches your entire pelvic region, including your abdominal muscles. Practice this restorative stretch in the evening after spending long hours of sitting during the day.

HOW TO DO IT

- Kneel with your buttocks resting lightly on your heels.

- Lean back gradually, and exhale, placing your hands on the floor behind you for support. Carefully lower yourself onto your elbows.

- Recline all the way back until your back reaches the floor. Move your arms to your sides, relaxing them, with your palms facing upward. Squeeze your knees together so that they don't separate wider than your hips or lift off the floor.

- Hold for the recommended time, release the stretch, and then return to the starting position.

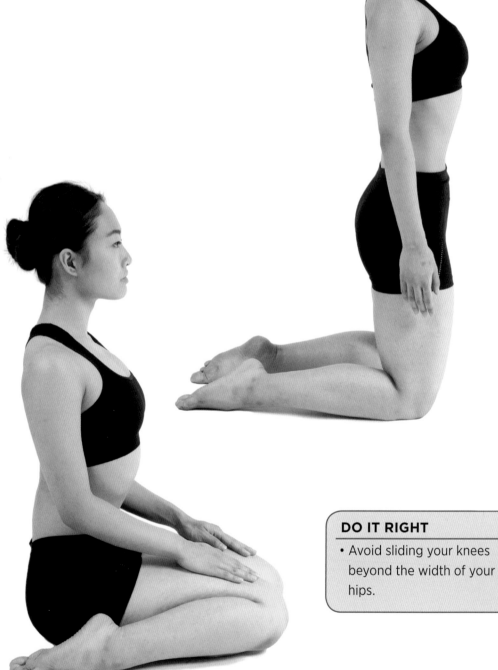

DO IT RIGHT

- Avoid sliding your knees beyond the width of your hips.

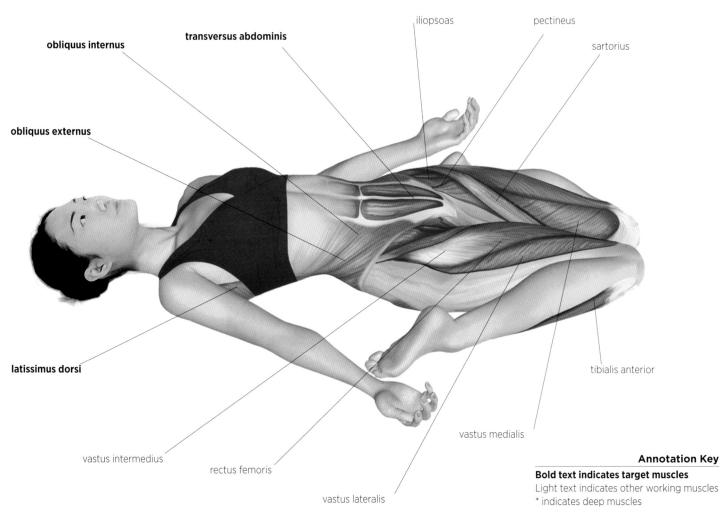

TARGETS
- Abdominals
- Thighs
- Groin
- Knees
- Ankles

TYPE
- Static

BENEFITS
- Loosens thighs, knees, hip flexors, and ankles
- Alleviates arthritis

CAUTIONS
- Knee injury
- Ankle injury
- Back issues

iliopsoas

pectineus

sartorius

obliquus internus

transversus abdominis

obliquus externus

tibialis anterior

latissimus dorsi

vastus medialis

vastus intermedius

rectus femoris

Annotation Key

Bold text indicates target muscles
Light text indicates other working muscles
* indicates deep muscles

vastus lateralis

Corkscrew Stretch

The Corkscrew targets your hips, thighs, and abdominals. This classic Pilates exercise really challenges your stamina as you move your legs together in a circular motion: the larger the circles, the harder the workout.

HOW TO DO IT

- Lie on the floor with your legs extended toward the ceiling.

- Press your legs and heels together, and point your toes.

- Inhale, as you lower your legs to your right.

- Continue circling, bringing your legs forward, then to your left, and back up to the center.

- Complete the circle, and bring your legs down to the floor, and then repeat in the opposite direction.

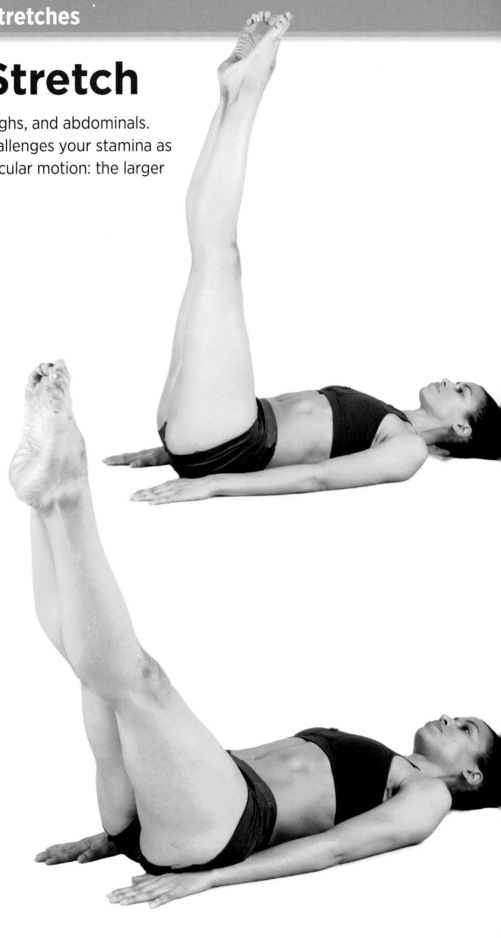

DO IT RIGHT
- Press your back and arms firmly into the floor.
- Pull your shoulder blades down your back.
- If you feel any strain in your joints, bend your knees slightly.
- Avoid hunching your shoulders.
- Avoid arching your back.

TARGETS
• Abdominals
• Obliques
• Hip flexors

TYPE
• Dynamic

BENEFITS
• Abdominal
  strengthener
• Hip stabilizer

CAUTIONS
• Hip pain
• Knee pain
• Neck
  problems

rectus abdominis

obliquus
internus*

iliopsoas*

pectineus*

sartorius

rectus femoris

transversus abdominis*

soleus

gastrocnemius

semimembranosus

vastus lateralis

tensor
fasciae latae

obliquus externus

Annotation Key

Bold text indicates target muscles
Light text indicates other working muscles
* indicates deep muscles

Jackknife Stretch

The Jackknife is a real test for the abdominal muscles. Your legs and hips will also benefit from this Pilates exercise, and you should find yourself becoming more flexible as you perfect this pose.

HOW TO DO IT

• Lie on your back with your legs straight up and your arms planted at your sides. Inhale, and engage your abdominals.

• As you exhale, lift your hips and spine from the floor, until you are supporting your weight on your upper back and shoulders, and your legs are at 45 degrees over your head.

• Extend your legs straight up and slowly roll your spine back down to the floor.

• Perform the recommended repetitions.

DO IT RIGHT

• Aim to keep your limbs as straight as possible throughout this stretch.
• Inhale while lowering your body and legs, and exhale as you lift.
• Avoid letting your hands leave the floor.

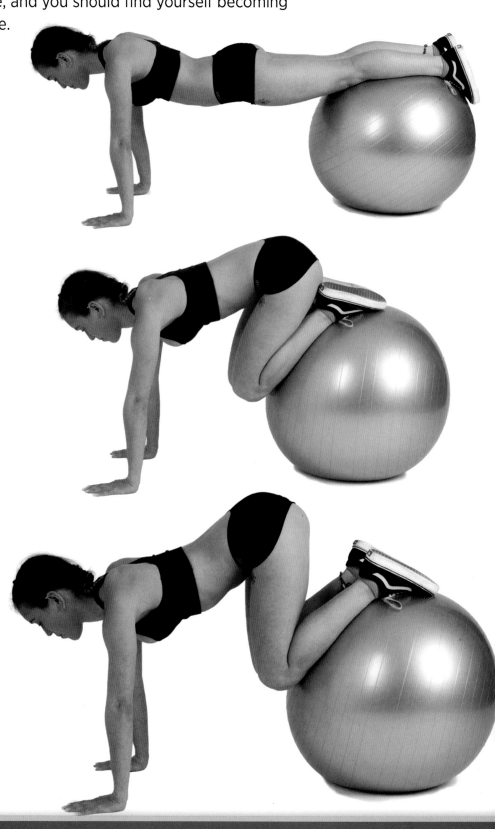

FACT FILE

TARGETS
• Abdominals
• Obliques
• Hip flexors

TYPE
• Dynamic

BENEFITS
• Abdominal
  strengthener
• Core stabilizer

CAUTIONS
• Neck
  problems
• Shoulder pain

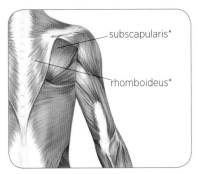

subscapularis*

rhomboideus*

rectus
abdominis

transversus
abdominis*

sartorius

Annotation Key

Bold text indicates target muscles
Light text indicates other working muscles
* indicates deep muscles

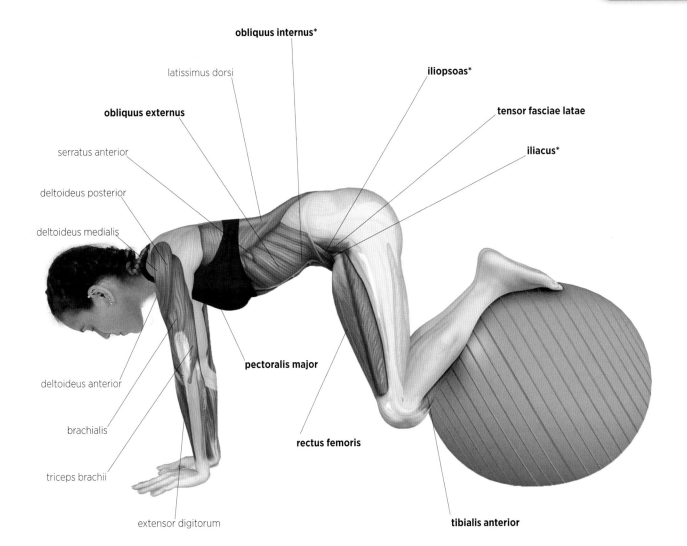

obliquus internus*

latissimus dorsi

iliopsoas*

obliquus externus

tensor fasciae latae

serratus anterior

iliacus*

deltoideus posterior

deltoideus medialis

pectoralis major

deltoideus anterior

brachialis

rectus femoris

triceps brachii

extensor digitorum

tibialis anterior

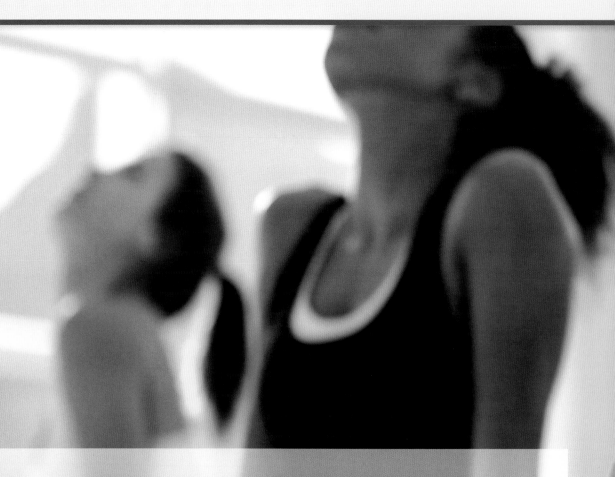

CHAPTER FIVE

LOWER-BACK STRETCHES

Back pain is a problem that affects just about everyone at some point in life. Learning to incorporate a range of stretches that target the spine's supporting muscles—especially those of the vulnerable lower-back—can help you relieve any tightness or pain that may arise if you spend too many hours sitting at a desk. Regularly practicing these stretches can also prevent back pain in the future.

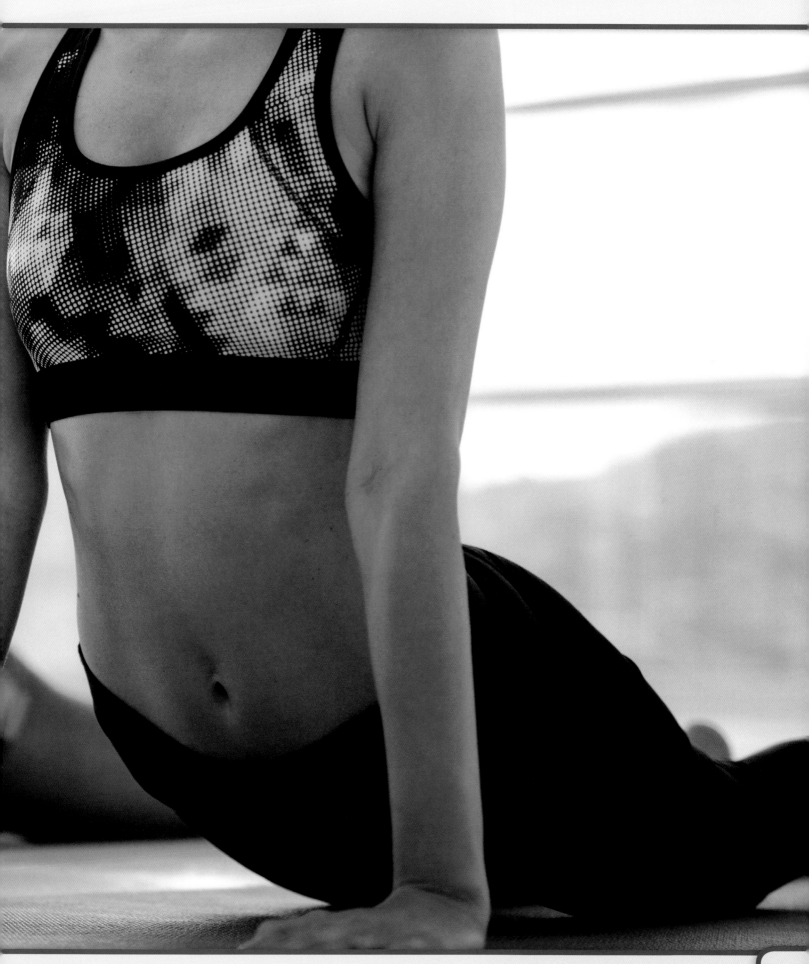

Lord of the Dance Yoga Stretch

In yoga, Lord of the Dance refers to the Hindu god Shiva. This graceful pose helps develop your balancing skills while deeply stretching your hips and shoulders.

HOW TO DO IT

• Begin by standing straight with your feet together. Bend your right knee, and draw your right heel toward your buttocks. Keep your left foot firmly planted into the floor.

• Turn your right palm outward, reach behind your back, and grasp the inside of your right foot. Lift through your spine from your tailbone to the top of your neck.

• Raise your right foot toward the ceiling, and push back against your right hand. At the same time, lift your left arm up toward the ceiling, and press your left thumb and index finger together in a gesture of unity.

• Lift your chest and left arm to help you stand upright and increase your flexibility rather than tilting your torso forward as you raise your back leg.

• Hold for the recommended breaths. Release your foot, and repeat on the opposite side.

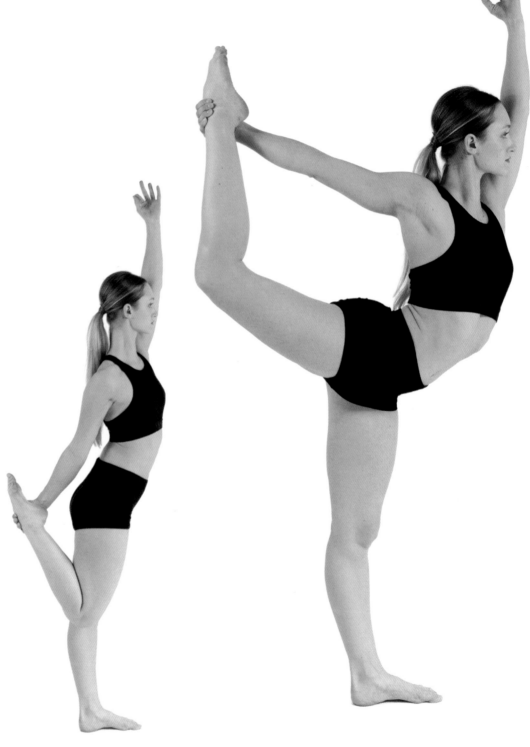

TARGETS
- Thighs
- Groin
- Chest
- Shoulders

TYPE
- Dynamic

BENEFITS
- Stretches thighs, groin, abdominals, shoulders, and chest
- Strengthens spine, thighs, hips, and ankles
- Improves balance

CAUTIONS
- Back injury
- Low blood pressure

Annotation Key

Bold text indicates target muscles
Light text indicates other working muscles
* indicates deep muscles

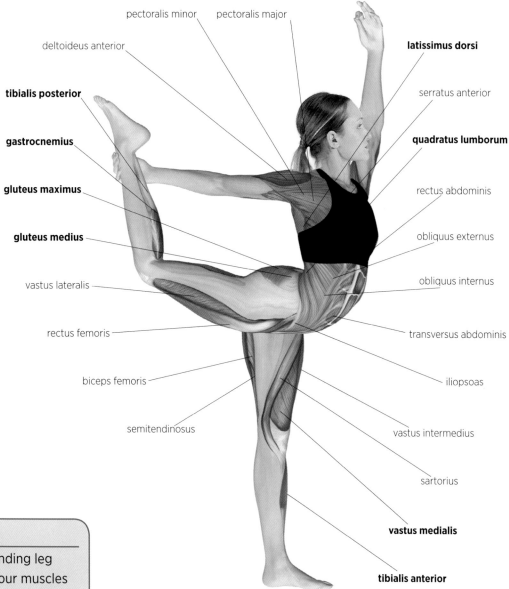

pectoralis minor
pectoralis major
deltoideus anterior
latissimus dorsi
serratus anterior
tibialis posterior
gastrocnemius
quadratus lumborum
rectus abdominis
gluteus maximus
obliquus externus
gluteus medius
vastus lateralis
obliquus internus
rectus femoris
transversus abdominis
biceps femoris
iliopsoas
semitendinosus
vastus intermedius
sartorius
vastus medialis
tibialis anterior

DO IT RIGHT
- Keep your standing leg straight and your muscles contracted.
- If at first you have trouble maintaining your balance, practice by placing your free hand on a wall for support.
- Avoid looking down at the floor, which can cause you to lose your balance.
- Avoid compressing your lower-back.

MODIFICATION
HARDER: Follow the first step. Turn your right palm outward, but instead of grasping the inside of your right foot, reach for the outside of your foot. Rotate your shoulder so that your right elbow points up toward the ceiling. Lift your leg and open your chest. Reach over your head with your left arm, bending your elbow, and grasp the top of your raised foot. Slowly walk your fingers back until both hands are holding your toes.

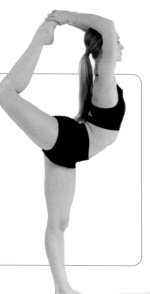

Half Lord of the Fishes Yoga Stretch

This exercise, most commonly known as Half Lord of the Fishes or Spine-Twisting Pose, offers a full-spine lateral twist. This is great for increasing the flexibility and function of the lower vertebrae of your spine.

Half Lord of the Fishes Pose is a deeper variation of Marichi's Pose (pages 60–61). This seated spinal twist, ideal for stretching your back, will help to open your hips and shoulders.

HOW TO DO IT

- Sit up straight with your legs extended in front of you and pressed together. Bend your right knee, and place your right foot on the outside of your left thigh, resting flat on the floor. Your left knee should point straight up toward the ceiling.

- Shift your weight slightly to your right as you bend your left leg inward and bring your heel close to your left hip.

- Extend your right hand on the floor behind your left hip, fingers pointing back. Inhaling, lift your left arm to find length on the left side of your body.

- Exhale, and twist your upper body to the right and bring your left elbow to the outside of your right knee. Ground down evenly through both sit bones.

- To deepen the twist, find resistance between your raised arm and your bent leg. If desired, turn your gaze over your left shoulder, and raise your left hand, palm turned away from your body. Hold for the recommended breaths and then repeat on the opposite side.

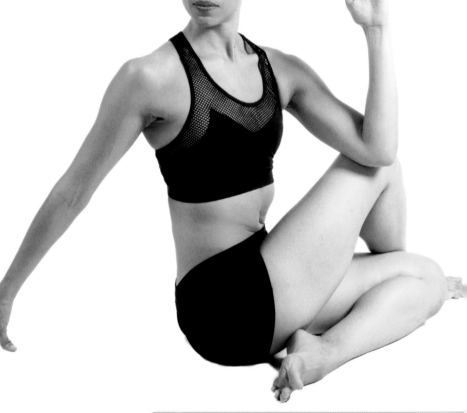

MODIFICATION

HARDER: Weave your left forearm back beneath your raised right knee, then draw your left arm behind your back toward your left hip until your hands meet. Clasp your hands together in this bound position.

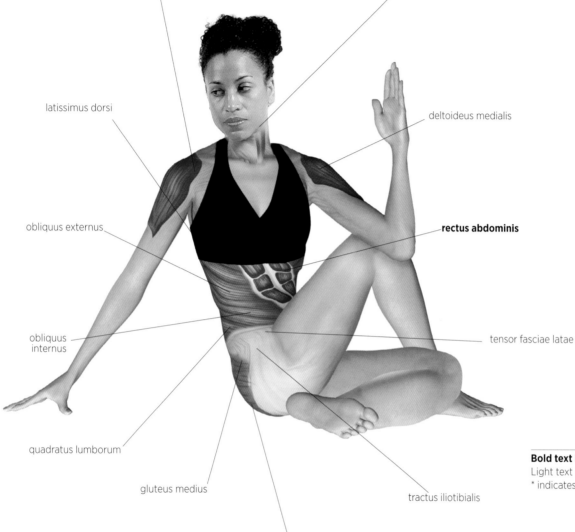

deltoideus anterior

sternocleidomastoideus

latissimus dorsi

deltoideus medialis

obliquus externus

rectus abdominis

obliquus internus

tensor fasciae latae

quadratus lumborum

gluteus medius

tractus iliotibialis

gluteus maximus

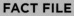

FACT FILE

TARGETS
• Upper body

TYPE
• Dynamic

BENEFITS
• Stretches
  spine,
  shoulders,
  hips, and neck
• Detoxifies
• Aids digestion

CAUTIONS
• Spine injury

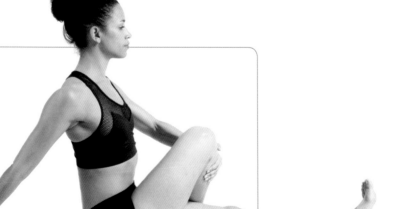

DO IT RIGHT

• Sit up tall and lengthen your
  spine as you twist.
• Distribute your weight evenly
  between both sit bones; if your
  hips feel uneven, try sitting on a
  block or a blanket.
• Broaden your collarbones as
  you draw your shoulder blades
  together.
• Avoid twisting your neck into
  an uncomfortable position.

Revolved Triangle Yoga Stretch

The Revolved Triangle exercise combines standing balance with a forward bend and a twist. It's a challenging standing pose that stretches the muscles of your outer hips and lengthens your hamstrings, while toning your legs, back, and obliques. Balancing your pelvis is essential to proper alignment.

HOW TO DO IT

• Stand in the middle of your mat and place your hands on your hips. Step your feet about 3 to 4 feet apart.

• Turn your right toes about 45 degrees to face the upper-right corner of your mat. Walk your left foot to the left several inches, coming into heel-to-heel alignment.

• Inhale both arms over your head into Upward Salute (pages 54–55). Exhale, and bring your left hand to your left hip.

• Inhale, and extend your right arm as high as possible, finding length along the right side of your body. Hinge forward with a flat back as you twist to your right.

• Place your left hand onto the floor on the outside of your right foot. Reach your right arm up to the ceiling, broadening across your collarbones.

• Exhale, twist your torso to the right, and gaze toward the thumb of your upper hand.

• Hold for the recommended breaths, and then repeat on the opposite side.

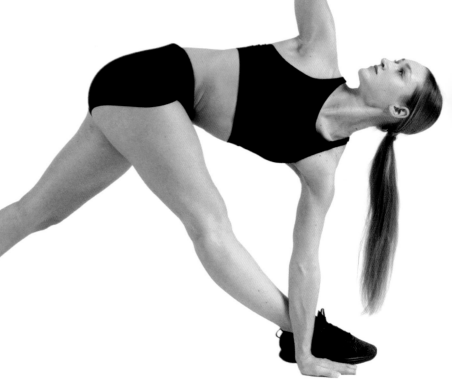

MODIFICATION

EASIER: If you find it difficult to reach the floor without rounding your spine, rest your hand on a block on the floor, outside of your front foot, directly beneath your shoulders. If needed, increase the height of the block by resting it on its side.

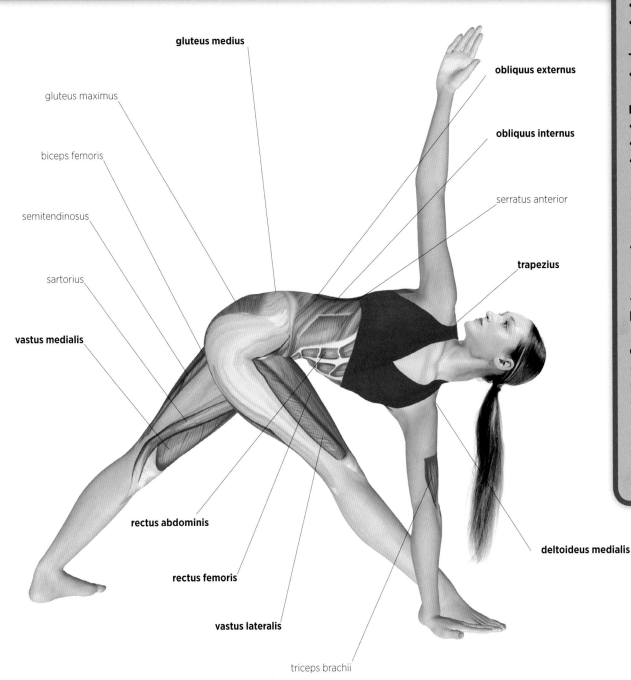

gluteus medius

gluteus maximus

biceps femoris

semitendinosus

sartorius

vastus medialis

rectus abdominis

rectus femoris

vastus lateralis

triceps brachii

obliquus externus

obliquus internus

serratus anterior

trapezius

deltoideus medialis

FACT FILE

TARGETS
• Hamstrings
• Spine
• Obliques

TYPE
• Dynamic

BENEFITS
• Detoxifies
• Aids digestion
• Stretches
  hamstrings,
  hips,
  shoulders, and
  arms
• Strengthens
  thighs and
  core
• Improves
  balance

CAUTIONS
• Diarrhea
• Headache
• High or
  low blood
  pressure
• Neck issues
• Pregnancy

DO IT RIGHT
• Keep your arms and legs straight.
• Use the inhalation to lengthen your spine, and the
  exhalation to twist.
• If you have tight hamstrings, widen your feet by
  walking your front foot closer to the edge of the mat,
  making sure that your feet are not lined up as if you
  were on a tightrope.
• Avoid rounding your spine.

Hip Circles

Performing hip circles on a Swiss Ball can help loosen your pelvic muscles, releasing any built-up tension in your hip joints. In addition, hip circles work the upper body and challenge your core, while relieving pain in your lower-back.

HOW TO DO IT

- Sit on a Swiss ball with your feet together and your hands on your hips.

- Tighten your abdominal muscles.

- Use your pelvis to rotate the ball slowly to the right in small counterclockwise circles.

- Return to the starting position, and then repeat in the opposite direction.

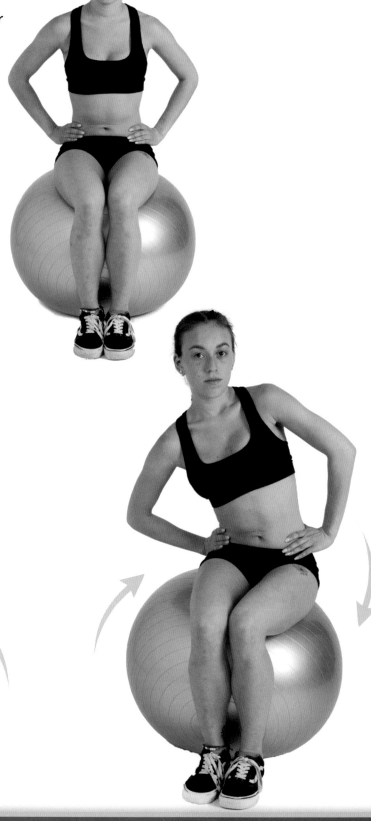

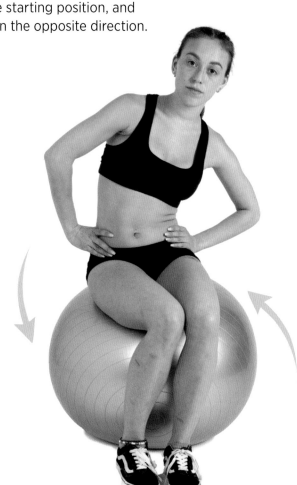

FACT FILE

TARGETS
- Lower-back
- Hips
- Abdominals

TYPE
- Dynamic

BENEFITS
- Stabilizes core
- Stretches lower-back
- Strengthens abdominals

CAUTIONS
- Severe lower-back pain
- Hip problems

Annotation Key

Bold text indicates target muscles
Light text indicates other working muscles
* indicates deep muscles

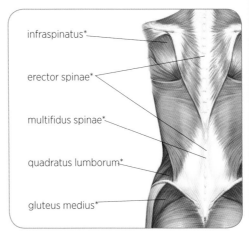

infraspinatus*

erector spinae*

multifidus spinae*

quadratus lumborum*

gluteus medius*

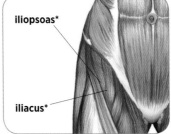

iliopsoas*

iliacus*

rectus abdominis

obliquus externus

transversus abdominis*

DO IT RIGHT

- Keep your circles small.
- If you feel a crunching in your neck, you are moving too widely.
- Avoid using your legs to initiate the movement.

Seated Russian Twist

This seated exercise works your abdominal muscles as you rotate from your midriff. This twisting motion is an effective way to relieve pain and tightness in your lower-back. The Seated Russian Twist also engages your obliques, which are crucial for rotational strength in your torso.

HOW TO DO IT

• Sit with your knees bent and your feet flat on the floor.

• Lift up through your torso.

• Extend your arms in front of you with your hands above your knees.

• Rotate your upper body to the right, keeping your arms parallel to the floor.

• Return to the center and rotate to the left.

• Repeat twisting from side to side for the recommended repetitions.

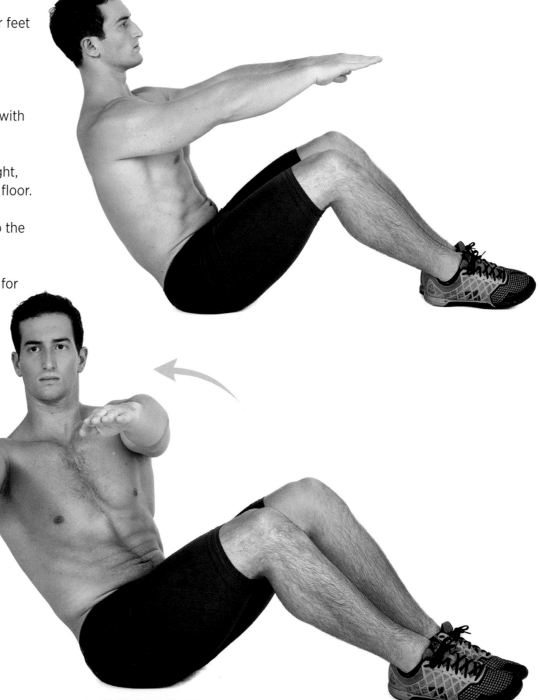

FACT FILE

TARGETS
• Abdominals
• Obliques

TYPE
• Dynamic

BENEFITS
• Increases
  abdominal
  endurance

CAUTIONS
• Shoulder pain
• Lower-back
  issues

Annotation Key

Bold text indicates target muscles
Light text indicates other working muscles
* indicates deep muscles

rectus abdominis

transversus abdominis*

tibialis anterior

latissimus dorsi

obliquus
internus*

obliquus externus

vastus intermedius*

iliacus*

iliopsoas*

rectus femoris

vastus lateralis

tensor fasciae latae

DO IT RIGHT

• Keep your back straight.
• Use your abs to perform the
  movement.
• Avoid shifting your feet or knees to
  the sides as you twist.

Cobra Stretch

The Cobra Stretch is a common back-bending movement in many yoga routines. It is best known for its ability to increase flexibility in the lower spine, while opening the chest and neck.

HOW TO DO IT

• Lie facedown, legs extended behind you with toes pointed. Position the palms of your hands on the floor near your shoulders, and rest your elbows on the floor.

• Push down into the floor, and slowly lift through the top of your chest as you straighten your arms.

• Pull your tailbone down toward the floor as you push your shoulders down and back.

• Elongate your neck and gaze forward.

DO IT RIGHT

• Pressure your hips into the floor.
• Relax your shoulders, and keep them down and away from your ears.
• Avoid tipping your head too far backward.
• Do not put excessive pressure on your lower-back by overdoing this stretch.

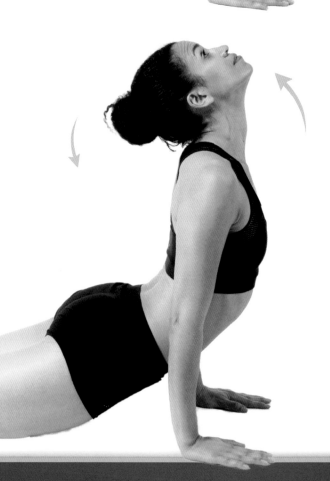

TARGETS
- Lower-back
- Abdominals

TYPE
- Static

BENEFITS
- Chest opener
- Arm strengthener
- Lower-back relief

CAUTIONS
- Lower-back problems
- Hip pain

MODIFICATION

EASIER: Lie facedown as you would for the full stretch, and lift up partway, keeping your elbows bent and your hands flat on the floor close to your body.

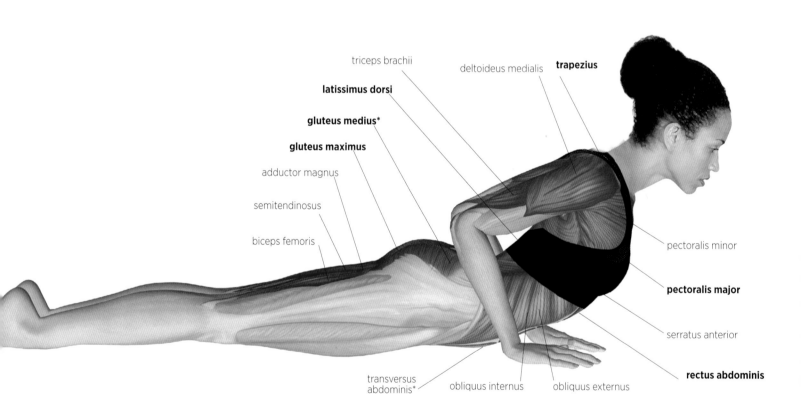

triceps brachii

deltoideus medialis

trapezius

latissimus dorsi

gluteus medius*

gluteus maximus

adductor magnus

semitendinosus

biceps femoris

pectoralis minor

pectoralis major

serratus anterior

rectus abdominis

transversus abdominis*

obliquus internus

obliquus externus

Annotation Key

Bold text indicates target muscles
Light text indicates other working muscles
* indicates deep muscles

Prone Trunk Raise

This is a more advanced variation of the Cobra Stretch (pages 176–177), in which you raise your torso up from the floor to conclude the stretch. This exercise not only strengthens the triceps and shoulders but also stretches the back and chest, while tightening the muscles in your abs and adductors.

HOW TO DO IT

- Lie prone on the floor. Bend your elbows, placing your hands flat on the floor on either side of your chest.

- Position your legs hip-width apart, and extend through your toes. The tops of your feet should be touching the floor.

- Inhale, and press against the floor with your hands and the tops of your feet, lifting your torso and hips off the floor.

- Contract your thighs, and tuck your tailbone toward your pubis.

- Lift through the top of your chest, fully extending your arms and creating an arch in your back from your upper torso.

- Push your shoulders down and back, and elongate your neck as you gaze slightly upward.

- Hold for the recommended time, then exhale as you lower yourself to the floor.

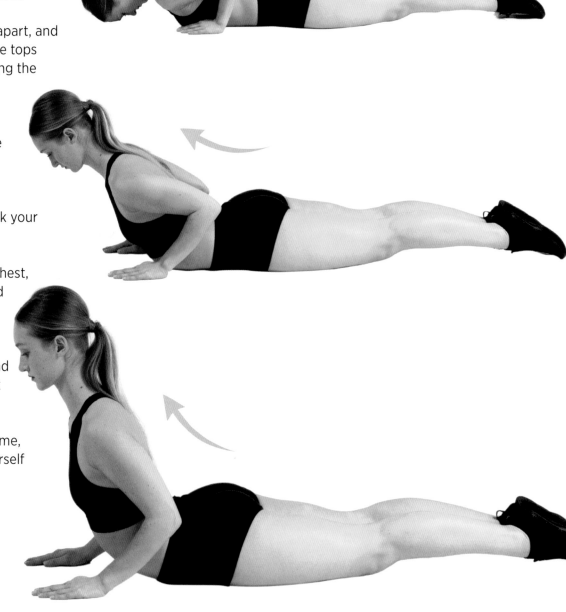

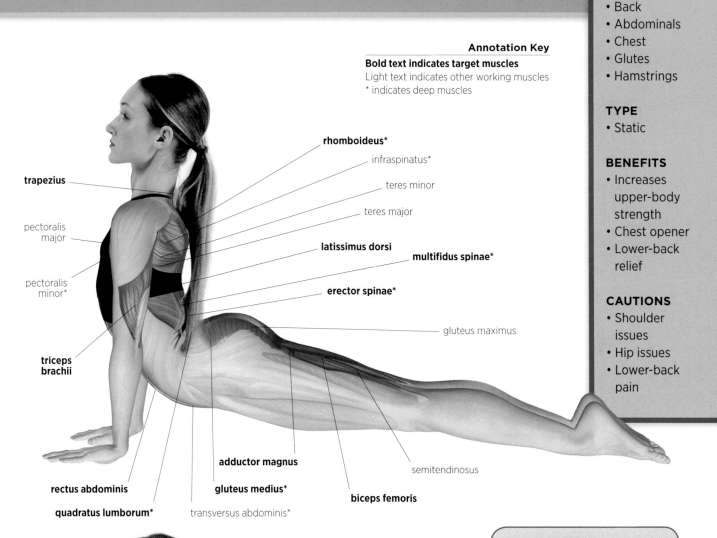

TARGETS
• Back
• Abdominals
• Chest
• Glutes
• Hamstrings

TYPE
• Static

BENEFITS
• Increases upper-body strength
• Chest opener
• Lower-back relief

CAUTIONS
• Shoulder issues
• Hip issues
• Lower-back pain

Annotation Key

Bold text indicates target muscles
Light text indicates other working muscles
* indicates deep muscles

rhomboideus*

infraspinatus*

teres minor

teres major

trapezius

pectoralis major

latissimus dorsi

multifidus spinae*

pectoralis minor*

erector spinae*

gluteus maximus

triceps brachii

adductor magnus

rectus abdominis

semitendinosus

gluteus medius*

quadratus lumborum*

biceps femoris

transversus abdominis*

DO IT RIGHT
• Keep your spine neutral as you progress through the motion.
• Gaze slightly upward as you lift your body.
• Move smoothly with control, not force.
• Avoid allowing your shoulders to lift up toward your ears.

Arm-Leg Extension

This stretching exercise strengthens your core and back as well as your glutes. The Arm-Leg Extension can also provide relief for a tense lower-back.

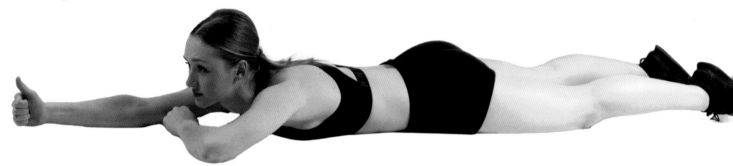

HOW TO DO IT

- Lie flat on the floor. Bend your left arm, and place your palm flat on the floor under your chin.

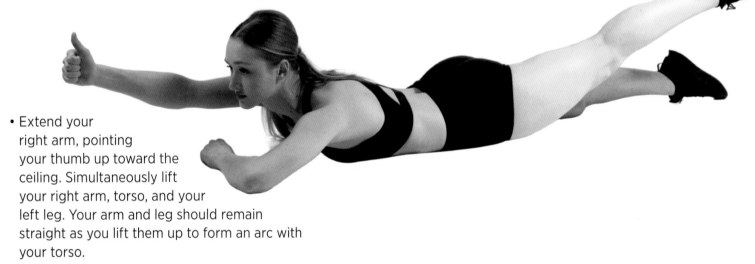

- Extend your right arm, pointing your thumb up toward the ceiling. Simultaneously lift your right arm, torso, and your left leg. Your arm and leg should remain straight as you lift them up to form an arc with your torso.

- Slowly lower your arm and leg back down, and then repeat to the opposite side.

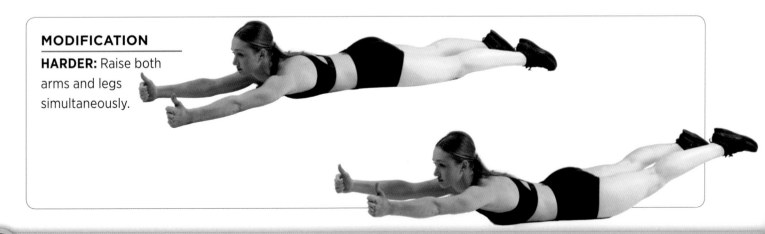

MODIFICATION

HARDER: Raise both arms and legs simultaneously.

TARGETS
• Spine
• Glutes

TYPE
• Static

BENEFITS
• Core exercise
• Glutes
  strengthener

CAUTIONS
• Lower-back
  pain
• Pelvic injury

Annotation Key

Bold text indicates target muscles
Light text indicates other working muscles
* indicates deep muscles

DO IT RIGHT

• Perform a simultaneous
  movement with your raised arm
  and leg.
• Keep your hip bones in contact
  with the floor.
• Avoid any rotation of your torso
  or hips from the floor.
• Avoid elevating your shoulder
  or bending your knee or elbow.

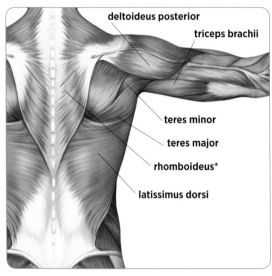

deltoideus posterior

triceps brachii

teres minor

teres major

rhomboideus*

latissimus dorsi

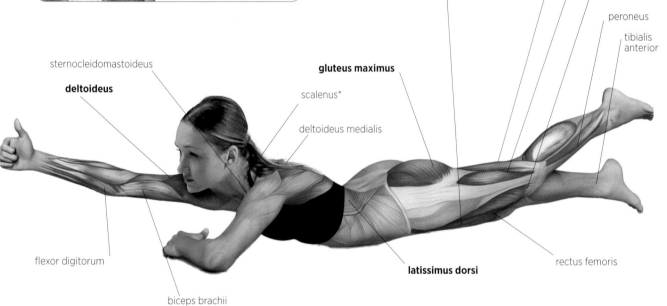

sternocleidomastoideus

deltoideus

scalenus*

deltoideus medialis

gluteus maximus

vastus intermedius*

biceps femoris

vastus lateralis

vastus medialis

peroneus

tibialis anterior

flexor digitorum

biceps brachii

latissimus dorsi

rectus femoris

MODIFICATION

HARDER: In a front
plank position, raise one
arm and the opposite
leg (stabilize with
all core muscles).

Rotated Back Extension

The Rotated Back Extension, performed on a Swiss ball, gives your back and sides a significant stretch. It requires an engaged core, making it a strengthening exercise as well.

HOW TO DO IT

• Lie facedown on a Swiss ball, so that your navel is on the center of the ball. Extend your legs behind you, resting on your toes.

• Place your hands behind your head, with your elbows out.

• Extend your back, lifting your chest away from the ball, and rotate your torso to the right.

• Hold for recommended time, and then return to the starting position.

• Repeat on the opposite side, alternating sides for the recommended repetitions.

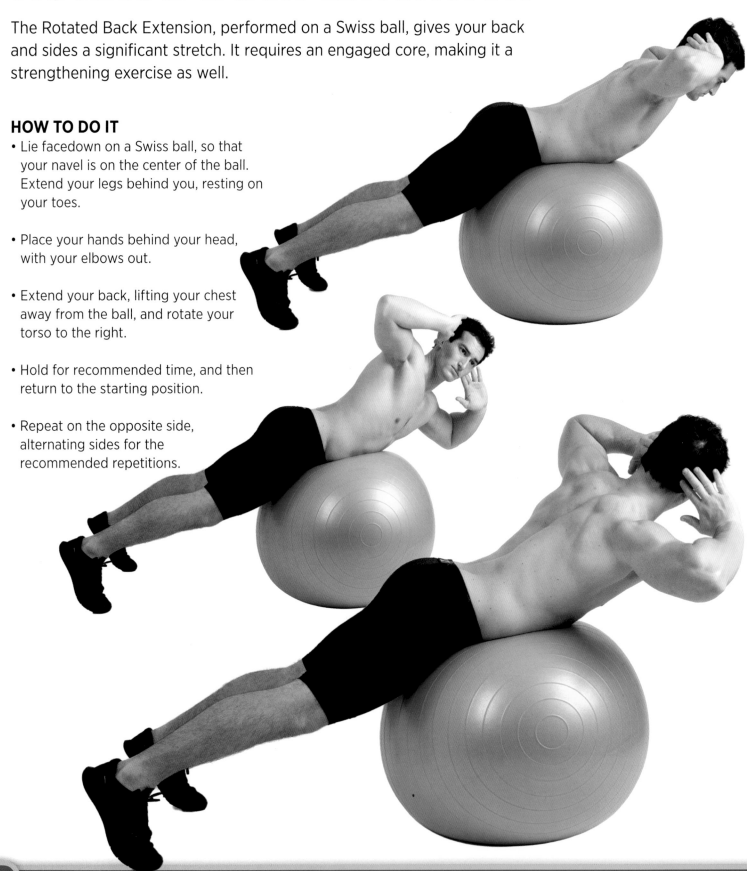

FACT FILE

TARGETS
• Middle back
• Lower-back
• Obliques

TYPE
• Dynamic

BENEFITS
• Stretches
  lower-back
  and obliques
• Strengthens
  core and back

CAUTIONS
• Neck issues
• Lower-back
  pain

Annotation Key

Bold text indicates target muscles
Light text indicates other working muscles
* indicates deep muscles

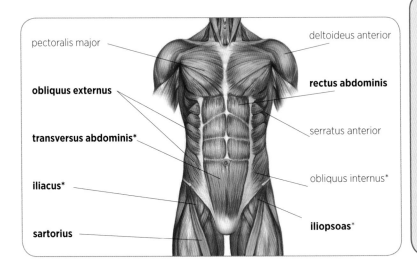

pectoralis major

deltoideus anterior

obliquus externus

rectus abdominis

transversus abdominis*

serratus anterior

iliacus*

obliquus internus*

sartorius

iliopsoas*

DO IT RIGHT
• Keep your toes firmly planted
  on the floor.
• Keep your arms out at a
  90-degree angle to your body
  with your elbows bent.
• Widen your feet for increased
  stability.
• Avoid shifting your hips as
  you rotate—hold them square
  to the ball throughout the
  movement.

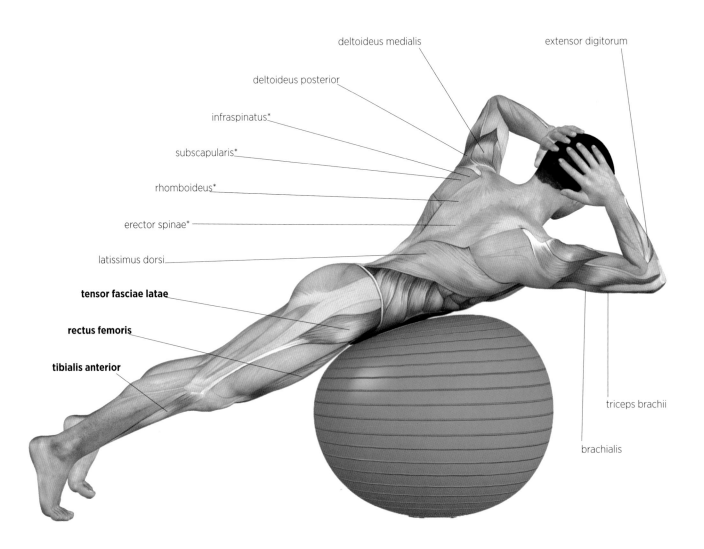

deltoideus medialis

extensor digitorum

deltoideus posterior

infraspinatus*

subscapularis*

rhomboideus*

erector spinae*

latissimus dorsi

tensor fasciae latae

rectus femoris

tibialis anterior

triceps brachii

brachialis

Abdominal Kick

When your hip flexors are tight, they pull on your lower spine, which can cause lower-back pain. Exercises like the reclining Abdominal Kick are a great way to keep your hip flexors limber, strengthen your core, and reduce tension in the lower vertebrae of your spine.

HOW TO DO IT

- Lie supine on the floor with your knees bent.

- Pull your right knee toward your chest and straighten your left leg, raising it about 45 degrees from the floor.

- Place your right hand on your right ankle, and your left hand on your right knee to maintain proper alignment of your leg.

- Alternate straightening and bending your legs, switching your hand placement at the same time.

- Repeat for the recommended repetitions.

DO IT RIGHT

- Place your outside hand on the ankle of your bent leg, and your inside hand on your bent knee.
- Lift the top of your sternum forward.
- Avoid allowing your lower-back to rise off the floor.
- Use your abdominals to stabilize your core while switching legs.

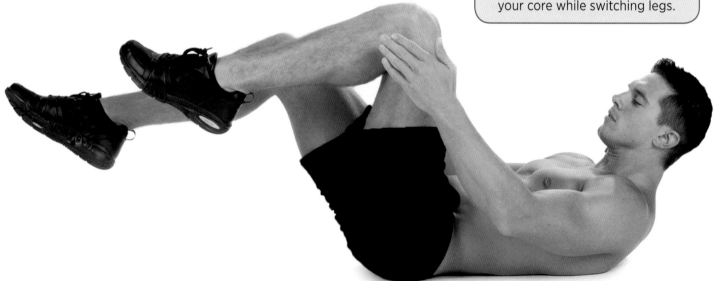

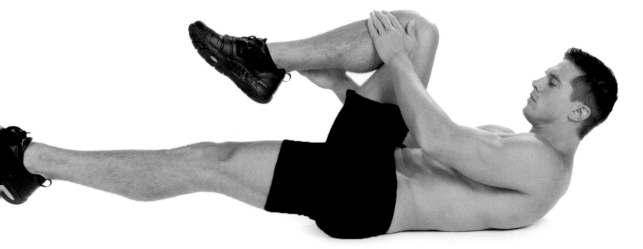

FACT FILE

TARGETS
• Spine
• Hip flexors
• Abdominals

TYPE
• Dynamic

BENEFITS
• Strengthens abdominals
• Stabilizes core and spine

CAUTIONS
• Neck issues
• Lower-back pain

Annotation Key

Bold text indicates target muscles
Light text indicates other working muscles
* indicates deep muscles

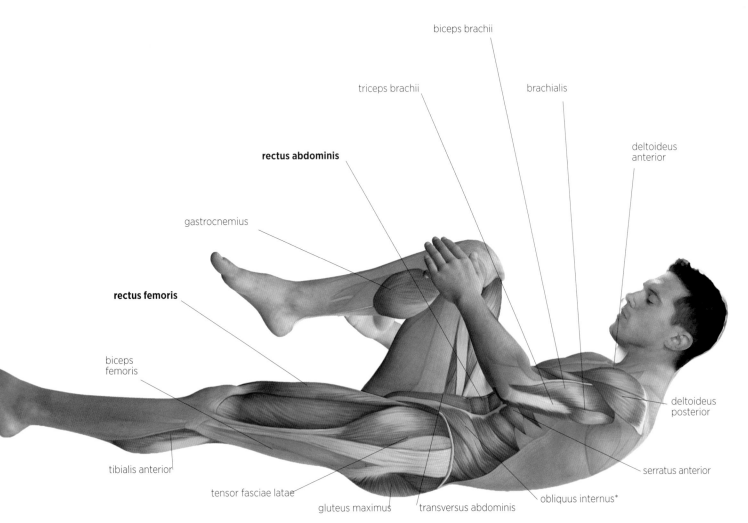

biceps brachii

triceps brachii

brachialis

deltoideus anterior

rectus abdominis

gastrocnemius

rectus femoris

deltoideus posterior

biceps femoris

tibialis anterior

serratus anterior

tensor fasciae latae

gluteus maximus

transversus abdominis

obliquus internus*

Inchworm Stretch

The Inchworm, also known as Monkey Walk, is a full-body stretch that really tests the limits of your flexibility. It is also a good gauge of overall fitness, requiring core and upper-body strength.

HOW TO DO IT

• Stand tall, and then carefully bend forward toward the floor until your palms are flat on the floor in front of you.

• Slowly walk your hands out to a plank position with your wrists directly under your shoulders. Keep your body parallel to the floor, legs hip-width apart, navel pressing toward your spine and shoulders pressing down your back.

• Pop your hips upward, and push your weight back onto your heels. Your body should be in the shape of an upside-down V. Hold for a few seconds before slowly walking your hands back toward your legs.

• Carefully rise back to a standing position. Pause, and then repeat for the recommended repetitions.

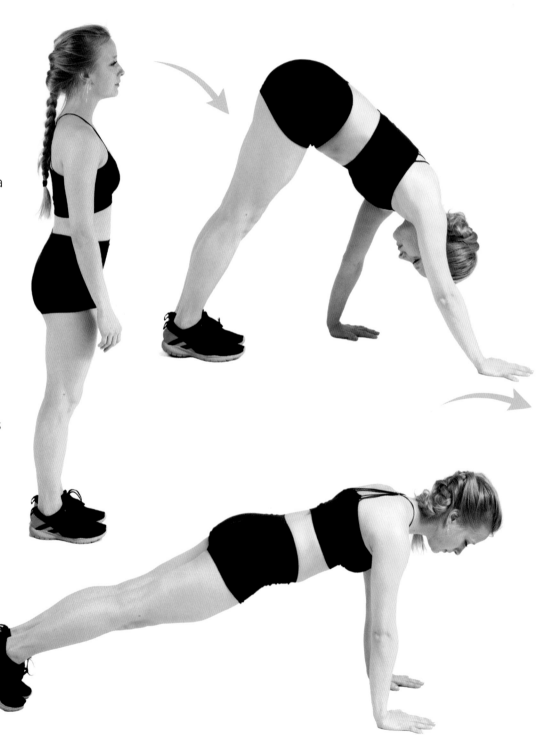

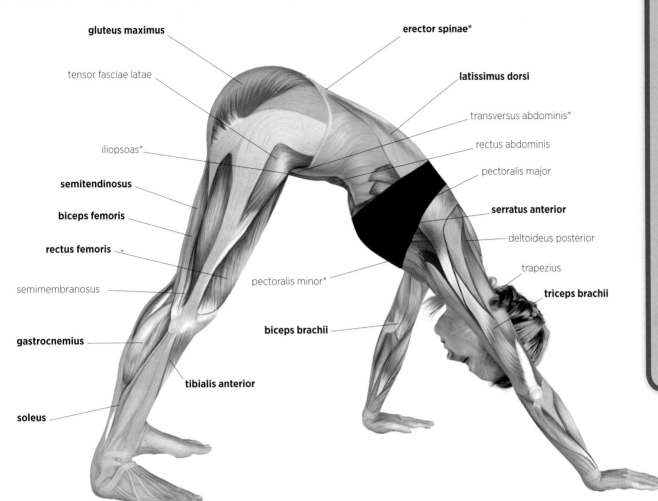

gluteus maximus

erector spinae*

tensor fasciae latae

latissimus dorsi

transversus abdominis*

iliopsoas*

rectus abdominis

pectoralis major

semitendinosus

serratus anterior

biceps femoris

deltoideus posterior

rectus femoris

trapezius

semimembranosus

triceps brachii

pectoralis minor*

gastrocnemius

biceps brachii

tibialis anterior

soleus

FACT FILE
TARGETS
- Upper arms
- Back
- Legs
- Glutes

TYPE
- Dynamic

BENEFITS
- Warms up muscles
- Stretches back and legs
- Tones arms, glutes, and back

CAUTIONS
- Lower-back issues
- Shoulder issues
- Wrist issues

Annotation Key

Bold text indicates target muscles
Light text indicates other working muscles
* indicates deep muscles

DO IT RIGHT
- Widen your stance if you have trouble reaching the floor with your hands.
- Keep your abdominals sleek and compact.
- Avoid rushing through the exercise.
- Avoid letting your stomach and spine sag while in the plank position.

Unilateral Knee-to-Chest Stretch

The Unilateral Knee-to-Chest exercise is an easy and relaxing way to get rid of back muscle tension. As a range-of-motion exercise, this movement increases your joint flexibility. The Knee to Chest stretch may also help reduce stiffness associated with spinal arthritis and spinal stenosis.

HOW TO DO IT

• Lie flat on your back, and bend your right knee in toward your chest.

• Placing your hands on your right hamstrings, gently hug your knee closer to your chest as you stretch.

• Release to the original position, and then repeat on the opposite side.

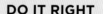

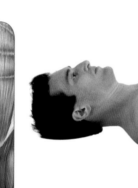

rectus abdominis

obliquus internus*

transversus abdominis*

tensor fasciae latae

iliopsoas

pectineus

sartorius

adductor longus

rectus femoris

DO IT RIGHT

• Keep your lower-back on the floor.
• Keep your back grounded.
• Avoid lifting your head or upper back.
• Avoid holding your breath.

MODIFICATION

HARDER: Place your hands on the top of your shin where it connects with your knee before hugging your knee into your chest.

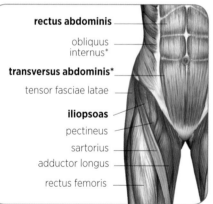

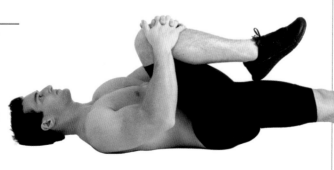

Unilateral Leg Raise

In this variation of the Unilateral Knee-to-Chest stretch, you straighten your leg upward as you bring your leg to your chest. This requires additional flexibility in the muscles running along the back of your leg and targets the lower-back more deeply.

HOW TO DO IT

- Lie on your back and bend your right knee in toward your chest.

- With your hands placed on your hamstrings near your knee, extend and straighten your right leg toward the ceiling.

- Point both feet.

- Switch your hand position, so your right hand is on your right calf muscle, and your left hand is on your hamstrings. Gently bring your thigh toward your chest, increasing the intensity of the stretch.

- Slowly release your leg back down to the starting position, and then repeat on the opposite side.

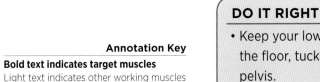

semimembranosus

semitendinosus

biceps femoris

soleus

gastrocnemius

erector spinae*

gluteus medius*

gluteus minimus*

gluteus maximus

Annotation Key

Bold text indicates target muscles
Light text indicates other working muscles
* indicates deep muscles

DO IT RIGHT

- Keep your lower-back on the floor, tucking in your pelvis.
- Keep your back grounded.
- Avoid lifting your head or upper back.
- Avoid holding your breath.

Latissimus Dorsi Stretch

The latissimus dorsi is a broad muscle that covers much of the lower-back. The lats draw your arms down and back. Reaching your arms overhead stretches them. You can stretch your lats while sitting, standing, or kneeling. Using a wall or table can help intensify the stretch.

HOW TO DO IT

• Stand upright, keeping your neck, shoulders, and torso straight.

• Raise both arms above your head and clasp your hands together, palms facing upward.

• Keeping your elbows straight, reach to the side to begin tracing a circular pattern with your torso.

• Lean forward and then to the opposite side as you slowly trace a full circle.

• Return to the starting position, and then repeat the sequence 3 times in each direction.

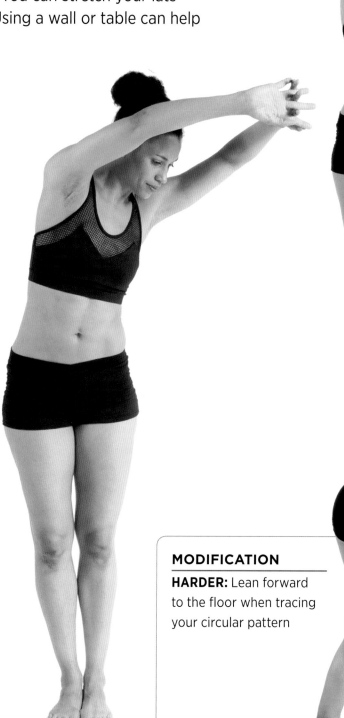

DO IT RIGHT
• Elongate your arms and shoulders as much as possible.
• Avoid leaning backward as you come to the top of the circle.

MODIFICATION
HARDER: Lean forward to the floor when tracing your circular pattern

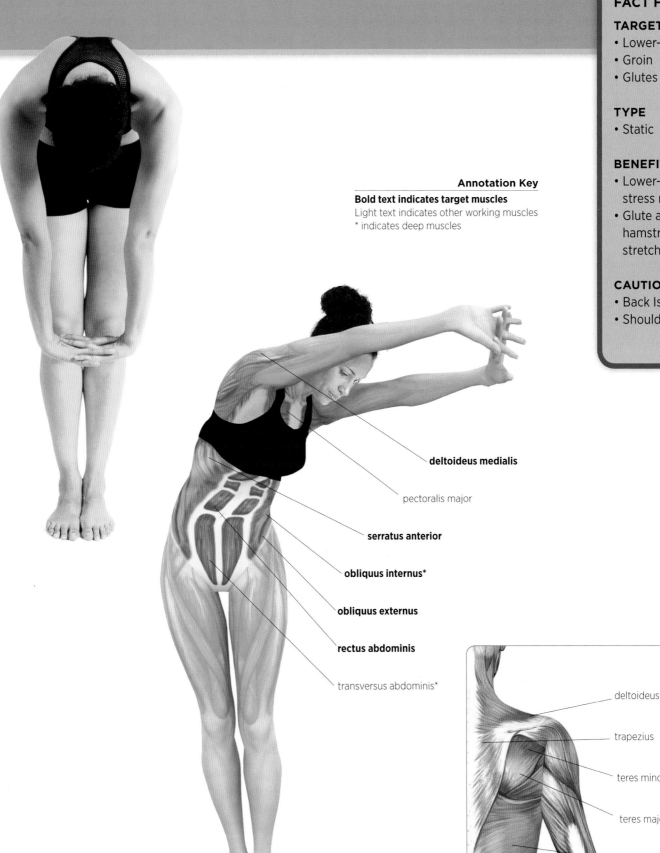

TARGETS
• Lower-back
• Groin
• Glutes

TYPE
• Static

BENEFITS
• Lower-back stress release
• Glute and hamstring stretch

CAUTIONS
• Back Issues
• Shoulder pain

Annotation Key

Bold text indicates target muscles
Light text indicates other working muscles
* indicates deep muscles

deltoideus medialis

pectoralis major

serratus anterior

obliquus internus*

obliquus externus

rectus abdominis

transversus abdominis*

deltoideus posterior

trapezius

teres minor

teres major

latissimus dorsi

Rollover Stretch

Borrowed from Pilates, the Rollover requires a strong core and a controlled, fluid progression. With time and practice, you can perfect this spinal stretch and core strengthener by engaging your abs, articulating your spine, and breathing deeply.

HOW TO DO IT

- Lie on your back with knees bent and arms at your sides.

- Inhale and elongate your spine.

- On exhale, raise your legs straight up and squeeze them together.

- Peel your spine off the mat and press into your palms for stability as you pull your legs overhead, parallel to the floor.

- Roll back down slowly.

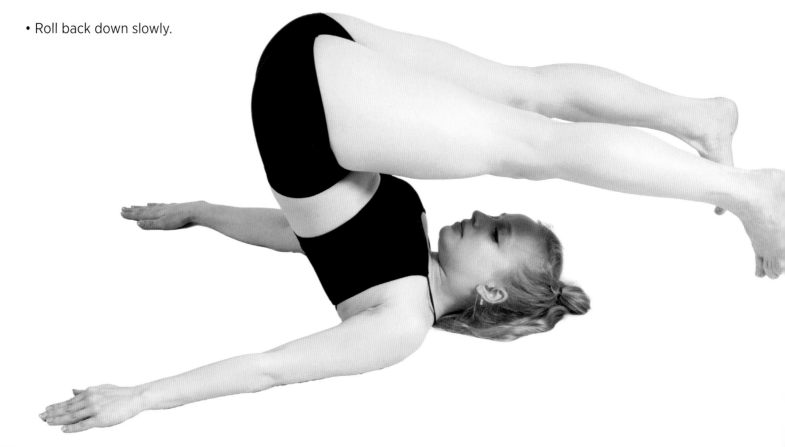

TARGETS
- Back
- Hamstrings
- Calves
- Abdominals

TYPE
- Dynamic

BENEFITS
- Hip strengthener
- Lower-back relief
- Core strength

CAUTIONS
- Neck pain
- Hip pain
- Lower-back problems

Annotation Key

Bold text indicates target muscles
Light text indicates other working muscles
* indicates deep muscles

DO IT RIGHT

- If you're having difficulty rolling over, bend your knees slightly or place a rolled-up towel under your hips.
- Avoid using momentum to push through the movement.

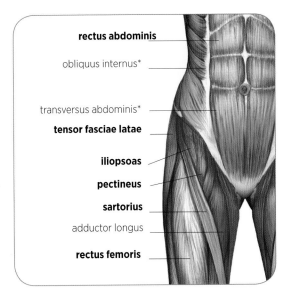

rectus abdominis

obliquus internus*

transversus abdominis*

tensor fasciae latae

iliopsoas

pectineus

sartorius

adductor longus

rectus femoris

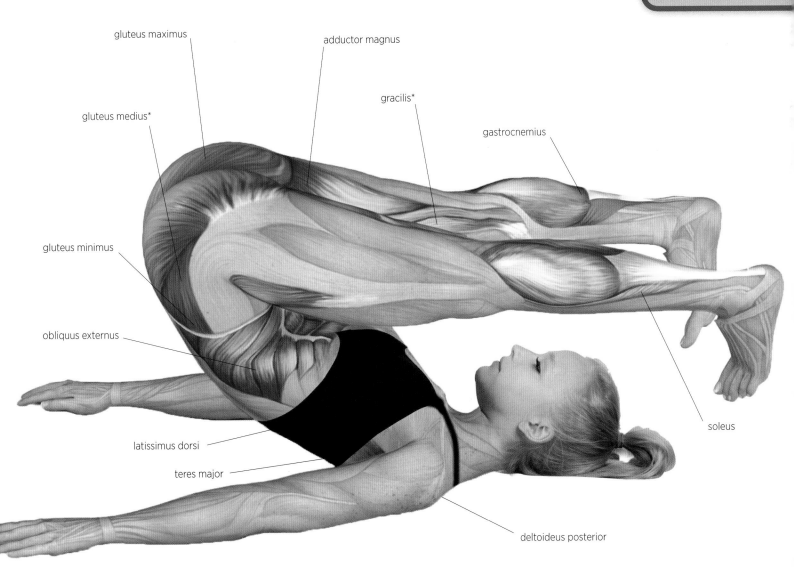

gluteus maximus

adductor magnus

gracilis*

gastrocnemius

gluteus medius*

gluteus minimus

obliquus externus

latissimus dorsi

teres major

soleus

deltoideus posterior

CHAPTER SIX

HIPS, GROIN, & GLUTES STRETCHES

A common problem affecting people with sedentary lifestyles is tightness in hip flexors and rotators. When your hips and glutes are tight, it can impact your gait, posture, spinal stability, and many major movement patterns. Aging also tends to create muscle imbalances around your hips. Performing a range of hip, groin, and gluteal stretches as part of a regular exercise regimen can address these problems and mitigate any current discomfort as well as prevent future injury.

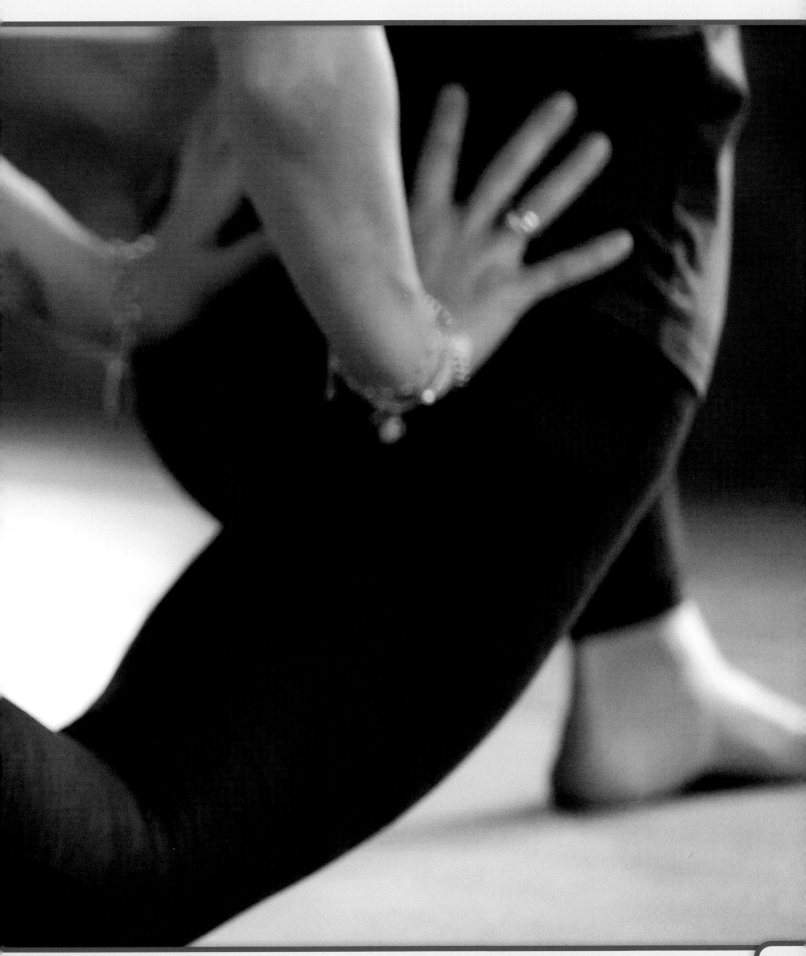

Hip and Iliotibial Band Stretch

The Hip and Iliotibial Band Stretch improves flexibility in your hips and keeps your iliotibial band supple. It also provides a full spinal and abdominal twist and boosts your overall mobility. If you're a runner or biker, this stretch can also help prevent sports-related injuries.

HOW TO DO IT

• Sit on the floor as straight as possible with your back flat and your legs extended in front of you. Your feet should be slightly flexed.

• Bend your right knee and cross it over to the outside of your left thigh. Keep your right foot flat on the floor.

• Wrap your left arm around your bent knee for stability as you rotate your torso.

• Hold this pose for the recommended amount of time. Slowly release, and then repeat on the opposite side.

FACT FILE

TARGETS
• Hips
• Iliotibial band
• Spine

TYPE
• Static

BENEFITS
• Stretches hip extensors and flexors
• Stretches obliques

CAUTIONS
• Severe lower-back pain

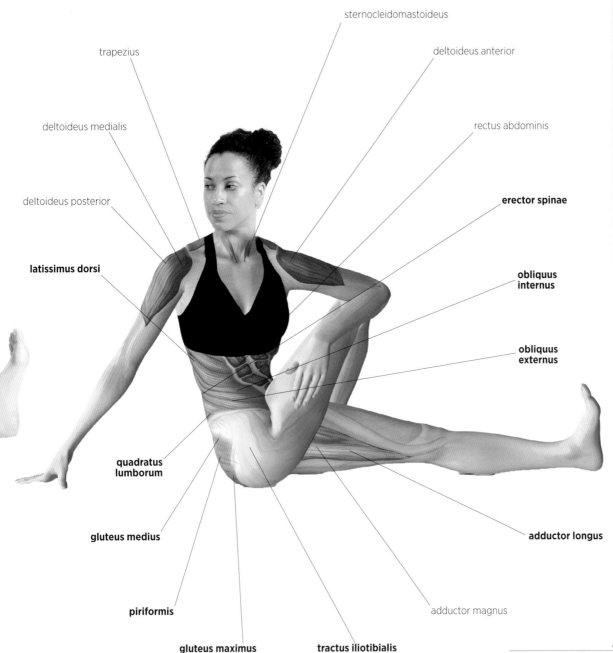

sternocleidomastoideus

trapezius

deltoideus anterior

deltoideus medialis

rectus abdominis

deltoideus posterior

erector spinae

latissimus dorsi

obliquus internus

obliquus externus

quadratus lumborum

gluteus medius

adductor longus

piriformis

adductor magnus

gluteus maximus

tractus iliotibialis

Annotation Key

Bold text indicates target muscles
Light text indicates other working muscles
* indicates deep muscles

DO IT RIGHT
• Apply even pressure to your leg with your active hand.
• Keep your torso upright as you pull your knee and torso together.
• Avoid lifting the foot of your bent leg off the floor.

Warrior II Yoga Stretch

Warrior II, a traditional yoga pose, offers hip-opening benefits and stretches your inner thighs. It also strengthens your legs and glutes, while engaging your core, chest, shoulder, and arm muscles.

HOW TO DO IT

- Stand straight with your hands on your hips. Step your feet about 3 to 4 feet apart.

- Extend your arms out to your sides, parallel to the floor, with your palms facedown.

- Turn your right foot out 90 degrees, positioning your feet in heel-to-heel alignment. Turn your torso to your right and bend your right knee, aligning your kneecap over your ankle.

- Keeping your left knee bent, lift your torso so that your shoulders line up over your hips. Keep a slight internal rotation to your back leg to keep your leg neutral.

- Continue to bend your left knee, externally rotating your left hip to open your thigh as you find a neutral pelvis. Turn your head toward your right and gaze past your fingers.

- Hold for the recommended time, and then repeat on the opposite side.

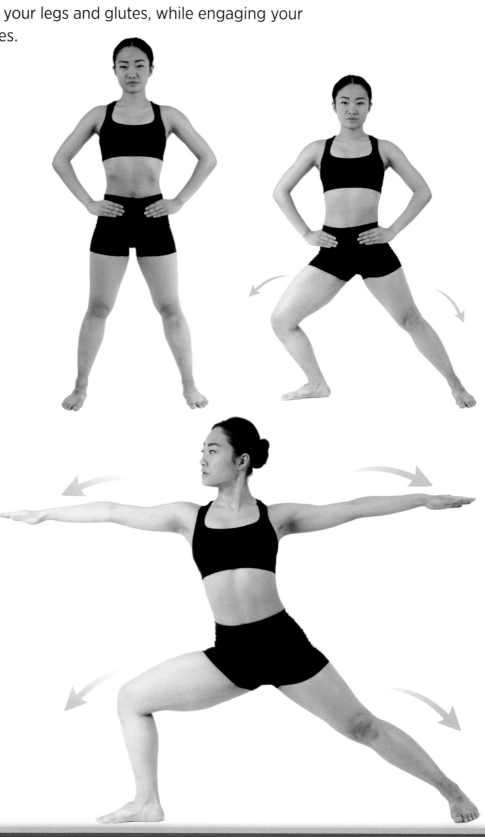

Annotation Key

Bold text indicates target muscles
Light text indicates other working muscles
* indicates deep muscles

rectus abdominis

obliquus externus

vastus intermedius

rectus femoris

obliquus internus

biceps femoris

transversus abdominis

vastus medialis

tensor fasciae latae

sartorius

vastus lateralis

adductor longus

adductor magnus

DO IT RIGHT

• Press your heels into the floor, engaging your inner-thigh muscles.
• Keep your shoulders directly above your hips.
• Keep your front knee in line with your ankle.
• Avoid arching your lower back.
• Avoid leaning over your front leg.

Tree Yoga Stretch

This elegant yoga stretch may look simple but requires steady focus and balance. Feel the stretch in your thighs, groin, and shoulders, as you tone your leg and abdominal muscles. Tree Yoga Stretch improves your balance and can relieve the symptoms of sciatica.

HOW TO DO IT

• Stand with your feet together and arms at your sides.

• Bend your right knee, and bring your right foot up to your left inner thigh, with toes pointing to the floor.

• Externally rotate your right thigh, allowing your right knee to point out to your right while keeping your hips level.

• Continue to open your right hip, rotating your inner thigh clockwise as you draw your tailbone downward to neutralize your pelvis. Press your right foot into your left inner thigh as you draw your left hip in for stability.

• Find your balance, exhale, and draw your hands together into prayer position at the heart.

• Hold for the recommended time, release the stretch, and then repeat on the opposite side.

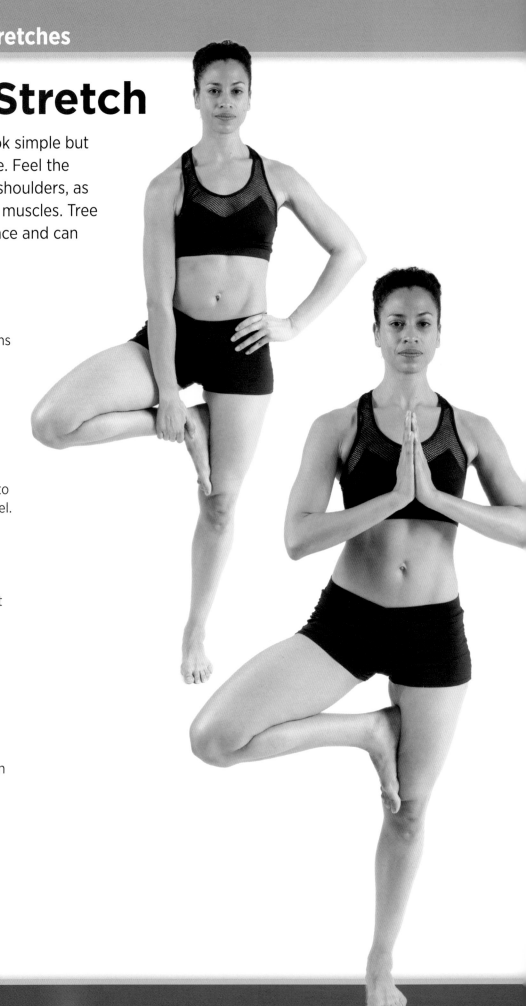

TARGETS
- Legs
- Groin

TYPE
- Static

BENEFITS
- Improves balance
- Strengthens legs, ankles, and feet
- Stretches inner thighs

CAUTIONS
- Groin issues
- Lower-back issues

MODIFICATION

HARDER: Bring your hands above your head, palms pressed together, as you balance.

Annotation Key
Bold text indicates target muscles
Light text indicates other working muscles
* indicates deep muscles

obliquus internus*

rectus abdominis

obliquus externus

tensor fasciae latae

transversus abdominis*

rectus femoris

gastrocnemius

iliopsoas*

pectineus*

vastus intermedius*

vastus lateralis

vastus medialis

soleus

tibialis anterior

DO IT RIGHT

- Keep your standing leg firming in place with your foot facing forward.
- If you need help placing your foot at your thigh, grasp your ankle with your hand; alternatively, you can rest your foot on the side of your shin.
- Ground down through all four corners of the raised foot to help you balance throughout the exercise.
- Avoid resting your foot on the sensitive kneecap area.

Forward Squat

The Forward Squat is an accessible and effective hip opener for beginners and experts alike. This position stretches your hips, thighs, and groin while enhancing your overall balance. The Forward Squat also lengthens your spine and releases tight calves and ankles.

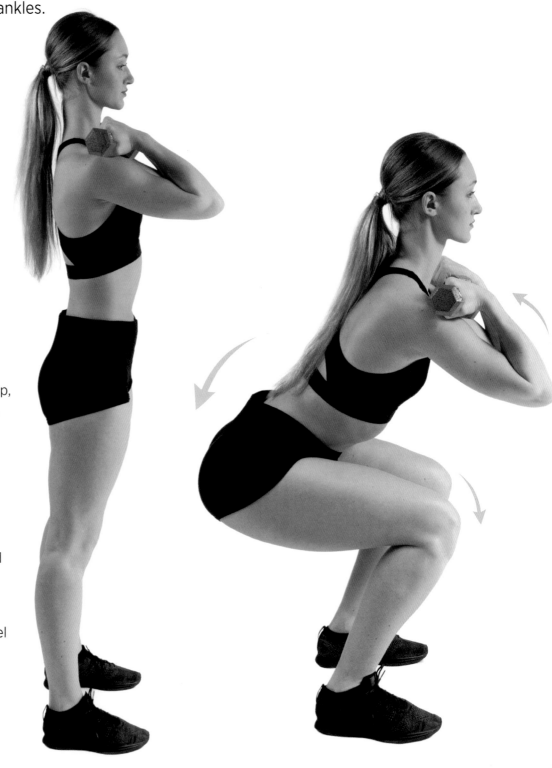

HOW TO DO IT

- Curl dumbells to your shoulders and hold.

- Stand with your chest and head up, and your arms extended forward.

- Keep your spine neutral and your feet slightly wider than shoulder-width apart.

- Retract your hips and bend your knees, keeping your head and chest up and your spine in neutral position.

- Lower your hips until your upper legs and thighs are at least parallel with the floor.

- Hold for the recommended time, and release the stretch.

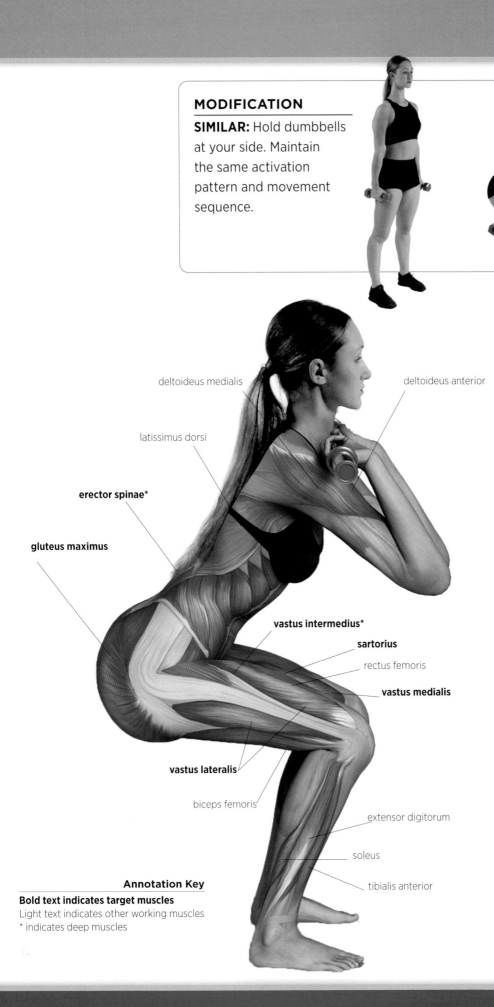

MODIFICATION

SIMILAR: Hold dumbbells at your side. Maintain the same activation pattern and movement sequence.

FACT FILE

TARGETS
• Thighs
• Hip flexors

TYPE
• Static

BENEFITS
• Enhances hip mobility
• Strengthens legs
• Engages abdominals

CAUTIONS
• Lower-back pain
• Leg weaknesses
• Knee problems

deltoideus medialis

deltoideus anterior

latissimus dorsi

erector spinae*

gluteus maximus

vastus intermedius*

sartorius

rectus femoris

vastus medialis

vastus lateralis

biceps femoris

extensor digitorum

soleus

tibialis anterior

Annotation Key
Bold text indicates target muscles
Light text indicates other working muscles
* indicates deep muscles

DO IT RIGHT
• Retract your shoulder blades.
• Keep your abdomen pulled up and in.
• Keep your knees parallel and in line with your feet.
• Avoid extending your knees beyond your toes.
• Avoid dropping your elbows; keep them and your upper arms parallel to the floor throughout.
• Avoid jutting your head forward or elevating your shoulder blades.

Sumo Squat

The wide-legged squatting stretch target your inner thighs. It opens the hips and groin area, and works your glutes, quadriceps, and hamstrings.

HOW TO DO IT

• Stand with your feet planted more than shoulder-width apart and your toes turned out 45 degrees.

• Bend your knees slightly, and tuck your pelvis forward.

• Lift your chest, and press your shoulders down and back.

• Place your hands on your thighs, and squat down until your thighs are parallel to the floor, keeping your weight on your heels.

• Push off with your heels at the bottom of the squat, squeezing your glutes and inner thighs as you rise back to the starting position. Perform the recommended repetitions.

DO IT RIGHT

• Try to sit rather than bend your legs to prevent straining your knees.
• Tuck in your pelvis and lift your chest throughout the stretch.
• Use your hands on your thighs to help open your legs and obtain greater turnout from your hips.
• Avoid letting your knees extend beyond your toes.
• Avoid hunching your shoulders.

TARGETS
• Groin
• Glutes
• Hip flexors
• Quadriceps
• Adductors

TYPE
• Static

BENEFITS
• Relieves tight
  groin muscles
• Opens the
  pelvic region

CAUTIONS
• Hip pain
• Knee issues

Annotation Key

Bold text indicates target muscles
Light text indicates other working muscles
* indicates deep muscles

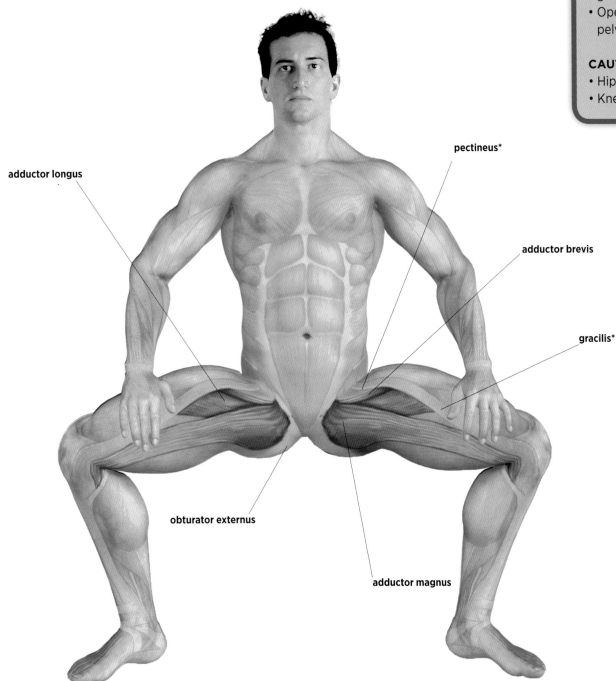

adductor longus

pectineus*

adductor brevis

gracilis*

obturator externus

adductor magnus

Side-Leaning Sumo Squat

The Side-Leaning Sumo Squat is a variation on the up-
down Sumo Squat that incorporates a deep oblique and
shoulder stretch. To increase the intensity of the stretch,
make sure your feet are grounded and your neck is long.

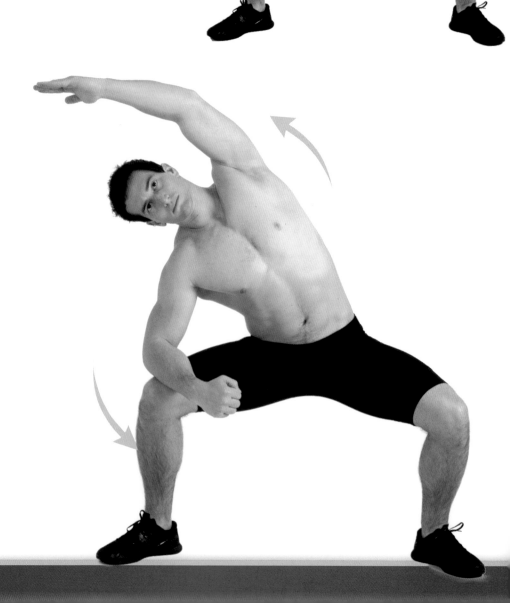

HOW TO DO IT

• Stand with your feet planted more than
  shoulder-width apart and your toes
  turned out 45 degrees.

• Lower yourself into the basic Sumo
  Squat (pages 204–205), with your
  knees bent and thighs parallel to the
  floor.

• Drop your right forearm onto your right
  thigh, just above your kneecap.

• Reach your left arm overhead to your
  right side.

• Hold this position for the recommended
  time, as you feel the stretch along your
  obliques.

• Round your left arm down so that both
  forearms are on your thighs, and bring
  your head back to the center.

• Push off with your heels at the bottom
  of the squat, squeezing your glutes and
  inner thighs to rise back to the starting
  position.

• Repeat on the opposite side.

FACT FILE

TARGETS
• Obliques
• Groin
• Hip flexors
• Adductors

TYPE
• Static

BENEFITS
• Opens the hips and groin
• Lengthens obliques
• Stretches shoulders and spine

CAUTIONS
• Hip pain
• Knee issues
• Spinal pain

Annotation Key

Bold text indicates target muscles
Light text indicates other working muscles
* indicates deep muscles

DO IT RIGHT

• Keep your upper body and back straight.
• Avoid leaning forward as you stretch to the side.
• Position your knees in line with your toes.
• Avoid tensing your jaw, as this will restrict your breathing.

pectineus*

obliquus externus

adductor brevis

gracilis*

obliquus internus*

obturator externus

adductor longus

adductor magnus

Side Adductor Stretch

The Side Adductor Stretch uses lateral movement to improve your stability, upper-leg strength, and overall flexibility. This exercise engages virtually all the muscles of your lower body.

HOW TO DO IT

• Stand upright and position your feet more than hip-width apart, toes turned slightly outward.

• Rest your hands on your lower thighs for support.

• Keeping your torso steady, gradually bend your knees outward.

• Without moving your torso, shift your weight to your left side, bending your knee while straightening your right leg.

• Hold for the recommended time, release the stretch, and repeat on the opposite side.

DO IT RIGHT
• Keep your spine neutral and your torso facing forward.
• Let your shoulders come slightly forward as you stretch.
• Anchor your feet to the floor.
• Avoid rounding your spine.
• Avoid hunching your shoulders and tensing your neck.
• Avoid letting either foot lift off the floor.
• Keep your bent knee in line with your foot.

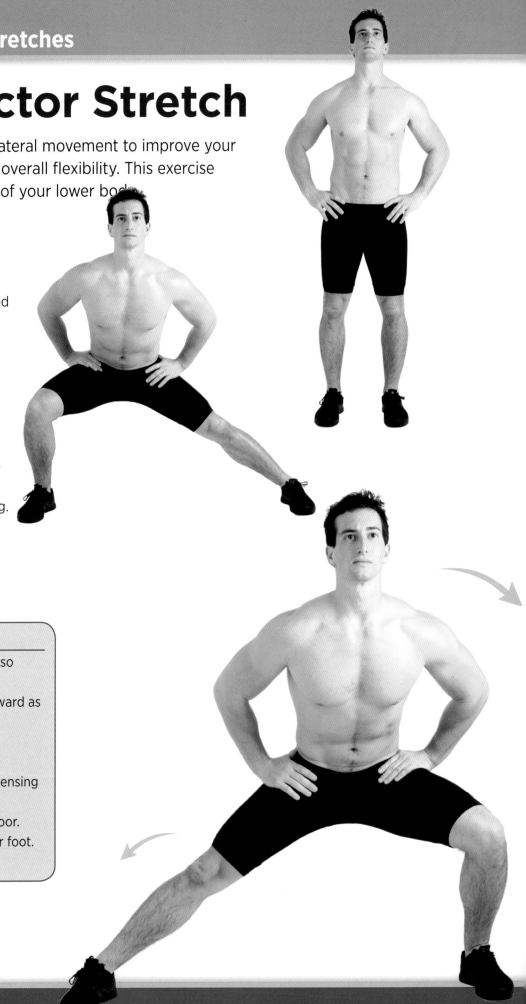

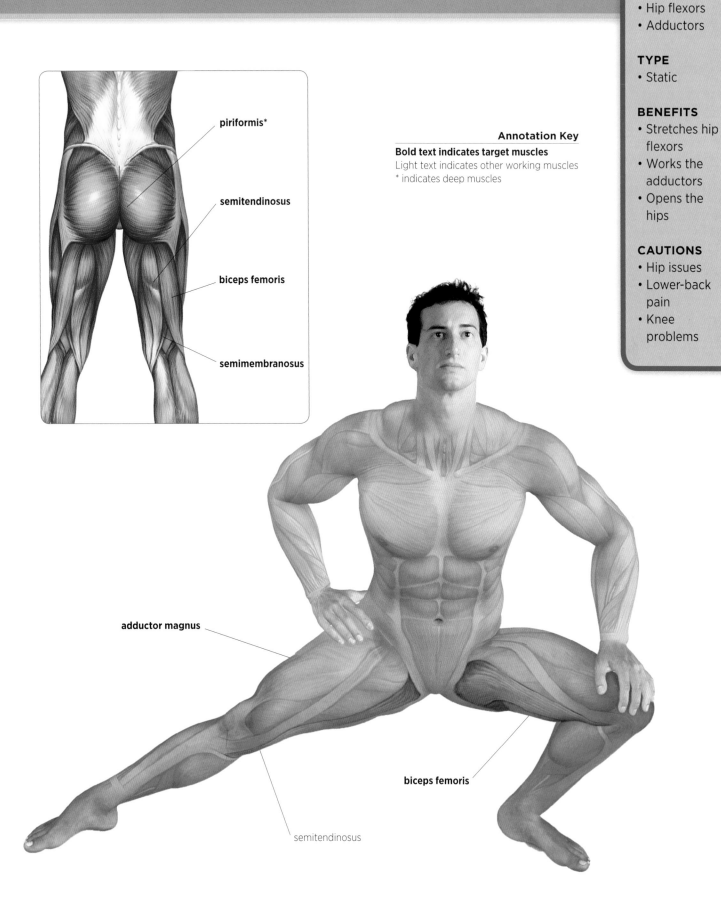

TARGETS
• Hip flexors
• Adductors

TYPE
• Static

BENEFITS
• Stretches hip flexors
• Works the adductors
• Opens the hips

CAUTIONS
• Hip issues
• Lower-back pain
• Knee problems

piriformis*

semitendinosus

biceps femoris

semimembranosus

Annotation Key
Bold text indicates target muscles
Light text indicates other working muscles
* indicates deep muscles

adductor magnus

biceps femoris

semitendinosus

Side Kick

Add a little cardio to your stretching routine with the Side Kick, which is also known as the Lateral Kick. It stretches your outer thigh muscles and your obliques, while also strengthening your lower body.

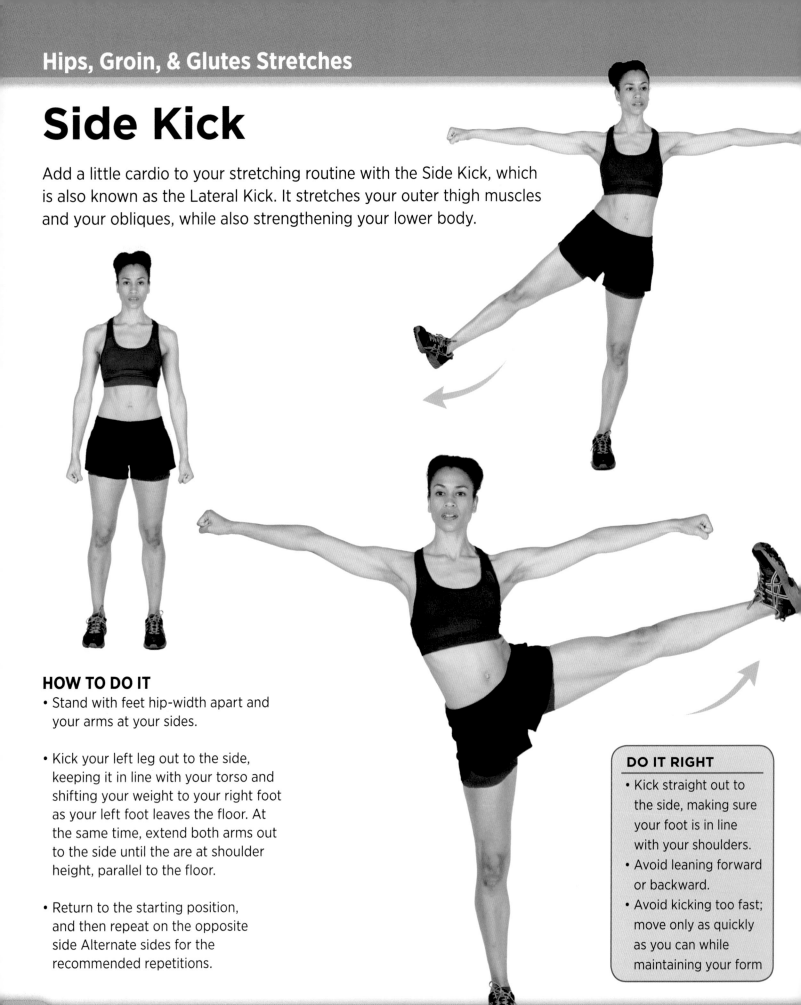

HOW TO DO IT

• Stand with feet hip-width apart and your arms at your sides.

• Kick your left leg out to the side, keeping it in line with your torso and shifting your weight to your right foot as your left foot leaves the floor. At the same time, extend both arms out to the side until the are at shoulder height, parallel to the floor.

• Return to the starting position, and then repeat on the opposite side Alternate sides for the recommended repetitions.

DO IT RIGHT

• Kick straight out to the side, making sure your foot is in line with your shoulders.
• Avoid leaning forward or backward.
• Avoid kicking too fast; move only as quickly as you can while maintaining your form

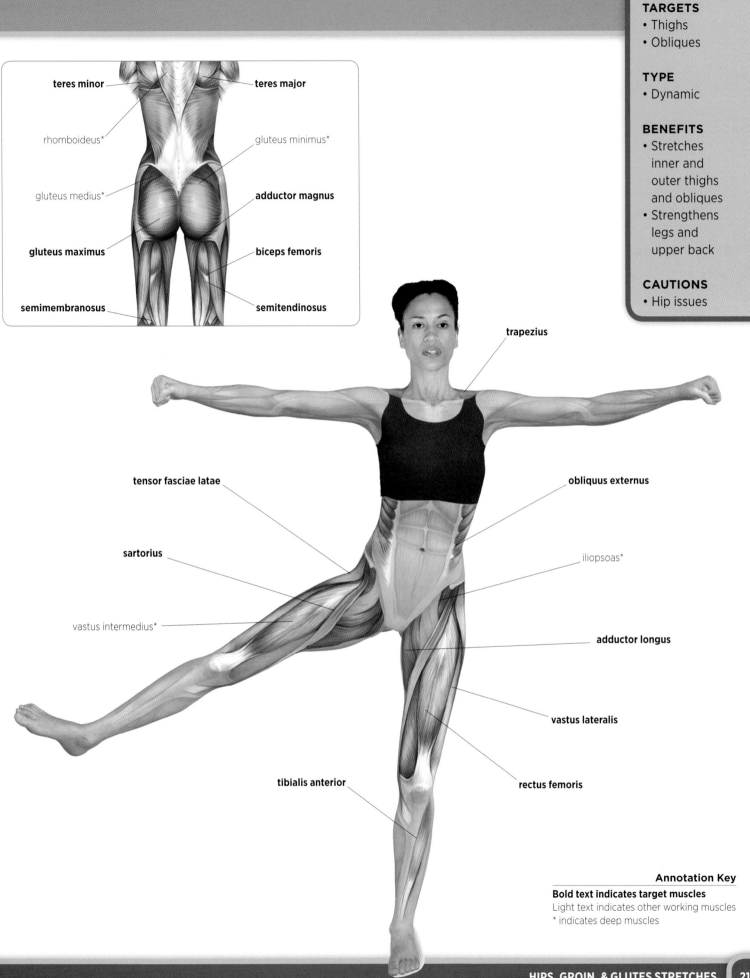

FACT FILE

TARGETS
• Thighs
• Obliques

TYPE
• Dynamic

BENEFITS
• Stretches inner and outer thighs and obliques
• Strengthens legs and upper back

CAUTIONS
• Hip issues

teres minor

teres major

rhomboideus*

gluteus minimus*

gluteus medius*

adductor magnus

gluteus maximus

biceps femoris

semimembranosus

semitendinosus

trapezius

tensor fasciae latae

obliquus externus

sartorius

iliopsoas*

vastus intermedius*

adductor longus

vastus lateralis

tibialis anterior

rectus femoris

Annotation Key

Bold text indicates target muscles
Light text indicates other working muscles
* indicates deep muscles

Garland Yoga Stretch

The Garland Yoga Stretch is a popular pose in many yoga routines that provides a more intense stretch than a traditional squat. This challenging position is a deep hip opener that also lengthens your spine and strengthens your core. It improves your balance as well.

HOW TO DO IT

- Stand with your feet turned out and wider than hip-width apart.

- Bend your knees as deeply as you can, squatting down until your hips are lower than your knees.

- Join your hands in prayer position in front of your heart. Hold for the recommended breaths.

DO IT RIGHT

- Apply gentle pressure between your elbows and your knees, encouraging your knees to open farther and deepening the inner-thigh stretch.
- Lengthen your spine, keeping your back straight.
- For added support, place a blanket under your heels.
- Broaden across your collarbones.
- Avoid rounding your shoulders forward.

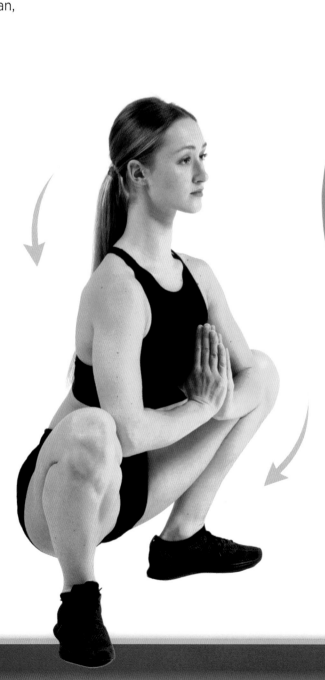

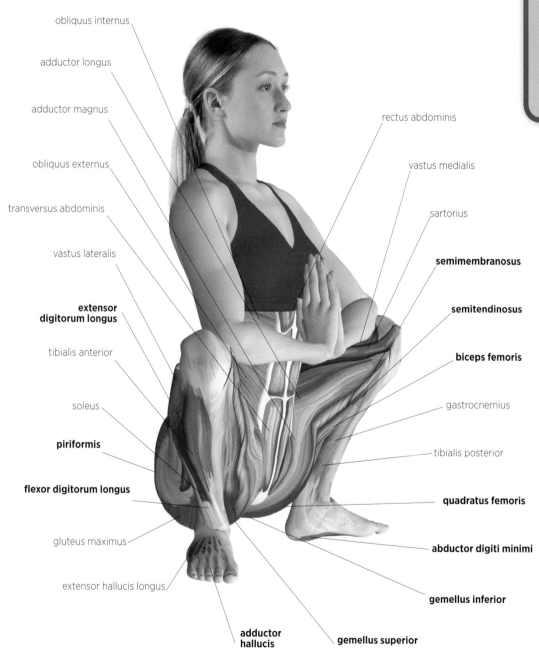

FACT FILE

TARGETS
• Inner thighs

TYPE
• Static

BENEFITS
• Stretches hips, groin, and ankles
• Lengthens spine
• Engages quadriceps and adductors

CAUTIONS
• Knee issues
• Lower-back issues

Annotation Key

Bold text indicates target muscles
Light text indicates other working muscles
* indicates deep muscles

obliquus internus

adductor longus

adductor magnus

obliquus externus

transversus abdominis

vastus lateralis

extensor digitorum longus

tibialis anterior

soleus

piriformis

flexor digitorum longus

gluteus maximus

extensor hallucis longus

adductor hallucis

gemellus superior

rectus abdominis

vastus medialis

sartorius

semimembranosus

semitendinosus

biceps femoris

gastrocnemius

tibialis posterior

quadratus femoris

abductor digiti minimi

gemellus inferior

Kneeling Side Lift

Tone your outer thighs and outer core with this Pilates-inspired stretching exercise. Take care not to let your extended foot touch the floor until the movement is complete.

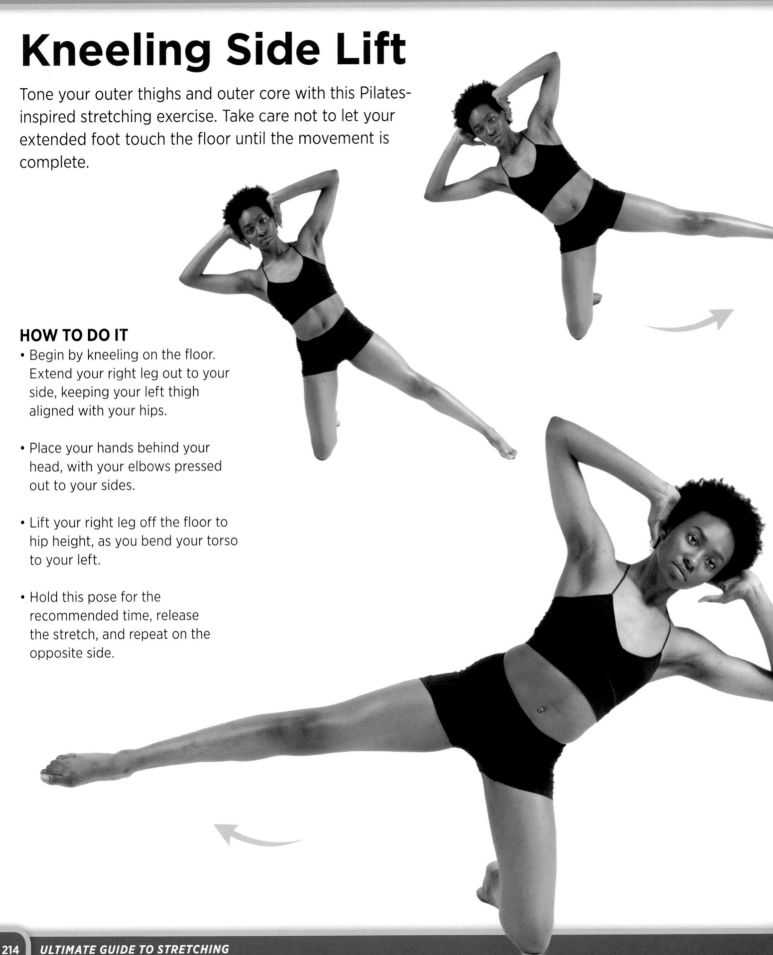

HOW TO DO IT

• Begin by kneeling on the floor. Extend your right leg out to your side, keeping your left thigh aligned with your hips.

• Place your hands behind your head, with your elbows pressed out to your sides.

• Lift your right leg off the floor to hip height, as you bend your torso to your left.

• Hold this pose for the recommended time, release the stretch, and repeat on the opposite side.

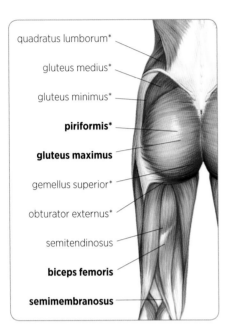

quadratus lumborum*

gluteus medius*

gluteus minimus*

piriformis*

gluteus maximus

gemellus superior*

obturator externus*

semitendinosus

biceps femoris

semimembranosus

TARGETS
• Hips
• Glutes
• Abdominal obliques
• Quadriceps

TYPE
• Static

BENEFITS
• Strengthens abdominal obliques, quadriceps, and hamstrings
• Improves posture

CAUTIONS
• Lower-back issues
• Knee issues

DO IT RIGHT
• Keep your torso facing forward and in line with your leg to help maintain your balance.
• Avoid sinking your neck into your shoulders.

Annotation Key
Bold text indicates target muscles
Light text indicates other working muscles
* indicates deep muscles

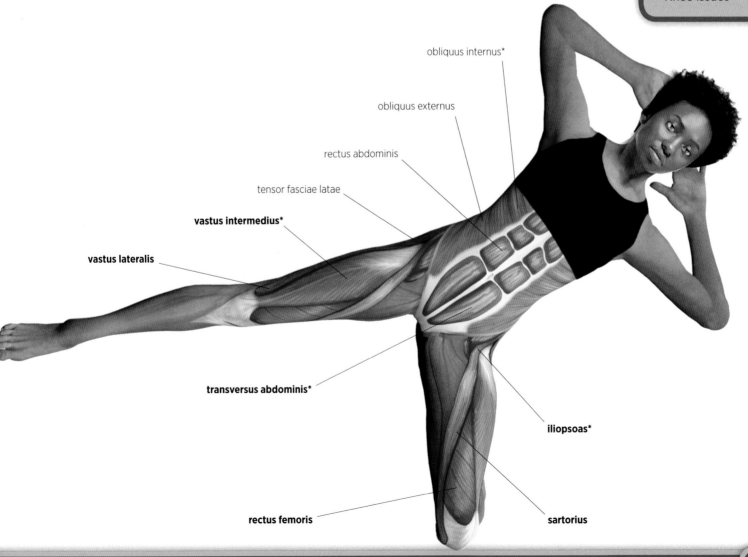

obliquus internus*

obliquus externus

rectus abdominis

tensor fasciae latae

vastus intermedius*

vastus lateralis

transversus abdominis*

iliopsoas*

rectus femoris

sartorius

Quadruped Leg Lift

This is a great stretch for lengthening your spine, arms, and leg. The Quadruped Leg Lift develops your core body strength and works your back, abdominals, and glutes, with the added bonus of improving your balance and coordination.

HOW TO DO IT

- Begin on all fours, with your back straight and your abdominals pulled in.

- Keeping your torso stable and your abdominals engaged, contract your left arm and your right leg.

- Extend your right arm and left leg outward, pulling them in opposite directions and lengthening along the spine. Hold this position for the recommended time, release, and repeat on the opposite side.

DO IT RIGHT

- Move slowly and with control.
- Keep your neck relaxed and your gaze toward the floor.
- Tuck your chin slightly while contracting your arm and leg inward.
- Keep your abs pulled in throughout the stretch.
- Avoid arching your back while your arm and leg are raised.
- Avoid twisting your torso.
- Avoid arching your neck.

MODIFICATION

HARDER: This variation will give your abs a greater challenge. Follow steps 1 and 2, and then draw your opposite knee and elbow inwards to touch. Repeat entire sequence on the other side.

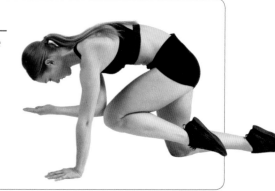

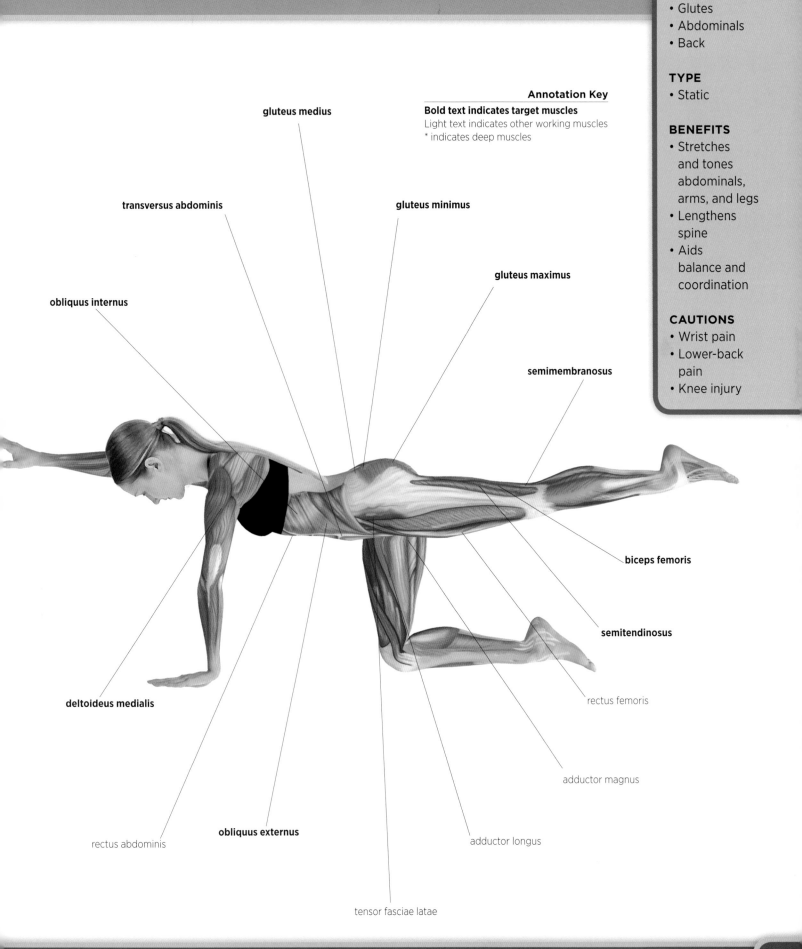

TARGETS
• Glutes
• Abdominals
• Back

TYPE
• Static

BENEFITS
• Stretches and tones abdominals, arms, and legs
• Lengthens spine
• Aids balance and coordination

CAUTIONS
• Wrist pain
• Lower-back pain
• Knee injury

Annotation Key
Bold text indicates target muscles
Light text indicates other working muscles
* indicates deep muscles

gluteus medius

transversus abdominis

gluteus minimus

gluteus maximus

obliquus internus

semimembranosus

biceps femoris

semitendinosus

deltoideus medialis

rectus femoris

adductor magnus

rectus abdominis

obliquus externus

adductor longus

tensor fasciae latae

Frog Straddle

The Frog Straddle offers a deep stretch in your inner-thigh muscles. Using the weight of your body, you can direct this stretch to target different muscle groups.

HOW TO DO IT

- Kneel on all fours.

- Bend your elbows, shift your weight forward, and lower your elbows and forearms onto the floor.

- Spread your knees apart, drawing your feet in slightly and putting some weight on them to take pressure off your knees.

- Lower your legs and buttocks down to the floor and bring the soles of your feet together to deepen the stretch.

MODIFICATION

HARDER: Move your forearms forward and lean into them. Try to keep both your pelvis and your heels on the floor as you stretch.

FACT FILE

TARGETS
• Adductors
• Hip flexors

TYPE
• Dynamic

BENEFITS
• Stretches hip
  flexors and
  adductors
• Opens hips

CAUTIONS
• Hip pain
• Knee issues

Annotation Key

Bold text indicates target muscles

Light text indicates other working muscles

* indicates deep muscles

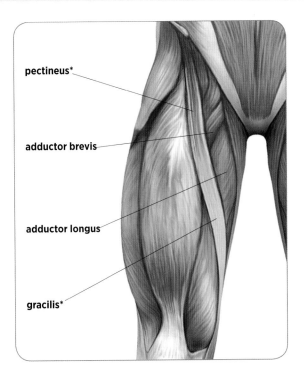

pectineus*

adductor brevis

adductor longus

gracilis*

DO IT RIGHT

• Stretch until you reach a
  challenging position but
  without pain.
• Avoid placing too much
  weight on your knees.
• Don't allow your lower
  back to sink.

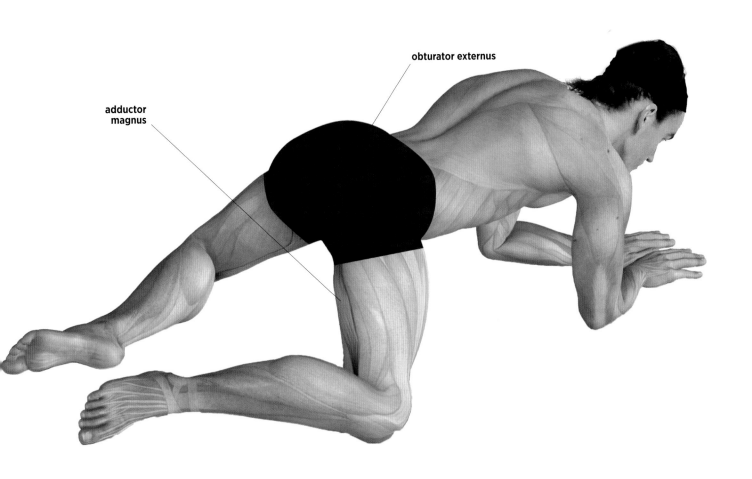

obturator externus

adductor
magnus

Pigeon Stretch

The Pigeon Stretch offers a deep stretch in your thighs, groin, and glutes. It also eases tension in your lower back and improves flexibility along your spine.

HOW TO DO IT

- Kneel with your buttocks resting lightly on your heels and your arms at your sides, supporting some of your weight.

- Straighten your left leg, extending it along the floor behind you, keeping your leg aligned with your body. Your right knee should be facing forward.

- Move your arms forward to rest slightly in front of your right knee. Your hands should be shoulder-width apart, and your palms flat on the floor.

- Keeping the rest of your body in alignment, move your right heel a few inches to your left so that it crosses the core of your body.

- Hold for the recommended time, release the stretch, and repeat on the opposite side.

DO IT RIGHT

- Avoid hyperextending your elbows; maintain a slight bend in your elbows.
- Lean primarily on your bent leg.
- Keep your shoulder blades pressed down.

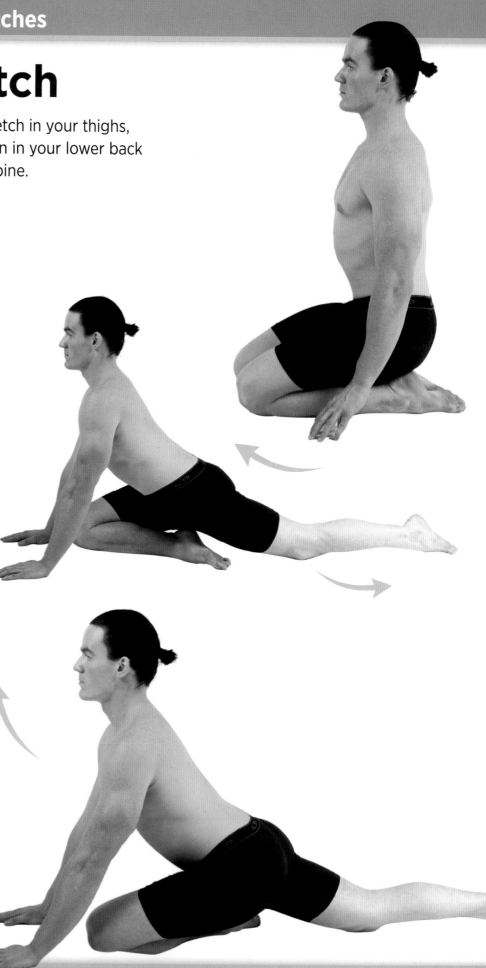

TARGETS
• Glutes
• Groin muscles
• Hamstrings
• Quadriceps

TYPE
• Static

BENEFITS
• Stretches gluteal area
• Loosens tight groin muscles
• Lengthens hamstrings and quadriceps

CAUTIONS
• Hip Pain
• Knee problems
• Lower-back pain

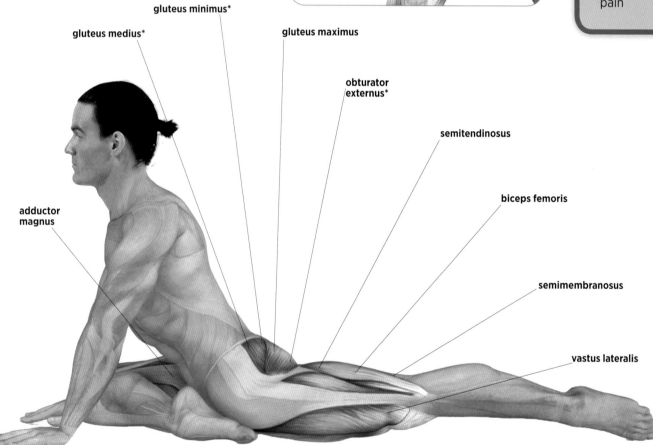

Annotation Key

Bold text indicates target muscles
Light text indicates other working muscles
* indicates deep muscles

iliopsoas*

pectineus*

adductor brevis

adductor longus

vastus intermedius*

rectus femoris

gracilis*

vastus medialis

gluteus minimus*

gluteus medius*

gluteus maximus

obturator externus*

semitendinosus

biceps femoris

semimembranosus

adductor magnus

vastus lateralis

Seated Leg Cradle

Seated Leg Cradle stretches your thighs, hamstrings, and calf muscles and releases tightness in your hip flexors. This stretch takes tension off your spine, increases your range of motion, boosts your circulation, and may help alleviate back pain.

HOW TO DO IT

• Sit on the floor with your legs extended in front of you.

• Bend your right knee and turn it outward. Place your right hand under your calf, and support your ankle with your left hand, hugging your leg it into your chest as if you were cradling a baby.

• Hold for the recommended time, release the stretch, and then repeat on the opposite side.

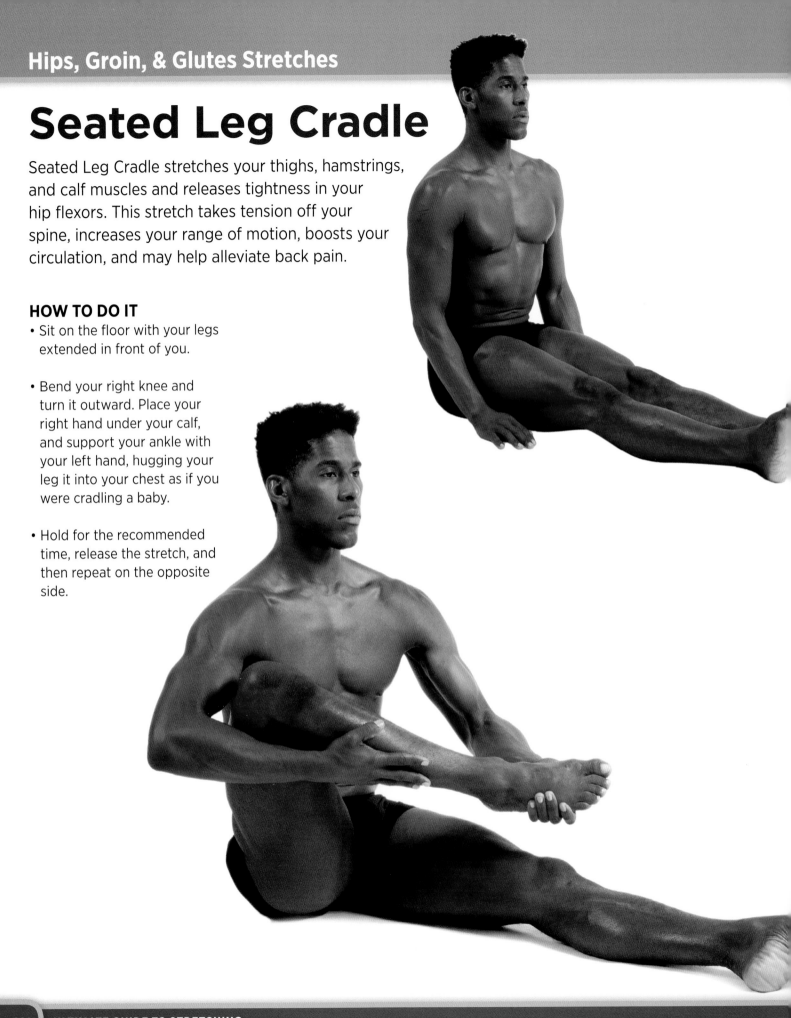

TARGETS
- Upper hamstrings
- Glutes

TYPE
- Passive

BENEFITS
- Opens hips
- Relieves hip flexor tightness
- Alleviate sore glutes

CAUTIONS
- Hip pain
- Knee injury
- Lower-back pain

Annotation Key

Bold text indicates target muscles
Light text indicates other working muscles
* indicates deep muscles

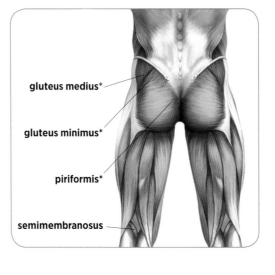

gluteus medius*

gluteus minimus*

piriformis*

semimembranosus

DO IT RIGHT
- Keep your chest lifted.
- Contract your gluteal muscles.
- Avoid holding your breath.

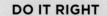

semitendinosus

biceps femoris

gluteus maximus

Front Split

Front and middle splits target the muscles in your hips, groin, and legs. Maximum flexibility in these areas offers several health benefits, including improved joint mobility, better posture, and protection against injury.

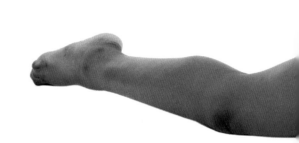

DO IT RIGHT

- Keep your chest open and lifted.
- Avoid forcing yourself down too soon; gradually work toward perfecting your form.

HOW TO DO IT

- Kneel on your left leg, with your right leg forward, making sure that your knee doesn't extend past your toes.

- Square your hips, and keep your left knee on the floor.

- Square your shoulders, using your hands on the floor for balance.

- Slowly, slide your right leg forward as you extend your left leg backward as far as you can without forcing the movement.

- Sit up tall, and hold for the recommended time.

- Release the stretch, and then repeat on the opposite side.

FACT FILE

TARGETS
- Hamstrings
- Quadriceps
- Inner thighs
- Calves
- Obliques

TYPE
- Dynamic

BENEFITS
- Deeply opens hips
- Strengthens pelvic floor
- Provides maximum flexibility in hips and upper legs

CAUTIONS
- Hip pain
- Lower-back pain

Annotation Key

Bold text indicates target muscles
Light text indicates other working muscles
* indicates deep muscles

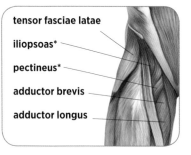

tensor fasciae latae
iliopsoas*
pectineus*
adductor brevis
adductor longus

gluteus medius*
gluteus minimus*
gluteus maximus*
obturator externus
semitendinosus
biceps femoris
semimembranosus

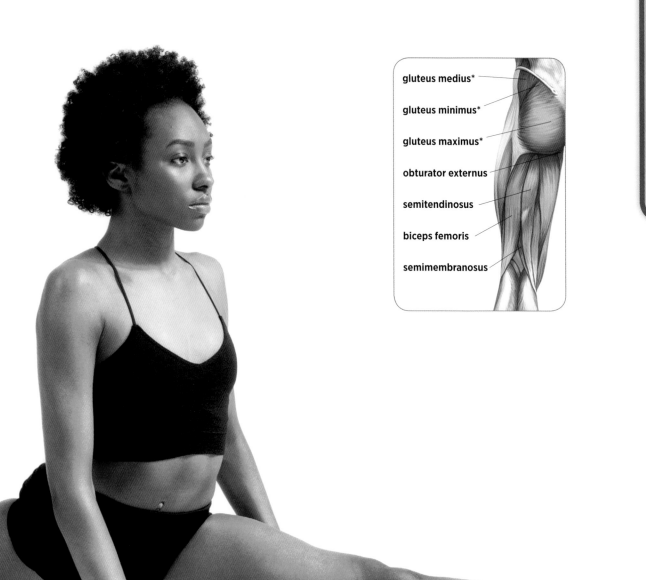

Chest-to-Floor Straddle Split

The Chest-to-Floor Straddle Split is an intense hip-opening stretch. It lengthens the muscles all along the front and back of your legs as well as your inner thighs.

HOW TO DO IT

• Begin by sitting upright with your legs extended out to your sides. Turn your legs out from your hips as far as you can comfortably reach.

• Your feet should be flexed with your toes pointing upward.

• Place your hands on the floor in front of you and slowly walk them forward as you lower your torso toward the floor.

• Hold for the recommended time, and then release the stretch.

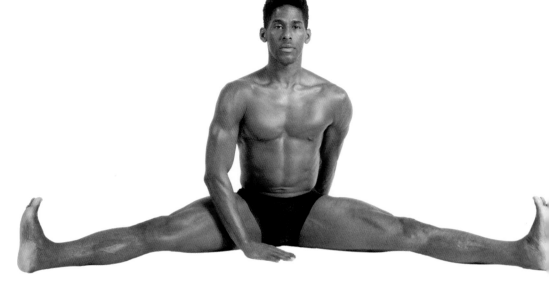

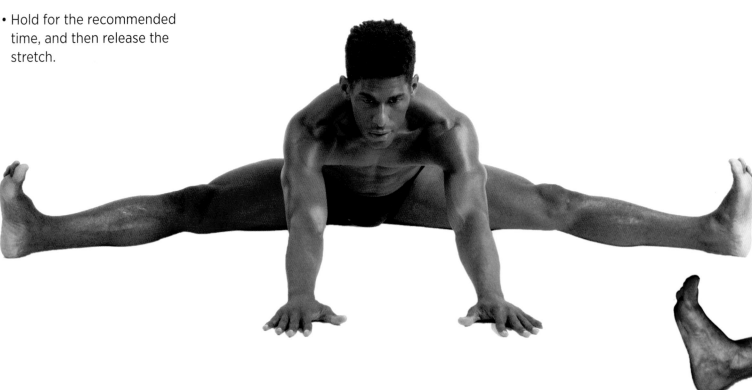

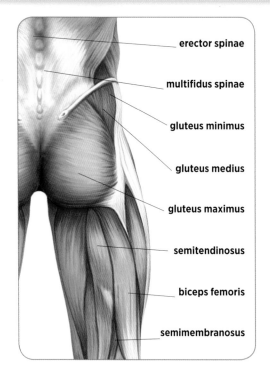

FACT FILE

TARGETS
- Hamstrings
- Quadriceps
- Inner thighs
- Calves
- Obliques

TYPE
- Dynamic

BENEFITS
- Opens hips
- Strengthens pelvic floor
- Provides maximum flexibility in hips and upper legs

CAUTIONS
- Hip pain
- Lower-back pain
- Knee pain

Annotation Key

Bold text indicates target muscles
Light text indicates other working muscles
* indicates deep muscles

DO IT RIGHT

- Keep your torso long and flat, and your chest lifted.
- Lengthen your spine as you bend forward.
- Keep your legs turned out from your hips.
- Avoid overdoing this stretch—move carefully and slowly.

erector spinae
multifidus spinae
gluteus minimus
gluteus medius
gluteus maximus
semitendinosus
biceps femoris
semimembranosus

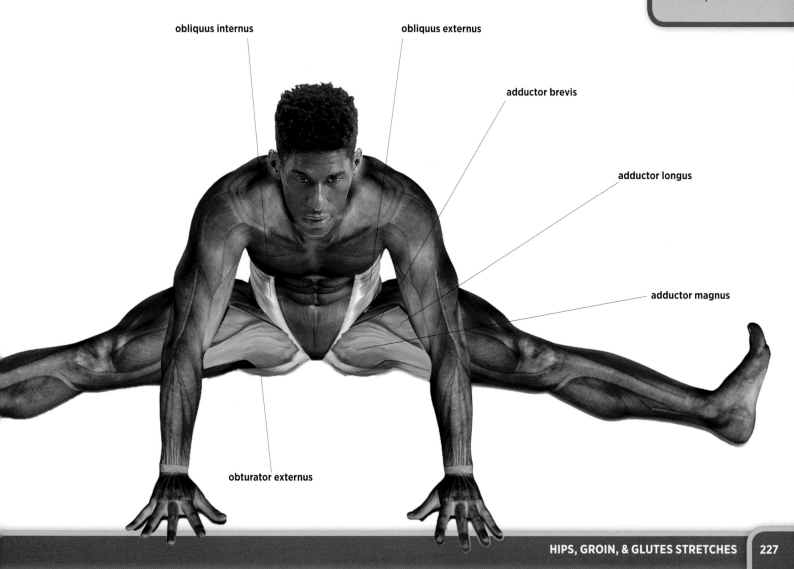

obliquus internus
obliquus externus
adductor brevis
adductor longus
adductor magnus
obturator externus

Double-Leg Straddle Split

The Double-Leg Straddle Split increases the flexibility in your ankles, leg joints, and lower back. It's a powerful hip opener and groin stretch. This can also improve your circulation in the pelvic region.

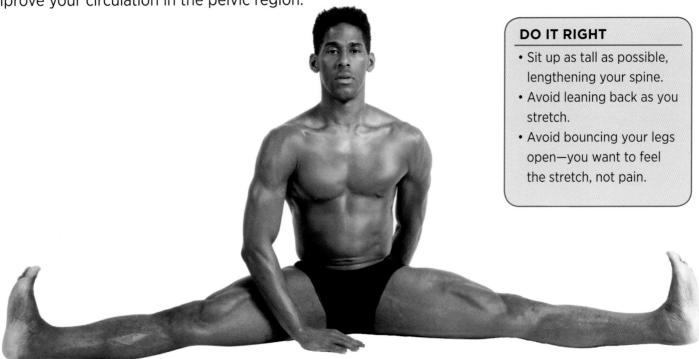

DO IT RIGHT
- Sit up as tall as possible, lengthening your spine.
- Avoid leaning back as you stretch.
- Avoid bouncing your legs open—you want to feel the stretch, not pain.

HOW TO DO IT
- Begin by sitting upright with your legs extended out to your sides. Turn your legs out from your hips as far as you can comfortably reach.

- Your feet should be flexed with your toes pointing upward.

- Place one hand on the floor directly in front of you and the other directly behind you.

- Align your hip bones on the floor, and lengthen your spine.

- Hold for the recommended time, and then release the stretch.

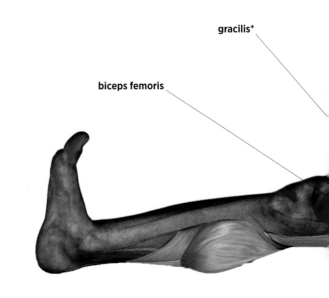

gracilis*

biceps femoris

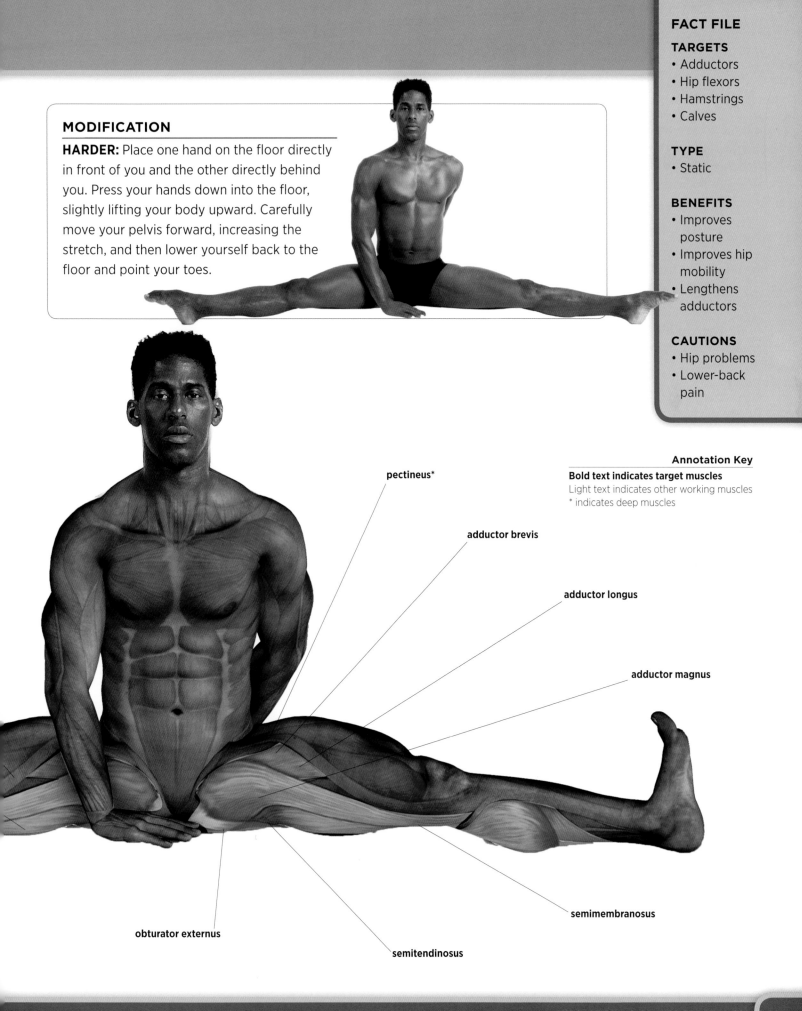

MODIFICATION

HARDER: Place one hand on the floor directly in front of you and the other directly behind you. Press your hands down into the floor, slightly lifting your body upward. Carefully move your pelvis forward, increasing the stretch, and then lower yourself back to the floor and point your toes.

Annotation Key

Bold text indicates target muscles
Light text indicates other working muscles
* indicates deep muscles

pectineus*

adductor brevis

adductor longus

adductor magnus

semimembranosus

obturator externus

semitendinosus

Chest-to-Thigh Straddle Split

The Chest-to-Floor Straddle Split, as other Straddle Splits, stretches all your leg muscles and lengthens your spine. This version adds a twist in your torso as you bend forward over your leg, targeting your abdominal obliques as well as your hip flexors.

HOW TO DO IT

• Begin by sitting upright with your legs extended out to your sides. Turn your legs out from your hips as far as you can comfortably reach.

• Your feet should be flexed with your toes pointing upward.

• Place your hands on either side of your right leg and walk them forward as you lower your torso toward your right leg.

• Hold for the recommended time, release the stretch, and repeat on the opposite side.

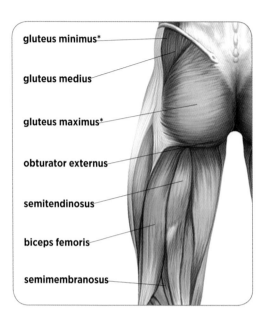

gluteus minimus*

gluteus medius

gluteus maximus*

obturator externus

semitendinosus

biceps femoris

semimembranosus

FACT FILE

TARGETS
• Inner thighs
• Hamstrings
• Glutes
• Rib cage
• Hip flexors

TYPE
• Static

BENEFITS
• Relieves tightness in inner thighs and hamstrings
• Intensely opens hips
• Targets abdominal obliques

CAUTIONS
• Hip pain
• Lower-back pain

DO IT RIGHT

• Keep the turnout in your legs, and aim your toes straight up.
• Avoid lifting your hip bones off the floor.
• Don't allow your legs to shift inward.

Annotation Key

Bold text indicates target muscles
Light text indicates other working muscles
* indicates deep muscles

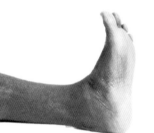

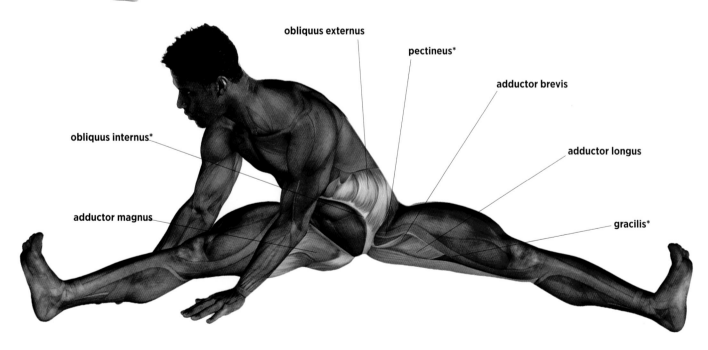

obliquus externus

pectineus*

adductor brevis

obliquus internus*

adductor longus

adductor magnus

gracilis*

Wide-Angle Seated Forward Bend

Wide-Angle Seated Forward Bend is a challenging pose that opens your hips and groin muscles and lengthens your spine. For those who are limber enough to relax into this stretch, it is a restful posture offering a full-body stretch.

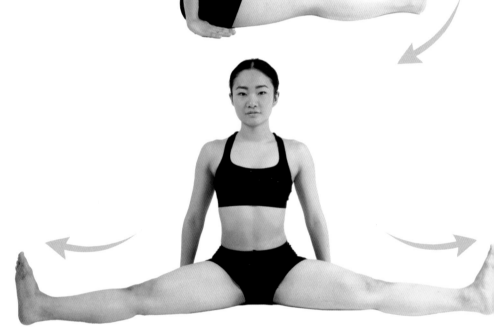

HOW TO DO IT

• Begin by sitting upright with your legs extended out to your sides. Turn your legs out from your hips as far as you can comfortably reach.

• Your feet should be flexed with your toes pointing upward.

• Place your hands on the floor behind your buttocks to push them forward, separating your legs even farther.

• Press the backs of your thighs and sit bones into the floor.

• Lift up through your torso and reach your hands to the floor in front of you.

• Slowly walk your hands forward as you lower your torso toward the floor. Stretch as far as possible without rounding your back.

• Hold for the recommended time, and then release the stretch.

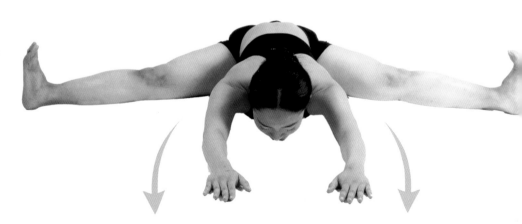

TARGETS
- Inner thighs
- Hamstrings
- Glutes
- Rib cage
- Hip flexors

TYPE
- Dynamic

BENEFITS
- Stretches groin and hamstrings
- Intensely opens hips
- Lengthens spine

CAUTIONS
- Back pain
- Hip pain
- Headache

DO IT RIGHT
- Keep the turnout in your legs, and aim your toes straight up.
- Avoid lifting your hip bones off the floor.
- Don't allow your legs to turn inward.

Annotation Key

Bold text indicates target muscles
Light text indicates other working muscles
* indicates deep muscles

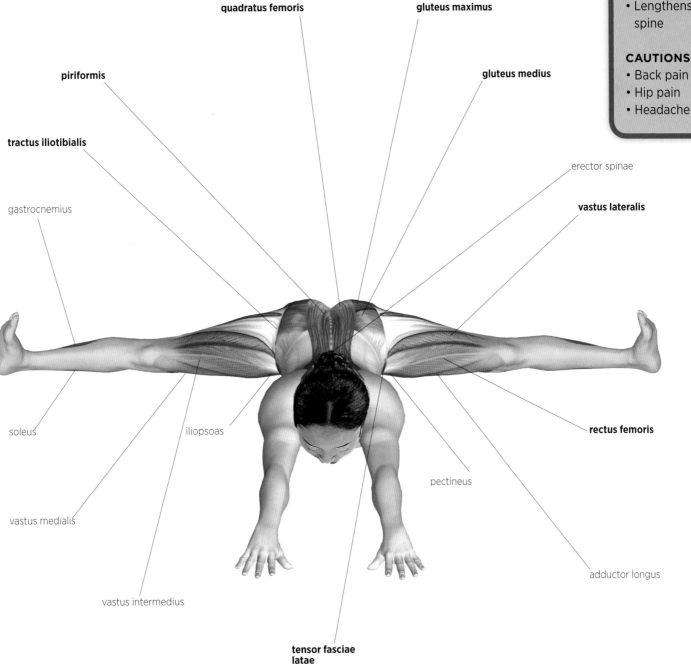

quadratus femoris

gluteus maximus

piriformis

gluteus medius

tractus iliotibialis

erector spinae

vastus lateralis

gastrocnemius

soleus

iliopsoas

rectus femoris

pectineus

vastus medialis

adductor longus

vastus intermedius

tensor fasciae latae

Lotus Yoga Stretch

For yogis, Lotus Yoga Stretch is the ultimate meditation pose. Entering this position can allow you to hold your body steady for long periods, and calm your mind. As well as facilitating meditation, this cross-legged sitting asana opens up your hips and stretches your ankles and knees. It looks simple, but beginners may find it difficult, so go at your own pace, honing your skills of concentration and focus.

HOW TO DO IT

• Sit up straight and cross your legs. With your hands, position your right foot on your left thigh.

• Position your left foot on your right thigh. Hook your ankles as far as possible up your thighs, drawing them toward your hips. Flex your feet to help keep your knees and ankles in alignment.

• Balance on your sit bones and press them evenly into the floor. Externally rotate your hips, feeling your inner knees opening away from each other. Find a neutral pelvis, drawing your tailbone toward the floor. Draw your abs in toward your spine.

• Sit up tall, lengthening your torso and broadening across your collarbones to lift your sternum and open your chest. Allow your arms to draw open, and position your hands either facing up, in a gesture of receiving, or facing down, in a gesture of grounding. Close your eyes as you hold for the recommended time.

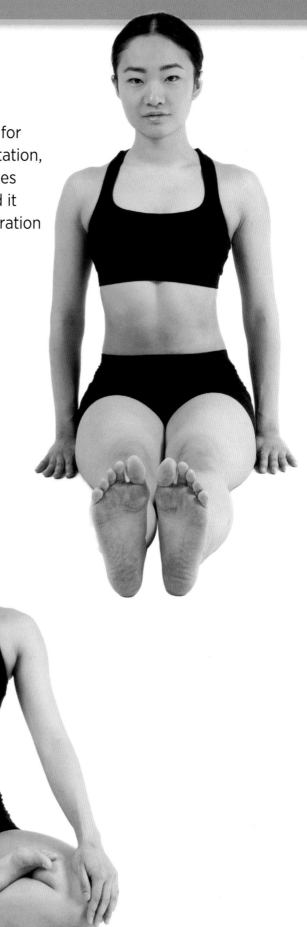

TARGETS
- Hips
- Glutes
- Legs

TYPE
- Static

BENEFITS
- Stretches lower body, knees, ankles, and buttocks
- Opens hips and groin
- Stimulates digestion
- Calms mind and body

CAUTIONS
- Ankle injuries
- Hip issues
- Knee issues

DO IT RIGHT

- Keep your back and upper body straight; if you have trouble sitting straight, place a folded blanket beneath your hips to raise them above your knees.
- Lengthen your spine.
- Avoid straining your knees; if you're not quite ready to perform the full pose, gradually ease into it with practice.
- Do not overextend your outer ankles.
- Avoid leaning or tilting your upper body to one side.

Annotation Key

Bold text indicates target muscles
Light text indicates other working muscles
* indicates deep muscles

obliquus externus

rectus abdominis

obliquus internus

transversus abdominis

iliopsoas

tibialis anterior

Seated Butterfly Stretch

The Seated Butterfly Stretch is a fairly simple exercise that targets the muscles in your groin and inner thighs. The hip opener also engages your abs and lengthens your spine.

HOW TO DO IT

- Sit up tall, with your knees out to your sides and the soles of your feet pressed together.

- Feel both sit bones firmly pressing into the floor, and find a neutral pelvis.

- Rest your hands on your ankles, and draw your heels in toward your groin.

- Pull your knees down toward the floor, and lift up along your spine.

- Hold for the recommended time, and release the stretch.

DO IT RIGHT

- Avoid slouching.
- Avoid holding your breath.
- Avoid rocking backward; instead, feel your sit bones anchored into the floor.

FACT FILE

TARGETS
- Hip flexors
- Adductors
- Lower back

TYPE
- Static

BENEFITS
- Stretches inner thighs
- Lengthens spine

CAUTIONS
- Hip issues
- Knee issues

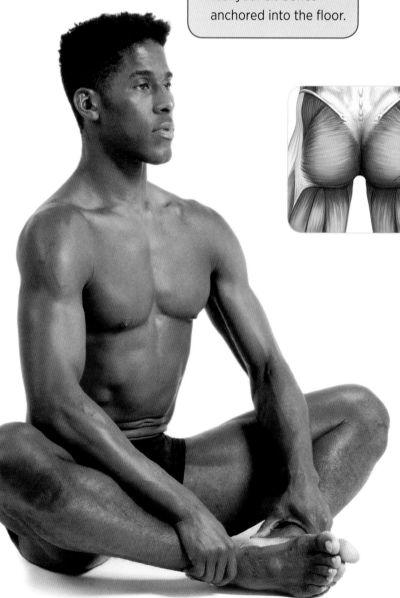

obturator externus*

Annotation Key
Bold text indicates target muscles
Light text indicates other working muscles
* indicates deep muscles

Folded Butterly Stretch

This variation of the Seated Butterfly incorporates a forward bend, adding a spinal stretch and opening the hips more deeply.

HOW TO DO IT

• From the Seated Butterfly (opposite page), place your forearms on your inner thighs, and grasp your feet. Keep your heels a comfortable distance from your groin.

• Fold your upper body forward until you feel a stretch in your upper inner thighs.

• Hold for the recommended time, and release the stretch.

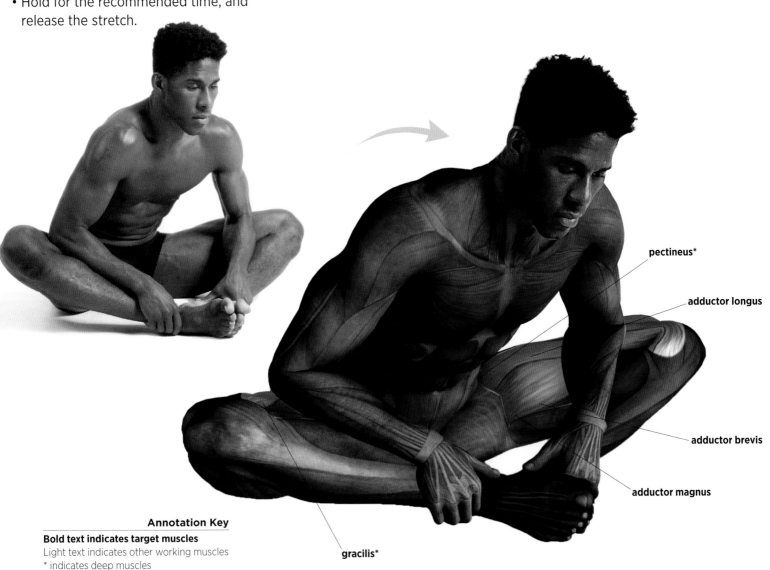

pectineus*

adductor longus

adductor brevis

adductor magnus

gracilis*

Annotation Key

Bold text indicates target muscles
Light text indicates other working muscles
* indicates deep muscles

Bound Angle Yoga Stretch

The restorative Bound Angle Yoga Stretch is an effective hip opener that can be adapted to any level of flexibility. This classic exercise also releases tension in your shoulders and along your back while improving hip mobility.

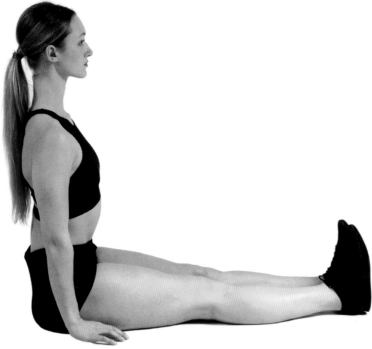

> **DO IT RIGHT**
> - To deepen the stretch, keep the outside of your feet on the floor and slightly lift your heels.
> - Avoid raising your lower back off the floor.
> - Do not bounce your legs open to achieve a deeper stretch.

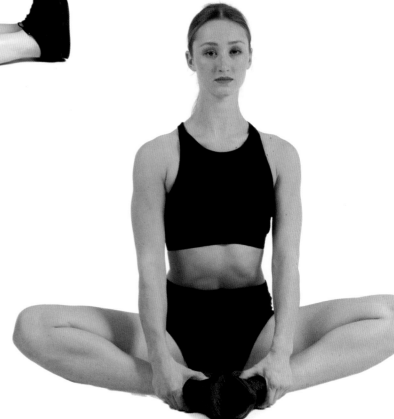

HOW TO DO IT

- Sit up tall, with your knees out to your sides and the soles of your feet pressed together.

- Feel both sit bones firmly pressing into the floor, and find a neutral pelvis.

- Wrap your hands around your ankles, and draw your heels in toward your groin.

- Pull your knees down toward the floor, and lift up along your spine.

- Hold for the recommended time, and release the stretch.

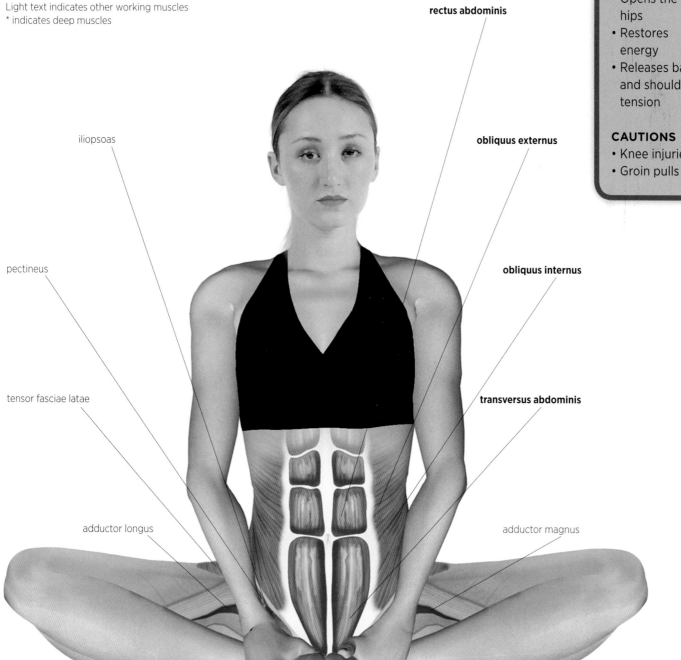

TARGETS
• Groin muscles
• Inner thighs
• Knees

TYPE
• Static

BENEFITS
• Opens the hips
• Restores energy
• Releases back and shoulder tension

CAUTIONS
• Knee injuries
• Groin pulls

Annotation Key

Bold text indicates target muscles
Light text indicates other working muscles
* indicates deep muscles

rectus abdominis

obliquus externus

iliopsoas

obliquus internus

pectineus

transversus abdominis

tensor fasciae latae

adductor longus

adductor magnus

biceps femoris

semimembranosus

semitendinosus

Clamshells

Clamshells strengthen your medial glutes and bring more power and stability to your hips. This exercise is commonly prescribed by physical therapists as a remedy for hip tightness and lower-back pain.

HOW TO DO IT

• Lie on your right side with your knees bent, aligning your shoulders, hips, and ankles. Bend your right arm and tuck your forearm under your head, keeping your head in line with your spine.

• Flex your feet, with your left toes pointing outward. Contract your glutes as you hinge open your hip and raise your left knee, keeping your heels together.

• Return to the starting position. Perform the recommended repetitions, and repeat on the opposite side.

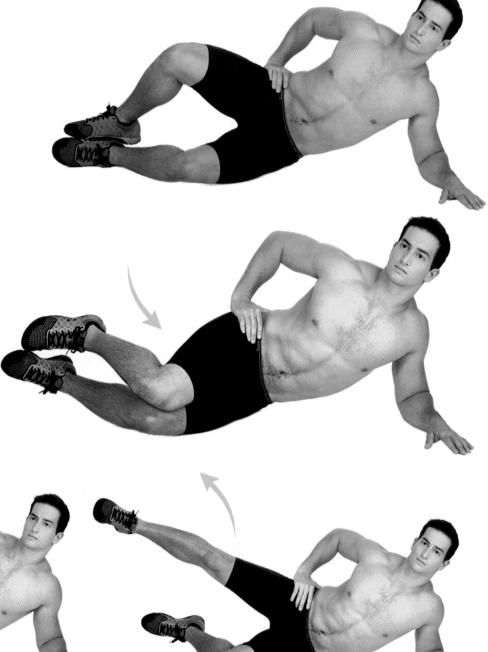

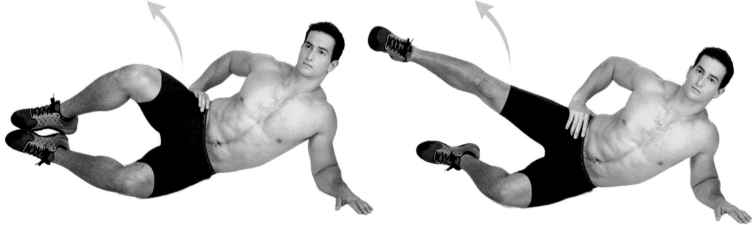

TARGETS
• Glutes
• Inner thighs

TYPE
• Dynamic

BENEFITS
• Increases hip
  stability
• Strengthens
  glutes and
  hamstrings
• Alleviates
  lower-back
  pain

CAUTIONS
• Lower-back
  injury
• Intense hip
  pain
• Intense knee
  pain

Annotation Key

Bold text indicates target muscles
Light text indicates other working muscles
* indicates deep muscles

DO IT RIGHT

• Focus on moving only
  your upper leg.
• Your upper leg should
  move as if it were on a
  hinge.
• Keep your spine stable.
• Avoid any pelvic
  movement.

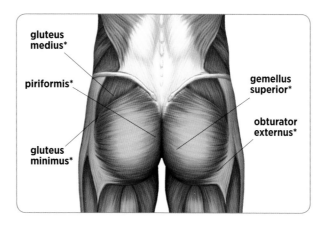

gluteus
medius*

piriformis*

gluteus
minimus*

gemellus
superior*

obturator
externus*

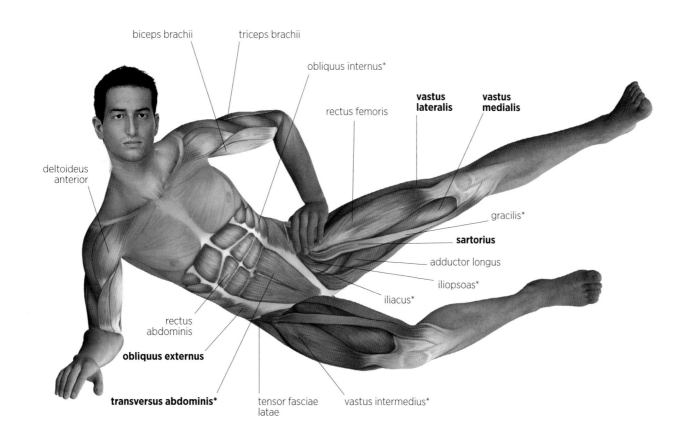

biceps brachii

triceps brachii

obliquus internus*

rectus femoris

**vastus
lateralis**

**vastus
medialis**

deltoideus
anterior

gracilis*

sartorius

adductor longus

iliopsoas*

iliacus*

rectus
abdominis

obliquus externus

transversus abdominis*

tensor fasciae
latae

vastus intermedius*

Piriformis Stretch

This excellent exercise targets the hard-to-reach piriformis muscle deep in the glutes. The piriformis laterally rotates and stabilizes your hip and is particularly important in sports that require sudden changes of direction. Keep this muscle flexible to help prevent against sciatica.

HOW TO DO IT

- Lie on your back with your knees bent and your feet planted on the floor.

- Cross your right ankle over your left thigh.

- Reach your hands behind your left thigh close to your knee, and gently pull your leg toward you.

- Hold for the recommended time, release the stretch, and repeat on the opposite side.

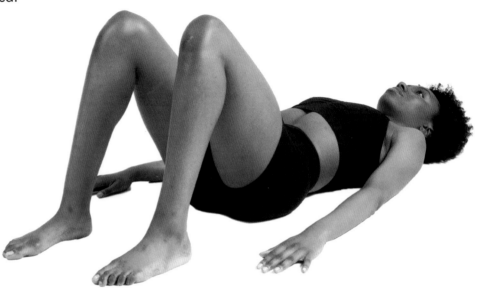

DO IT RIGHT

- Be sure to ease into the movement slowly.
- Try to relax your hips to enable a deeper stretch.
- Avoid pulling your thigh to your chest forcefully.

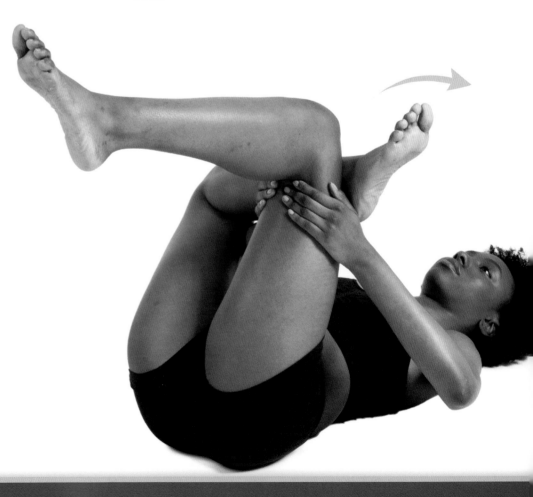

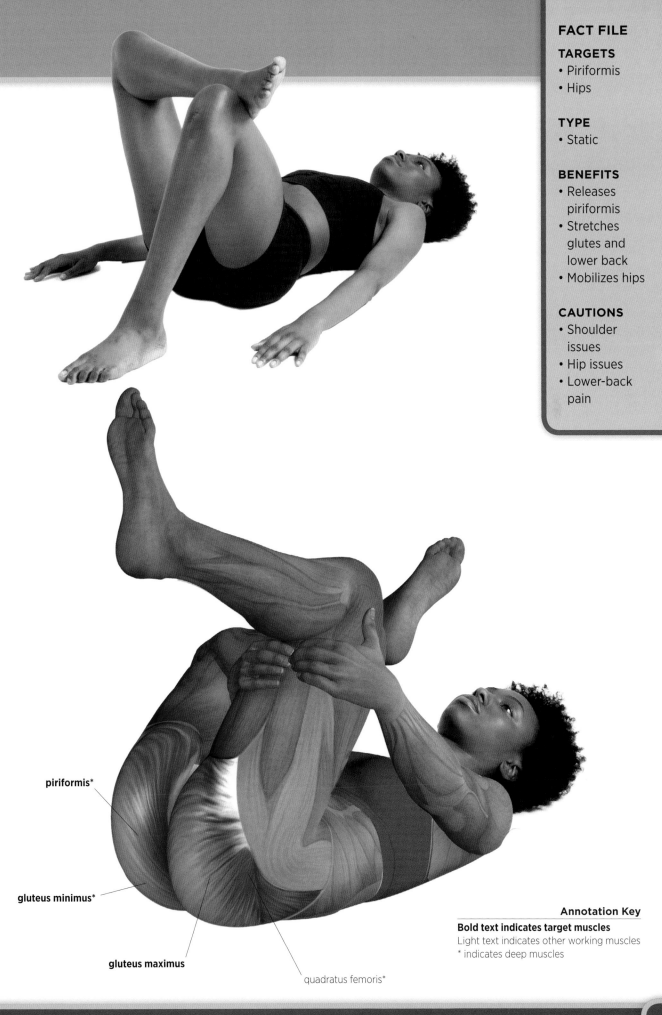

piriformis*

gluteus minimus*

gluteus maximus

quadratus femoris*

Annotation Key
Bold text indicates target muscles
Light text indicates other working muscles
* indicates deep muscles

Piriformis Bridge

This exercise stretches the muscles in your hips and glutes, especially the deep piriformis muscle. A tight piriformis can lead to excruciating pain along your sciatic nerve, so add these bridges to your stretching routine to prevent against injury.

HOW TO DO IT

• Lie on your back with your knees bent and your feet planted on the floor.

• Cross your right ankle over your left thigh.

• Press your palms into the floor and engage your abdominal muscles as you lift your hips. Your body should form a diagonal line from your shoulders to your knees.

• Slowly and with control, return to the starting position. Release the stretch, and repeat on the opposite side.

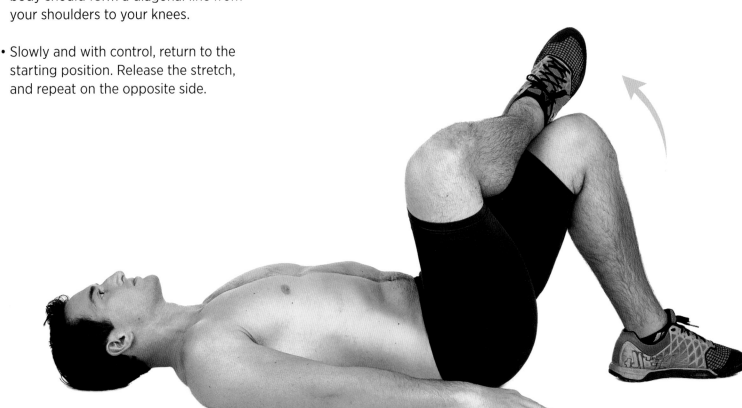

DO IT RIGHT

• Squeeze your buttocks as you lift and lower your hips and back.
• Draw your navel toward your spine.
• Avoid tensing your neck.
• Avoid lifting your shoulders to your ears.

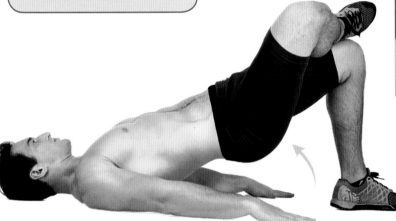

erector spinae*

multifidus spinae*

quadratus lumborum*

gluteus medius*

gluteus minimus*

gluteus maximus

piriformis*

biceps femoris

semitendinosus

semimembranosus

Annotation Key
Bold text indicates target muscles
Light text indicates other working muscles
* indicates deep muscles

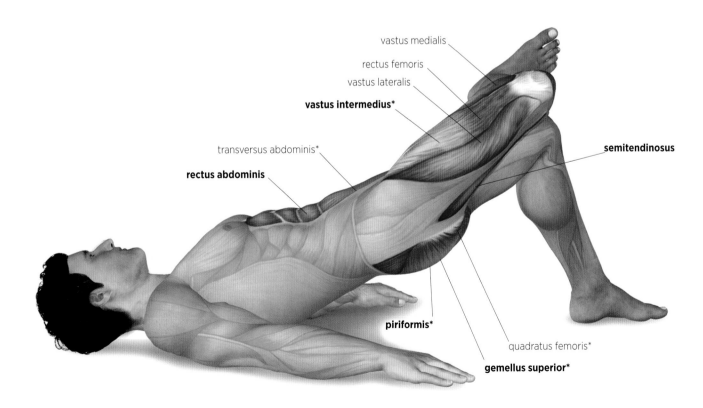

vastus medialis

rectus femoris

vastus lateralis

vastus intermedius*

transversus abdominis*

rectus abdominis

semitendinosus

piriformis*

quadratus femoris*

gemellus superior*

Lying-Down Groin Stretch

This reclining groin-stretching exercise is a fairly straightforward way to create space in your hips and loosen the groin muscles. You can allow gravity to pull your legs gently downward, or use your hands to add more pressure to stretch the adductors of your inner thighs.

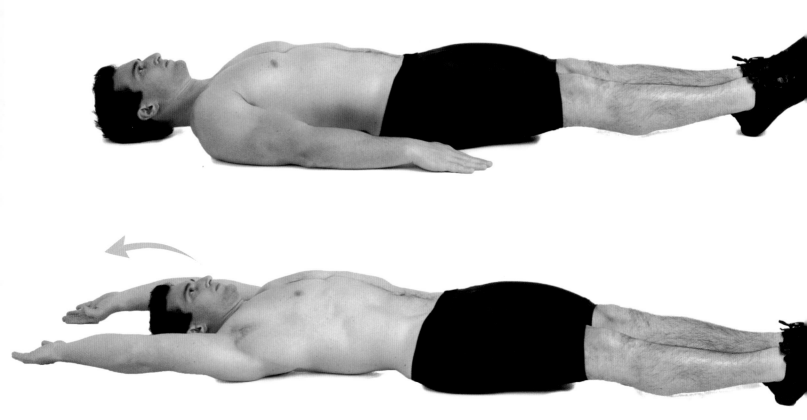

HOW TO DO IT

- Lie flat on your back with your knees bent.

- Lower your knees out to your sides, turning from your hips, and press the soles of your feet together.

- Place your hands on your inner thighs to deepen the stretch.

- Hold for the recommended time, and release the stretch.

DO IT RIGHT

- To deepen the stretch, keep the outside of your feet on the floor and slightly lift up your heels.
- Avoid raising your lower back off the floor.
- Do not flutter your legs open to achieve a deeper stretch.

Annotation Key

Bold text indicates target muscles
Light text indicates other working muscles
* indicates deep muscles

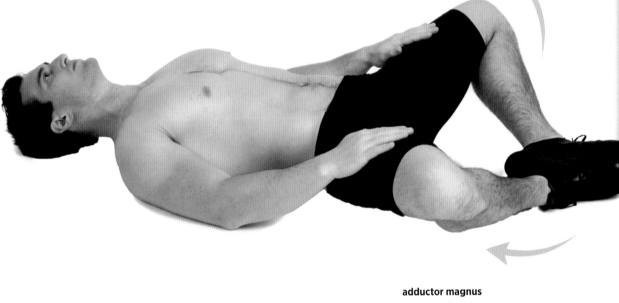

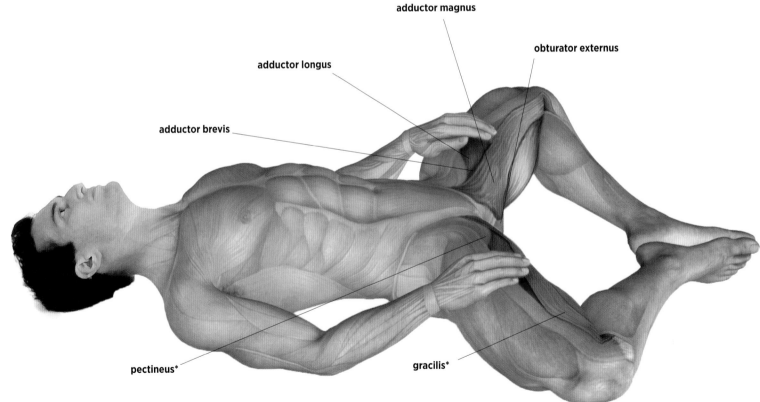

adductor magnus

obturator externus

adductor longus

adductor brevis

pectineus*

gracilis*

Hip Adductor Stretch

This reclining Hip Adductor Stretch incorporates a lateral opening movement with your leg extended out to your side. It's a welcome a counterpoint to day-to-day movements, and can provide targeted relief to tight groin, or adductor, muscles.

HOW TO DO IT

• Lie on your back, and bend your right knee in toward your chest.

• Place your hands on your hamstrings just below your knee, and extend your right leg straight toward the ceiling, pointing your toes.

• Release your left hand from your hamstrings, and lower your left arm to the floor.

• Move your right hand under your right calf muscle, and extend your leg out to your side, pointing your foot.

• Release the stretch, and repeat the on the opposite side.

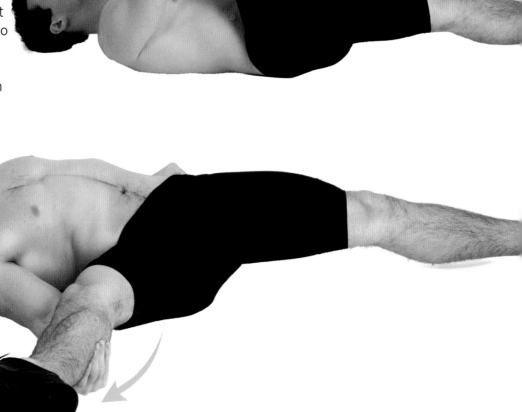

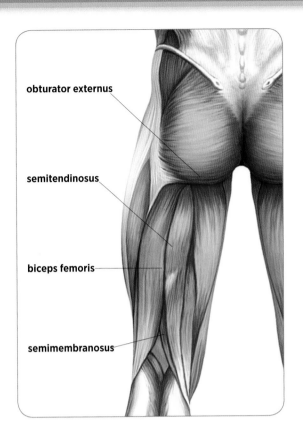

FACT FILE

TARGETS
- Groin muscles
- Glutes
- Hamstrings
- Lower back

TYPE
- Dynamic

BENEFITS
- Opens hips
- Stretches adductors

CAUTIONS
- Hip pain
- Shoulder pain
- Lower-back pain

Annotation Key

Bold text indicates target muscles

Light text indicates other working muscles

* indicates deep muscles

obturator externus

semitendinosus

biceps femoris

semimembranosus

DO IT RIGHT

- Flex the foot of your extended leg to ensure a deep stretch.
- Avoid lifting your lower back off the floor or twisting your torso.
- Breathe deep; don't hold your breath.

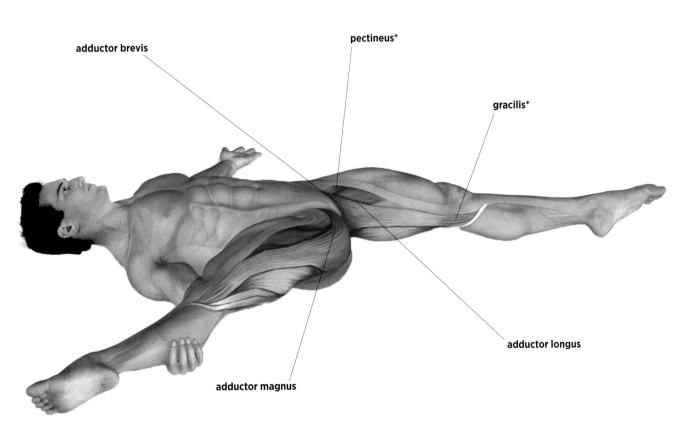

adductor brevis

pectineus*

gracilis*

adductor longus

adductor magnus

Lying-Down Figure 4 Stretch

Figure 4 Stretch gently opens your hips, stretches the piriformis, glutes, and lower back, and relieves tension in the muscles surrounding the sacrum. This stretch is used to mobilize your hip joints and stretch your hip muscles. Since tight hips can cause back stiffness, this stretch can also be used to prevent and relieve back pain.

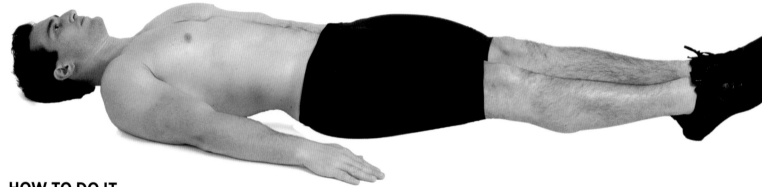

HOW TO DO IT

• Lie on your back with your legs extended. Point both toes.

• Bend your right knee and turn your leg out so that your right ankle rests on your left thigh just above your knee, creating a figure 4.

• Bend your left leg, drawing both legs in toward your chest as you grasp the back of your left thigh.

• Push your right elbow against your right inner thigh, turning out your right leg slightly to increase the intensity of the stretch.

• Hold for the recommended time, release the stretch, and repeat on the opposite side.

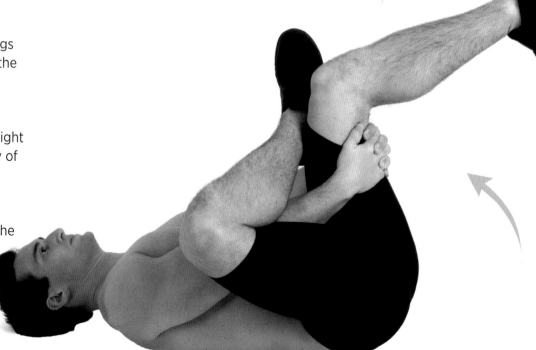

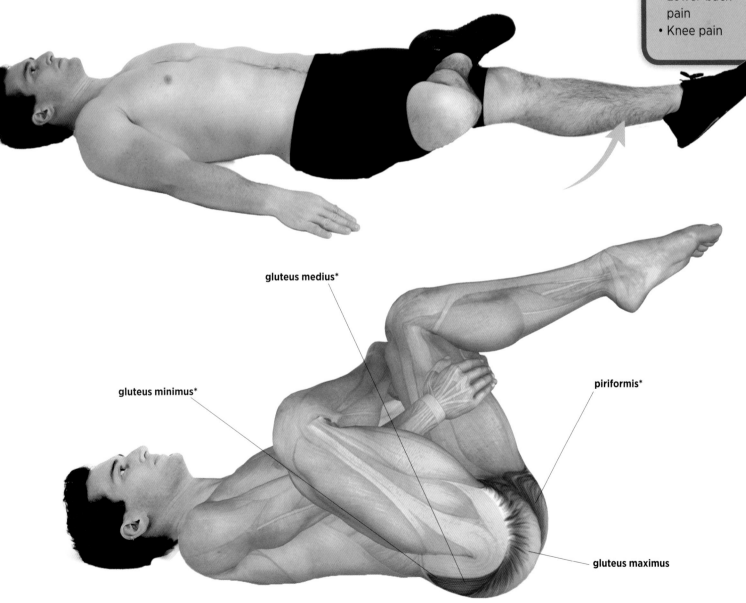

FACT FILE

TARGETS
• Glutes
• Adductors

TYPE
• Static

BENEFITS
• Mobilizes hip joints
• Relieves back pain
• Increases flexibility in glutes and hamstrings

CAUTIONS
• Hip pain
• Lower-back pain
• Knee pain

Annotation Key

Bold text indicates target muscles
Light text indicates other working muscles
* indicates deep muscles

DO IT RIGHT

• Keep your head and shoulder blades on the floor.
• Avoid twisting your lower body; instead, keep your hips square.

gluteus medius*

gluteus minimus*

piriformis*

gluteus maximus

Internal Hip Rotator Stretch

A sedentary lifestyle can lead to tight hip flexors and rotators as well as weak gluteal muscles. This can affect your gait, posture, spinal stability, and movement patterns. Simple hip stretches such as this one can ensure that your body stays functional, limber, and healthy.

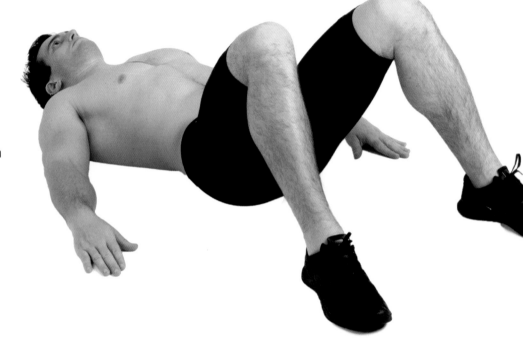

HOW TO DO IT

• Lie on your back with your arms extended at your sides.

• Bend your knees, planting your feet generously more than shoulder-width apart.

• Keeping the rest of your body still, rotate your right hip inward, bringing your knee toward the floor.

• Slowly return to the starting position, and repeat on the opposite side.

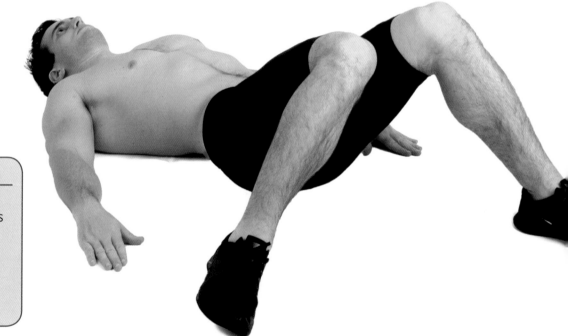

DO IT RIGHT
• Keep your abdominals tight and rest your hands on the floor to support your lower back.
• Avoid lifting your lower back and glutes.

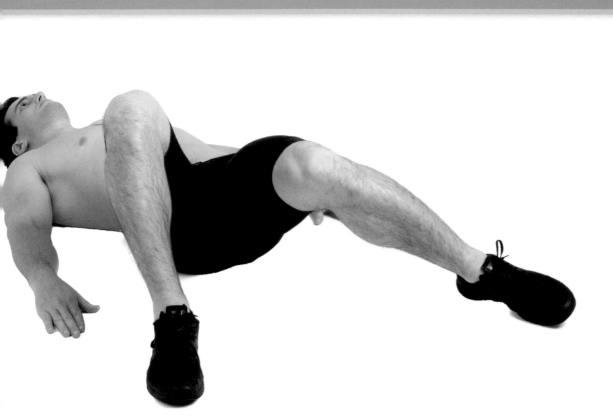

FACT FILE

TARGETS
- Hip rotators
- Glutes

TYPE
- Dynamic

BENEFITS
- Increases range of motion in hip rotators and hip flexors
- Relieves lower-back pain
- Engages glutes

CAUTIONS
- Hip pains
- Lower-back pain

Annotation Key

Bold text indicates target muscles
Light text indicates other working muscles
* indicates deep muscles

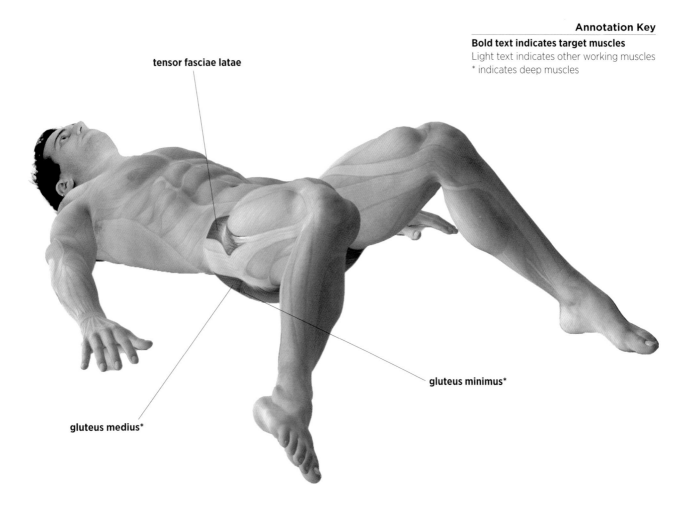

tensor fasciae latae

gluteus minimus*

gluteus medius*

Happy Baby Stretch

Performed on your back, this gentle stretch engages your hamstrings and inner thighs. A relaxing exercise for your back, it also opens your hips, shoulders, and chest.

HOW TO DO IT

• Lie on your back.

• Bend your knees in toward your chest and grasp the outside of your feet.

• Lower your knees toward the floor as you open your legs.

• Pull into your heels to deepen the intensity of the stretch.

• Hold for the recommended time, and then release the stretch.

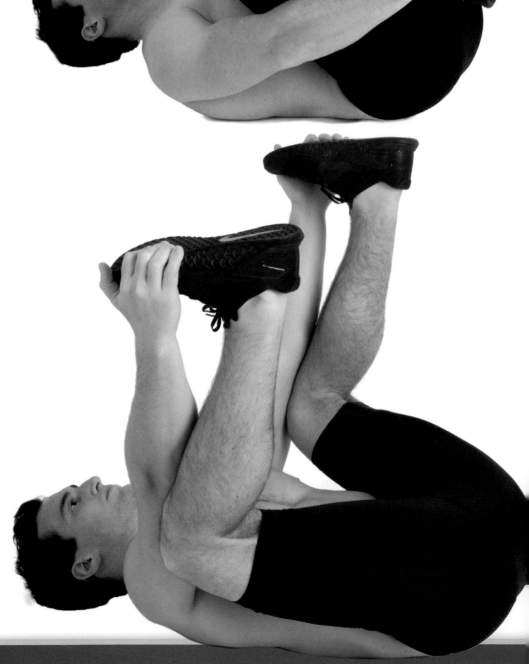

DO IT RIGHT

• Keep your elbows slightly bent.
• Draw your shoulders toward the floor.
• Tuck your pelvis forward to engage your abdominals and keep your lower back anchored.
• Avoid lifting your head or shoulder blades off the floor.

TARGETS
- Glutes
- Hamstrings
- Lower back

TYPE
- Static

BENEFITS
- Releases lower back and sacrum
- Opens hips and inner thighs
- Stretches hamstrings
- Relieves lower-back pain
- Elongates spine

CAUTIONS
- Neck or knee injury
- Hip pain

Annotation Key

Bold text indicates target muscles
Light text indicates other working muscles
* indicates deep muscles

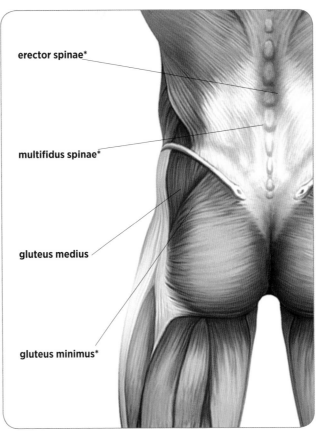

erector spinae*

multifidus spinae*

gluteus medius

gluteus minimus*

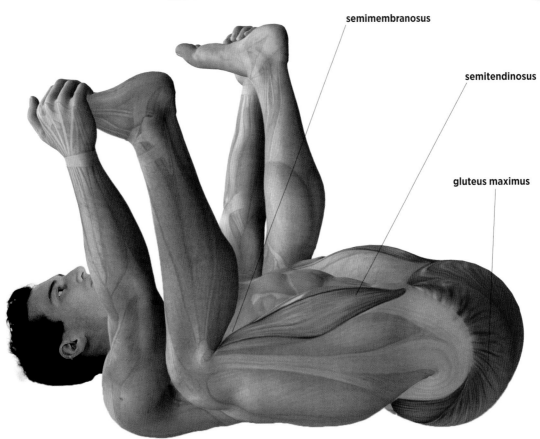

semimembranosus

semitendinosus

gluteus maximus

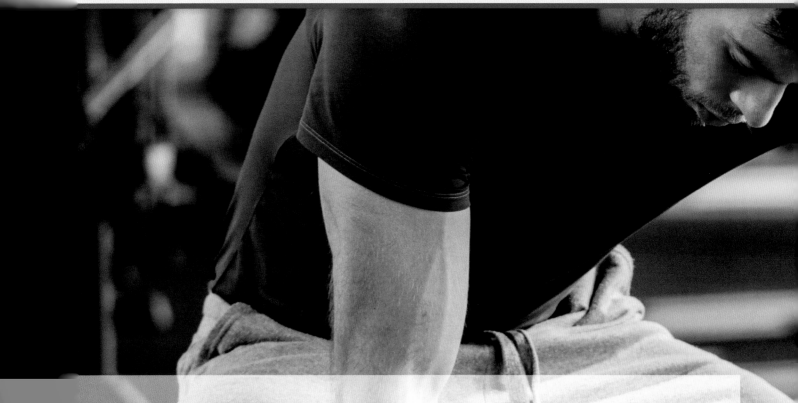

CHAPTER SEVEN

LEG, ANKLE, & FOOT STRETCHES

One of the primary reasons to practice stretching is to work on your flexibility. All forms of stretching help improve your mobility, but leg stretches in particular allow you to achieve the deeper flexibility exercises. The main leg muscles that people stretch to reduce tightness are the hamstrings, quadriceps, and calves. Focusing on each of these major leg muscle groups not only lengthens these muscles but also improves the range of motion in your joints. Add these leg exercises to your stretching routine to help perform simple daily tasks such as bending to tie your shoes or running to catch the train.

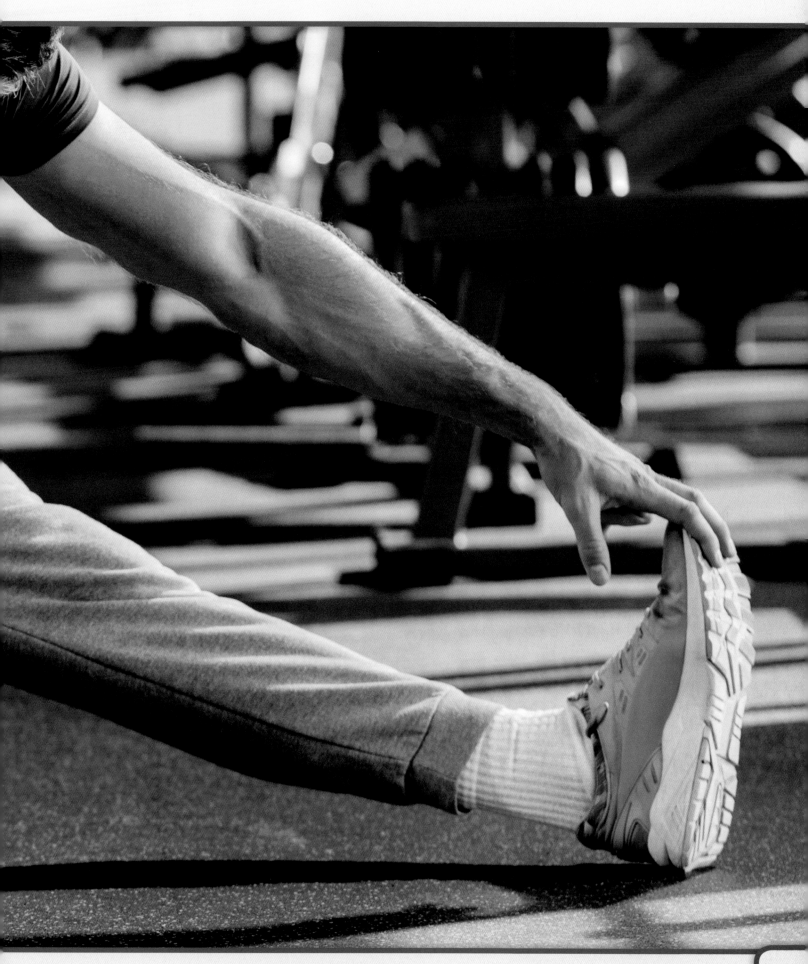

Standing Forward Bend

The Standing Forward Bend lengthens your hamstrings and calves and stretches your entire back. This basic inversion exercise, a common first step in many yoga sequences, also benefits your circulation as you lower your head below your heart.

HOW TO DO IT

- Stand straight with your feet together and arms at your sides. Inhale, and raise your arms toward the ceiling. Exhale, as you hinge at your hips to fold forward, bringing your arms down. Try to reach your fingertips to the floor in line with your toes.

- Straighten your legs and arms as you draw in your abdominals. Press your heels into the floor as you lift your tailbone up toward the ceiling, keeping your hips in line with your heels.

- Inhale, and lengthen your spine, as you fold further from your hips and rest your palms on the floor.

- Lengthen your torso as you bring your belly closer to your thighs.

- Hold for the recommended time, inhaling to lengthen your spine and exhaling to fold deeper.

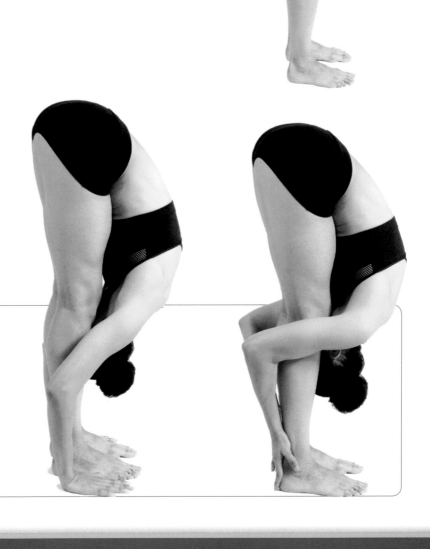

MODIFICATION

HARDER: Bend forward so your head is between your knees and your palms down flat to the floor—or reach behind your ankles for stability.

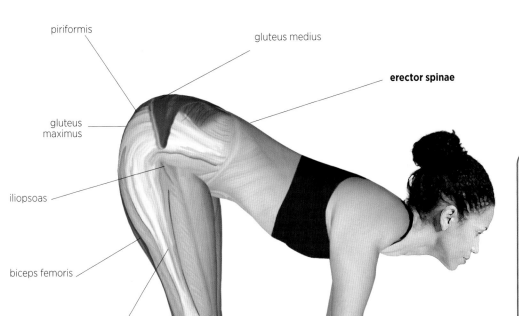

FACT FILE

TARGETS
- Spine
- Core
- Lower body

TYPE
- Static

BENEFITS
- Stretches hamstrings, hips, and spine
- Strengthens thighs and knees
- Improves circulation
- Reduces stress
- Improves posture
- Aids digestion

CAUTIONS
- Lower-back issues
- Neck pain
- Osteoporosis

Annotation Key

Bold text indicates target muscles
Light text indicates other working muscles
* indicates deep muscles

piriformis

gluteus medius

erector spinae

gluteus maximus

iliopsoas

biceps femoris

tractus iliotibialis

gastrocnemius

soleus

DO IT RIGHT

- Bend from your hips, not your waist.
- Keep a slight bend in your knees if your lower back or hamstrings are tight.
- If you cannot reach your fingertips to the floor, place your hands on your shins or cross your arms.
- Avoid shifting your weight backward and positioning your hips behind your heels.
- Avoid compressing your neck.
- Avoid rolling your spine into or out of the pose.

Toe Touch

The ability to touch one's toes is a mainstay for those who hope to maintain flexibility. Pushing your fingertips slightly farther through the Standing Forward Bend (pages 258–259), you can feel an even deeper stretch in your hamstrings and calf muscles.

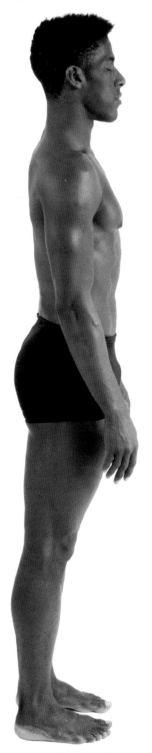

HOW TO DO IT

• Stand straight with your feet shoulder-width apart. Bend your knees slightly.

• Slowly round your spine downward, from your neck through your lower back, and lower your arms along the sides of your legs.

• Continue to lower downward as you bend at the waist. Let the weight of your body draw your head toward the floor as you stretch.

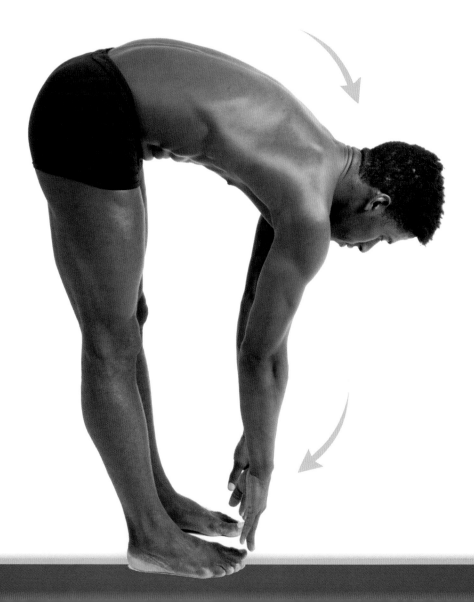

FACT FILE

TARGETS
• Hamstrings
• Back

TYPE
• Static

DO IT RIGHT

• Relax your neck and jaw.
• Breathe naturally and steadily throughout the stretch.
• Avoid letting your knees touch—keep your thighs slightly apart to help your gluteal muscles engage and stretch.

BENEFITS
• Stretches spine, hips, hamstrings, and calves
• Strengthens back and thighs
• Improves posture
• Benefits circulation and energy
• Relieves stress

CAUTIONS
• Back issues
• Neck injury
• Osteoporosis

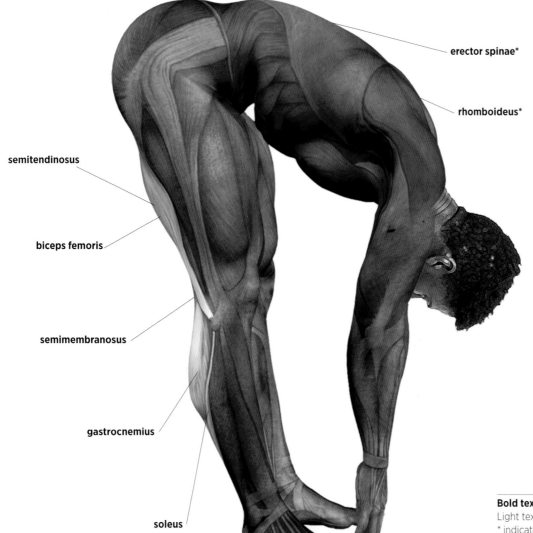

erector spinae*

rhomboideus*

semitendinosus

biceps femoris

semimembranosus

gastrocnemius

soleus

Annotation Key
Bold text indicates target muscles
Light text indicates other working muscles
* indicates deep muscles

Standing Splits

Standing Splits tone your entire body and provide an effective stretch from neck to ankle. They are also particularly beneficial for firming and lifting your glutes. To feel the deepest stretch in your hamstrings and calves, try to pull your feet away from each other rather than just lifting up your back foot.

HOW TO DO IT

• Stand straight with your feet together and arms at your sides.

• Lift your arms above your head, and hinge from your hips to bend forward, bringing your hands to the floor.

• Shift your weight onto your left leg, keeping your hips square. Contract your leg muscles as you fold your torso onto your left thigh.

• Lift your right heel toward the ceiling, extending both legs in opposite directions as far as you are able.

• Hold for the recommended breaths, and then repeat on the opposite side.

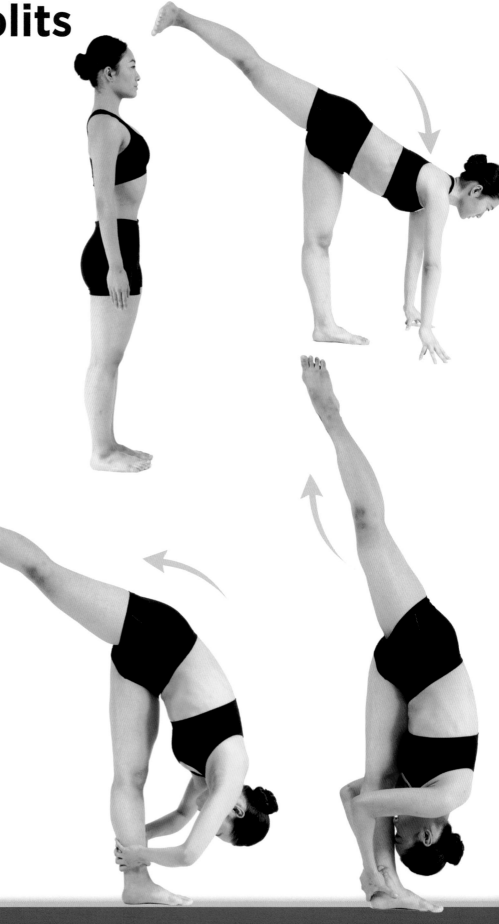

TARGETS
- Thighs
- Groin
- Glutes

TYPE
- Static

BENEFITS
- Stretches lower body
- Strengthens thighs, knees, calves, and ankles
- Improves balance

CAUTIONS
- Ankle issues
- Knee injury
- Lower-back pain

DO IT RIGHT

- Contract your leg muscles, and ground your standing foot throughout the exercise.
- If you have trouble reaching the floor with your hands, place blocks on the floor for support.
- Avoid compressing the back of your neck while holding the pose.

Annotation Key

Bold text indicates target muscles
Light text indicates other working muscles
* indicates deep muscles

semitendinosus

vastus intermedius

biceps femoris

vastus lateralis

gluteus maximus

rectus femoris

tractus iliotibialis

adductor magnus

gluteus medius

sartorius

tensor fasciae latae

gracilis

vastus medialis

soleus

gastrocnemius

Standing Quadriceps Stretch

Stretching the quadriceps muscles improves flexibility in this large muscle group at the front of your thighs. This single-leg standing stretch adds an additional challenge, requiring you to focus on balancing on one leg while performing the stretch on your other leg. For an easier version of this stretch, use a towel or resistance band to pull in your raised foot.

HOW TO DO IT

- Stand with your legs together and feet shoulder-width apart. Bend your knees slightly, and tuck your pelvis slightly forward. Lift your chest, and press your shoulders downward and back.

- Bend your right knee behind you, so that your ankle is raised toward your buttocks.

- Reach down with your right hand to grab your foot just below your ankle, and gently pull as you stretch.

- Release the stretch, and then repeat on the opposite side.

DO IT RIGHT

- Avoid bringing your foot closer to your buttocks than you can comfortably reach. Unless you are very limber, this can compress the knee joint.

MODIFICATION

EASIER: Wrap a small towel around your ankle, and pull the ends to aid in raising your foot.

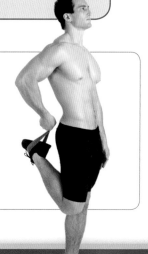

FACT FILE

TARGETS
- Quadriceps

TYPE
- Static

BENEFITS
- Deep quadriceps stretch
- Improves balance
- Improves circulation

CAUTIONS
- Knee pain
- Ankle weakness
- Shoulder stiffness

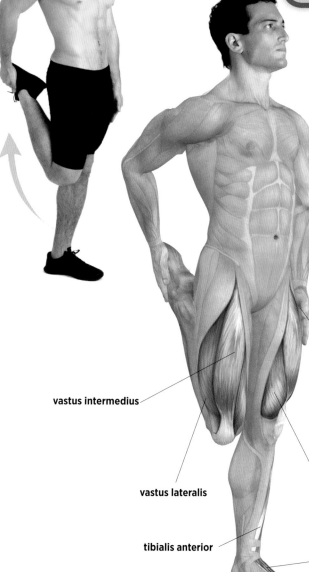

rectus femoris

vastus intermedius

vastus medialis

vastus lateralis

tibialis anterior

extensor digitorum brevi

Kneeling Sprinter Stretch

Tight ankles or tight IT bands often contribute to knee pain. The Kneeling Sprinter Stretch is a simple but effective exercise that can improve mobility—not just in the targeted muscles but also in the entire posture of the body.

HOW TO DO IT

• Kneel on the floor, with your toes pointed behind you.

• Bring your right leg up and place your right foot flat on the floor next to your left knee.

• Position your palms flat on the floor slightly in front of your legs, just beyond shoulder-width apart.

• Sit back on your right heel as you lean slightly forward.

• Hold for the recommended time, release the stretch, and then repeat on the opposite side.

FACT FILE

TARGETS
• Calves
• Achilles tendon
• Quadriceps

TYPE
• Static

BENEFITS
• Stretches calves
• Lengthens Achilles tendon
• Strengthens quadriceps and glutes

CAUTIONS
• Knee pain

DO IT RIGHT

• Keep the sole of your front foot and the top of your back foot on the floor.
• Lean your chest farther forward over your raised upper leg to increase the intensity of the stretch.
• Avoid rolling your front foot inward.

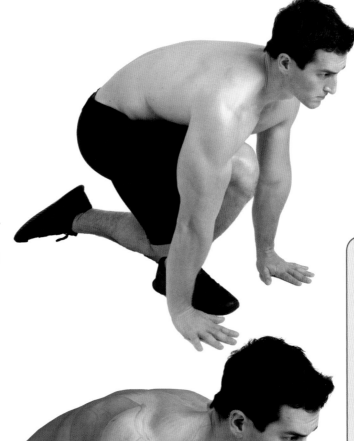

Annotation Key

Bold text indicates target muscles
Light text indicates other working muscles
* indicates deep muscles

tendo calcaneus

extensor digitorum brevis

soleus

Warrior I Yoga Stretch

Warrior I, a classic yoga pose, is especially effective at increasing flexibility in your hip flexors, the muscles at the front of your hips that pull your leg upward.

HOW TO DO IT

- Stand straight with your feet together and your hands on your hips. Step your feet about 3 to 4 feet apart.

- Turn your right toes outward about 45 degrees, and walk your left foot to your left several inches until your feet are in heel-to-heel alignment.

- Keeping your right leg straight, bend your left knee. Inhale, lifting your torso and arms above your head so that your upper body and arms form a straight line. Externally rotate your arms with palms facing each other, and push energy up through your fingertips.

- Hold for the recommended time, and then repeat on the opposite side.

DO IT RIGHT

- Keep your bent knee in line with your toes and your front thigh parallel to the floor.
- Reach up through your arms as you ground your feet down.
- Find a slight bend in your upper back.
- Keep your shoulders directly above your hips.
- Avoid twisting the knee of your back leg.

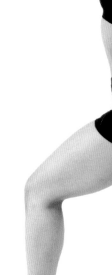

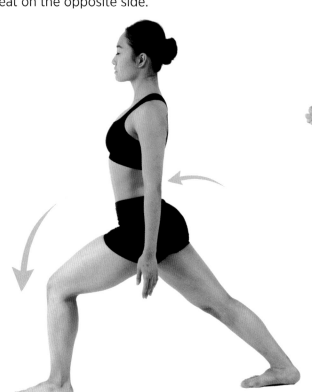

TARGETS
- Hips
- Legs
- Shoulders

TYPE
- Static

BENEFITS
- Increases stamina
- Strengthens shoulders, arms, thighs, ankles, and calves
- Stretches groin, abdominals, chest, and shoulders

CAUTIONS
- Knee injury
- Lower-back issues
- Shoulder pain

Annotation Key

Bold text indicates target muscles

Light text indicates other working muscles

* indicates deep muscles

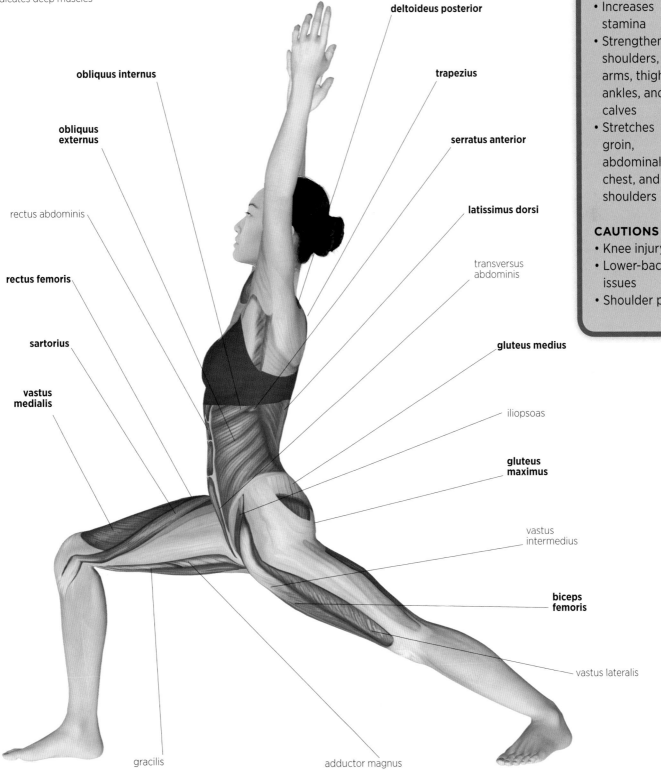

obliquus internus

obliquus externus

rectus abdominis

rectus femoris

sartorius

vastus medialis

deltoideus posterior

trapezius

serratus anterior

latissimus dorsi

transversus abdominis

gluteus medius

iliopsoas

gluteus maximus

vastus intermedius

biceps femoris

vastus lateralis

gracilis

adductor magnus

Inverted Hamstring Stretch

This is an advanced muscle toning and stretching exercise that primarily targets the hamstrings and, to a lesser degree, the glutes. The Inverted Hamstring is also excellent for improving balance and core strength and stability.

HOW TO DO IT

• Stand straight with your feet shoulder-width apart. Bend your knees slightly, and raise your arms above your head.

• Bend forward at the waist while simultaneously spreading your arms out to your sides for balance and lifting your left leg behind you.

• Continue to bend forward until your torso and raised leg are roughly parallel to the floor.

• Return to the standing position, and then repeat on the opposite side.

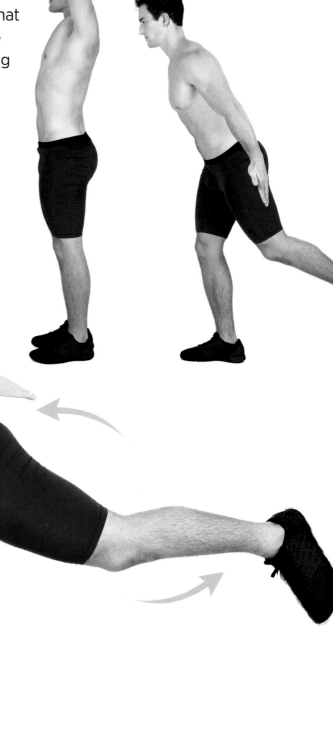

DO IT RIGHT

• Keep your spine neutral as you progress through the motion.
• Align your knees over your ankles.
• Move slowly through the stretch.
• Avoid letting your back foot touch the floor.
• Avoid using your arms to move your body.

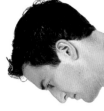

TARGETS
• Hamstrings
• Glutes

TYPE
• Static

BENEFITS
• Helps stabilize
  the body
• Strengthens
  the core

CAUTIONS
• Back issues
• Shoulder pain

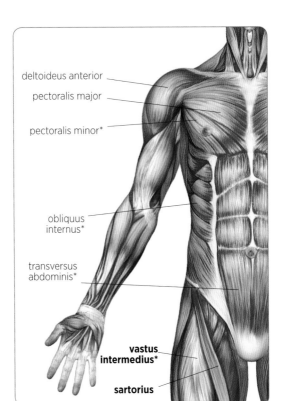

deltoideus anterior

pectoralis major

pectoralis minor*

obliquus
internus*

transversus
abdominis*

**vastus
intermedius***

sartorius

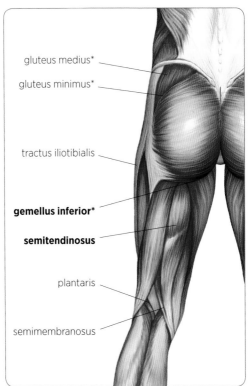

gluteus medius*

gluteus minimus*

tractus iliotibialis

gemellus inferior*

semitendinosus

plantaris

semimembranosus

Annotation Key

Bold text indicates target muscles
Light text indicates other working muscles
* indicates deep muscles

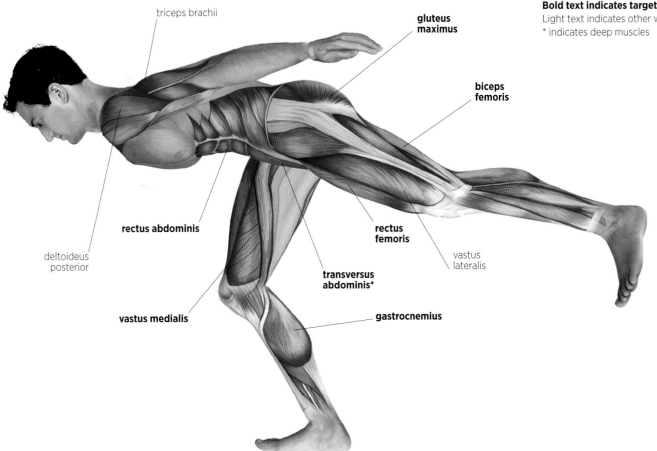

triceps brachii

**gluteus
maximus**

**biceps
femoris**

rectus abdominis

deltoideus
posterior

**rectus
femoris**

vastus
lateralis

**transversus
abdominis***

vastus medialis

gastrocnemius

Hip Flexor Stretch

The hip flexors are a group of muscles around your upper and inner thighs and pelvic region. Hip flexors draw together your leg and hip bones at your hip joints. Running, jumping, and standing call on these muscles, so keep them toned and supple with this targeted stretch.

HOW TO DO IT

• Kneel on the floor, and place your right foot in front of you so that your knee is bent less than 90 degrees.

• Bring your torso forward, bending your right knee so that it shifts toward your toes.

• Keeping your torso in neutral position, press your left hip forward and downward to create a stretch over the front of your thigh. Raise your arms toward the ceiling, keeping your shoulders relaxed.

• Bring your arms down, and move your hips backward. Straighten your right leg, and bring your torso forward. Place your hands on either side of your right leg for support.

• Hold for recommended time, and then repeat on the opposite side.

MODIFICATION

HARDER: During the backward movement, raise your back knee off the floor and straighten your back leg. Keep your hands on the floor.

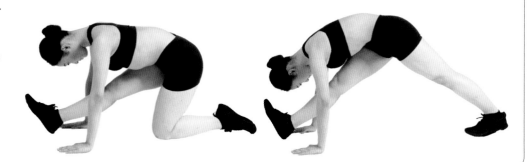

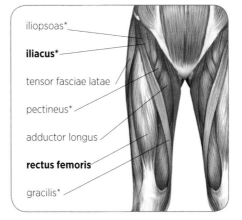

FACT FILE

TARGETS
• Hip flexors
• Adductors
• Quadriceps

TYPE
• Dynamic

BENEFITS
• Strengthens and stretches hip flexors
• Conditions hips for running and jumping

CAUTIONS
• Hip issues
• Knee pain

DO IT RIGHT

• Keep your shoulders and neck relaxed.
• Move your entire body as one unit throughout the stretch.
• Avoid extending your front knee too far over your planted foot.
• Try not to rotate your hips.
• Avoid shifting the knee of your back leg outward.

iliopsoas*
iliacus*
tensor fasciae latae
pectineus*
adductor longus
rectus femoris
gracilis*

Annotation Key
Bold text indicates target muscles
Light text indicates other working muscles
* indicates deep muscles

obliquus externus

latissimus dorsi

biceps femoris

vastus lateralis

semimembranosus

gastrocnemius

rectus abdominis

adductor magnus

vastus intermedius*

vastus medialis

semitendinosus

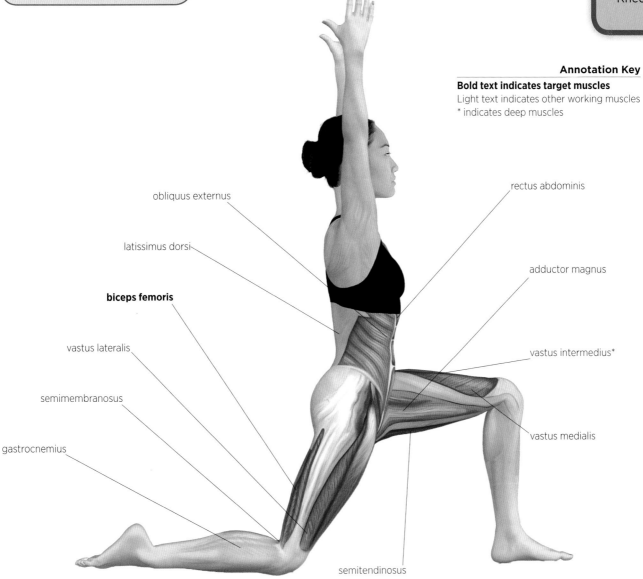

Hip-to-Thigh Stretch

Your glutes and hamstrings are the primary muscles that open your hip joints. The Hip-to-Thigh Stretch will keep these muscles in top shape, making everyday movements easier.

HOW TO DO IT

• Kneel on the floor, and step your right foot in front of you. Keep your right foot flat on the floor and your left foot flexed.

• Shift your weight and gradually bring your torso forward, bending your right knee more deeply so that your knee shifts toward your toes.

• Extend your arms straight in front of you.

• Keeping your torso stable, press your left hip forward until you feel a stretch over the front of your thigh.

• Raise your arms toward the ceiling.

• Hold for recommended time, release the stretch, and the repeat on the opposite side.

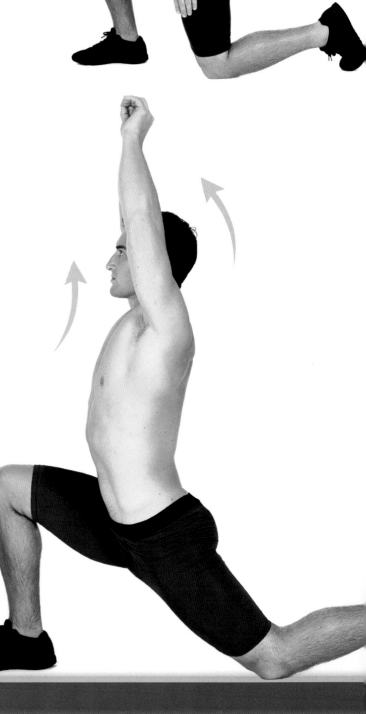

TARGETS
- Glutes
- Hamstrings
- Quadriceps

TYPE
- Static

BENEFITS
- Stretches hips and thighs
- Improves range of motion in legs

CAUTIONS
- Hip or groin problems
- Knee issues

Annotation Key
Bold text indicates target muscles
Light text indicates other working muscles
* indicates deep muscles

DO IT RIGHT

- Relax your shoulders.
- Keep your upper body stable.
- Reach up but do not force the stretch.
- Avoid extending your front knee too far over your planted foot.
- Avoid overstretching your thigh.

rectus femoris

gluteus medius*

gluteus minimus*

gluteus maximus

vastus intermedius*

vastus lateralis

Chair Plié

The Chair Plié is a squatting stretch that primarily targets your inner thighs, quadriceps, and, to a lesser degree, your glutes, hamstrings, and hip flexors. As long as you have a sturdy chair at hand, this exercise can be performed anywhere.

HOW TO DO IT

• Stand facing the back of a sturdy chair. Position your feet more than shoulder-width apart, and turn out your toes.

• Use the chair for balance as you bend your knees and lower your body into a squat position. Keep your knees aligned over your toes.

• Return to the starting position, and perform the recommended repetitions.

DO IT RIGHT
• Keep your upper body stable.
• Don't depend on the chair too much to move through the exercise.
• Move smoothly rather than swinging with momentum.
• Avoid lowering your buttocks past your knees.
• Avoid stressing your lower back.

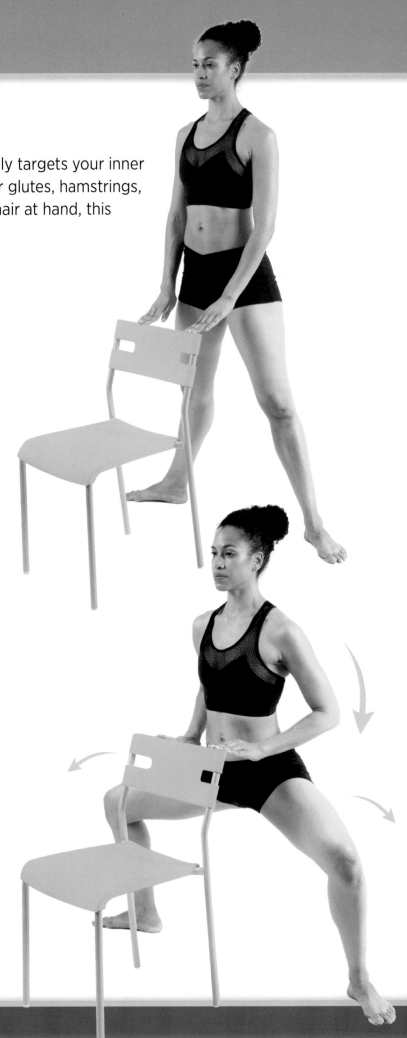

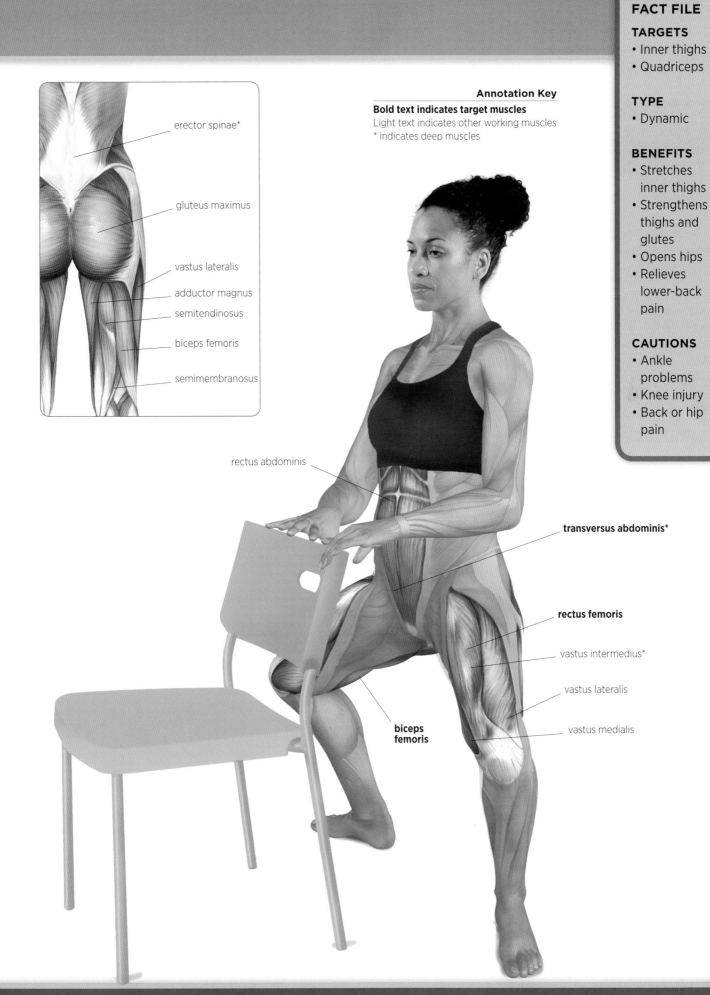

TARGETS
- Inner thighs
- Quadriceps

TYPE
- Dynamic

BENEFITS
- Stretches inner thighs
- Strengthens thighs and glutes
- Opens hips
- Relieves lower-back pain

CAUTIONS
- Ankle problems
- Knee injury
- Back or hip pain

erector spinae*

gluteus maximus

vastus lateralis

adductor magnus

semitendinosus

biceps femoris

semimembranosus

Annotation Key

Bold text indicates target muscles
Light text indicates other working muscles
* indicates deep muscles

rectus abdominis

transversus abdominis*

rectus femoris

vastus intermedius*

vastus lateralis

vastus medialis

biceps femoris

LEG, ANKLE, & FOOT STRETCHES   275

Chair Squat

Chair Squats are particularly beneficial for beginners who are learning proper squatting technique. This stretching exercise is also useful for anyone with conditions that affect balance or coordination.

HOW TO DO IT

• Stand upright with a sturdy chair behind you.

• Clasp your hands, and position them in front of your chest.

• Slowly lower your body into a squat position.

• Continue lowering until you are resting on the chair.

• With control, rise back up to the starting position.

• Perform the recommended repetitions.

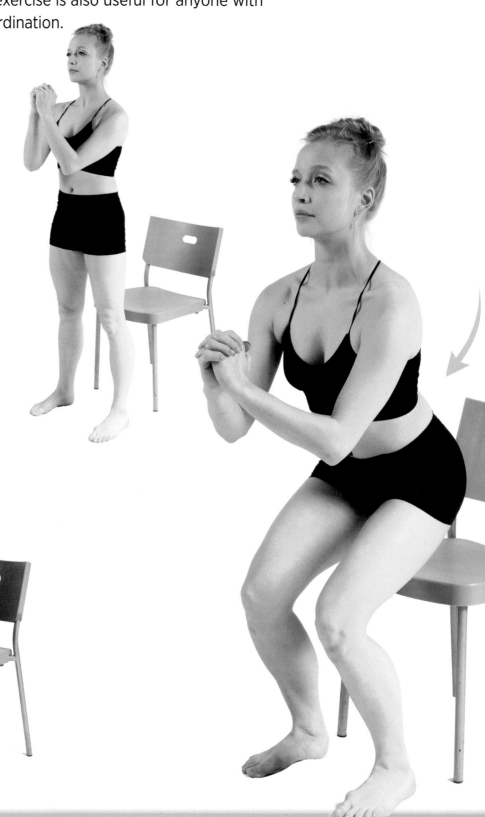

TARGETS
- Quadriceps
- Glutes

TYPE
- Dynamic

BENEFITS
- Stretches thighs and glutes
- Counteracts sedentary lifestyle

CAUTIONS
- Hip issues
- Knee injury
- Lower-back pain

DO IT RIGHT
- Gaze forward and keep your back straight.
- Avoid arching your back or hunching forward.

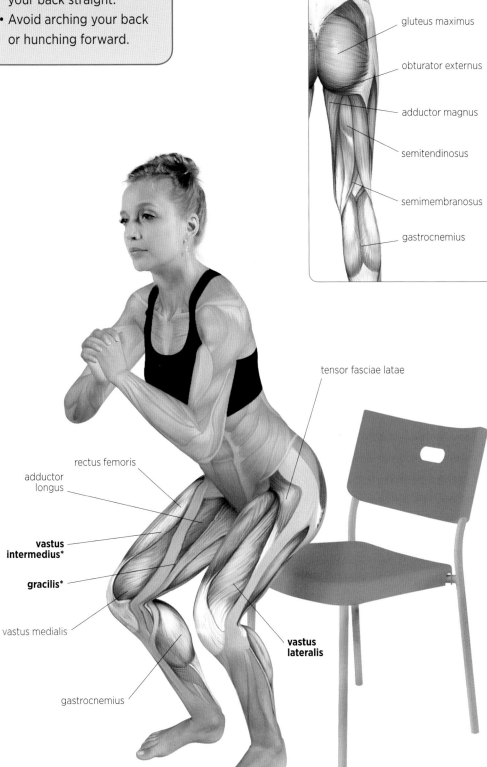

erector spinae*

gluteus maximus

obturator externus

adductor magnus

semitendinosus

semimembranosus

gastrocnemius

tensor fasciae latae

rectus femoris

adductor longus

vastus intermedius*

gracilis*

vastus medialis

vastus lateralis

gastrocnemius

Annotation Key
Bold text indicates target muscles
Light text indicates other working muscles
* indicates deep muscles

Forward Lunge

The Forward Lunge is useful as a warm-up or cooldown exercise. It helps to stretch tight hamstrings and hip flexors, which may result from sitting, running, or cycling. When performed correctly, lunges work all your lower-body muscles and improve your balance.

HOW TO DO IT

- Begin in the Sumo Squat (pages 204–205).

- Drop your hands onto the floor in front of you, transferring some of your weight onto your arms.

- Carefully walk your hands to your right as you pivot your right foot forward.

- Step your left leg back behind your body, extending it straight. Keep your right knee bent.

- Place your hands on your right knee, and hold for the recommended time.

- Return to the Sumo Squat, and repeat on the opposite side.

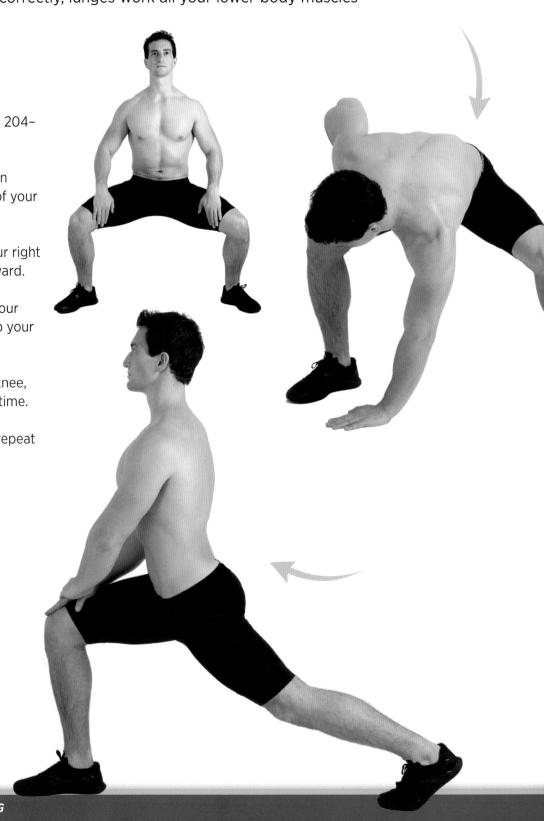

DO IT RIGHT
- Keep your back leg extended and in line with your hips to form one long straight line.
- Keep your bent knee directly above your ankle.
- Avoid dropping your back leg to the floor.
- Relax your shoulders.

TARGETS
- Quadriceps
- Glutes
- Inner thighs
- Hamstrings

TYPE
- Dynamic

BENEFITS
- Reduces tightness in hips and hamstrings
- Engages abdominals and glutes
- Reduces risk of sports-related injuries

CAUTIONS
- Hip pain
- Knee issues
- Lower-back pain

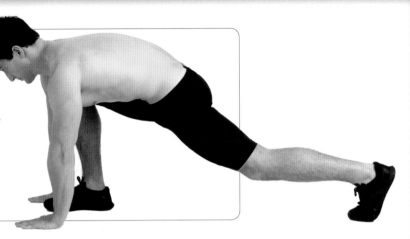

MODIFICATION

HARDER: Place your palms or fingertips on the floor on either side of your front foot. Keep your head in line with your spine, focusing your gaze forward a few feet in front of you.

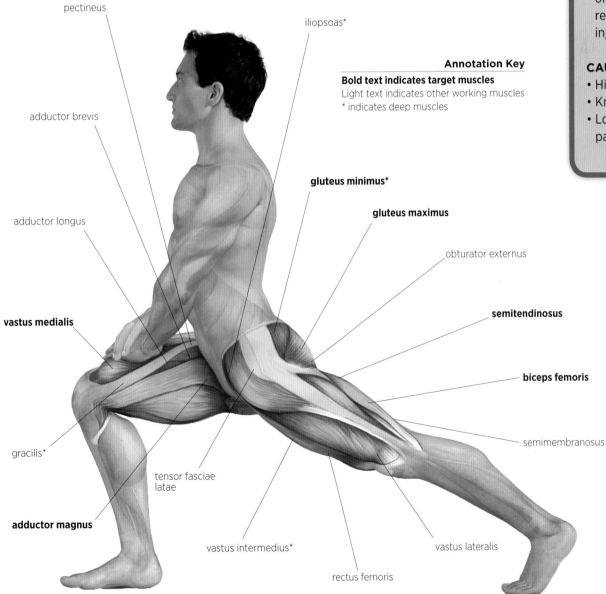

pectineus

iliopsoas*

adductor brevis

Annotation Key

Bold text indicates target muscles
Light text indicates other working muscles
* indicates deep muscles

adductor longus

gluteus minimus*

gluteus maximus

obturator externus

vastus medialis

semitendinosus

biceps femoris

gracilis*

semimembranosus

tensor fasciae latae

adductor magnus

vastus intermedius*

vastus lateralis

rectus femoris

Forward Lunge with Twist

This deep forward lunge incorporates a lateral spinal twist, which augments the benefits of the standard lunge by adding both a chest opener, and more targeted stretch of the hips.

HOW TO DO IT

• Begin in the Forward Lunge (pages 278–279) with your right leg forward.

• Place your hands on the floor on either side of your right foot.

• Balancing your weight over your left hand, carefully and slowly guide your right arm up toward the ceiling, twisting your torso upward.

• Return to the starting position, and repeat on the opposite side.

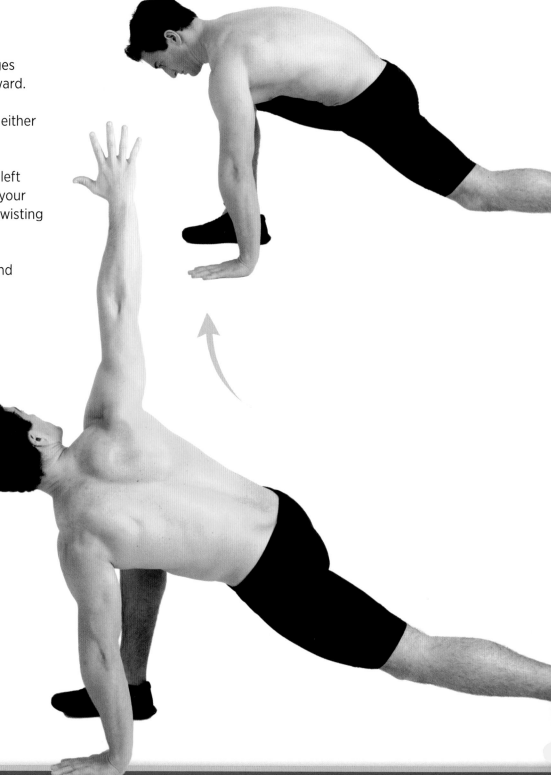

DO IT RIGHT

• Gaze up toward your elevated arm and hand, and stretch your raised fingers upward.

• Keep your chest slightly elevated.

• Keep your legs and feet parallel.

• Avoid holding your breath.

• Avoid rounding your back.

Annotation Key

Bold text indicates target muscles
Light text indicates other working muscles
* indicates deep muscles

TARGETS
- Quadriceps
- Glutes
- Hip adductors
- Hamstrings
- Obliques
- Rib cage
- Chest
- Shoulders

TYPE
- Dynamic

BENEFITS
- Opens hips
- Engages all the leg muscles
- Relieves lower-back pain
- Opens chest

CAUTIONS
- Lower-back injury
- Hip pain
- Ankle weakness

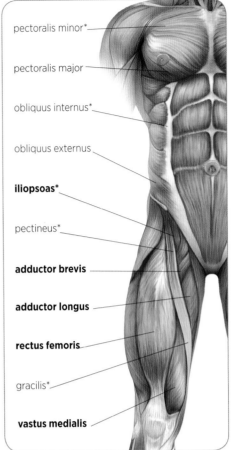

pectoralis minor*

pectoralis major

obliquus internus*

obliquus externus

iliopsoas*

pectineus*

adductor brevis

adductor longus

rectus femoris

gracilis*

vastus medialis

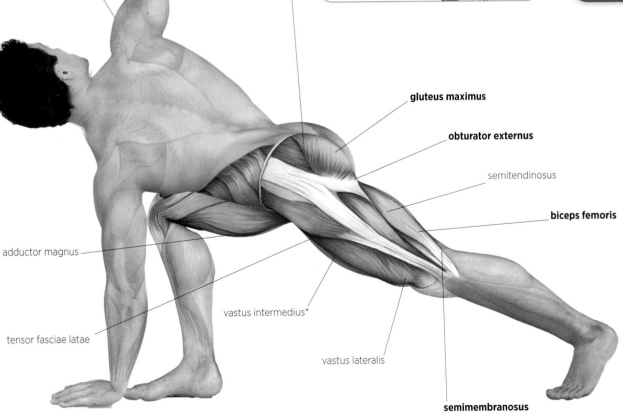

deltoideus anterior

gluteus minimus*

gluteus maximus

obturator externus

semitendinosus

biceps femoris

adductor magnus

vastus intermedius*

tensor fasciae latae

vastus lateralis

semimembranosus

Reverse Lunge with Lateral Extension

Reverse Lunge stretches require more complex body movements compared with forward lunges. Reverse Lunges, however, place less stress on your knees while still toning the entire length of your legs and torso.

HOW TO DO IT

- Stand straight with your feet together and arms at your sides. Step your right leg back, resting your toes on the floor.

- Bend your knees as you move into a lunge position.

- Lower your body, flexing your left knee and hip until your right lower leg is almost in contact with the floor.

- Raise your arms out to your sides to shoulder height.

- Return to the starting position, and then repeat on the opposite side.

DO IT RIGHT

- Keep your shoulders pressed downward.
- Relax your neck and shoulders; don't hunch.
- Make sure your upper body remains upright throughout the stretch.
- Avoid arching your back.
- Avoid twisting your hips.

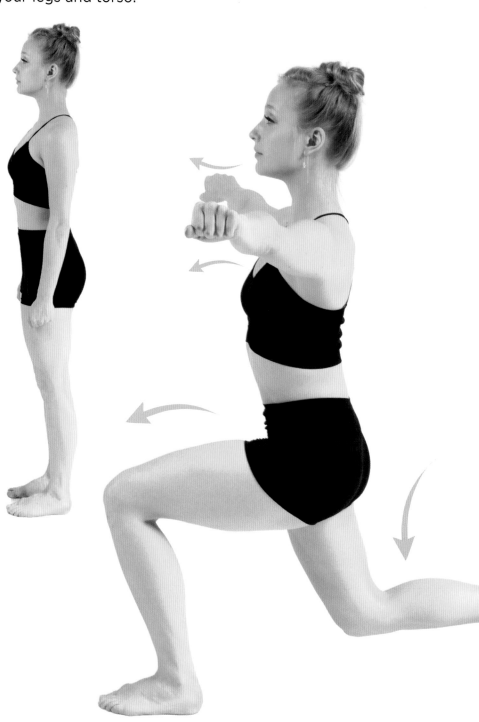

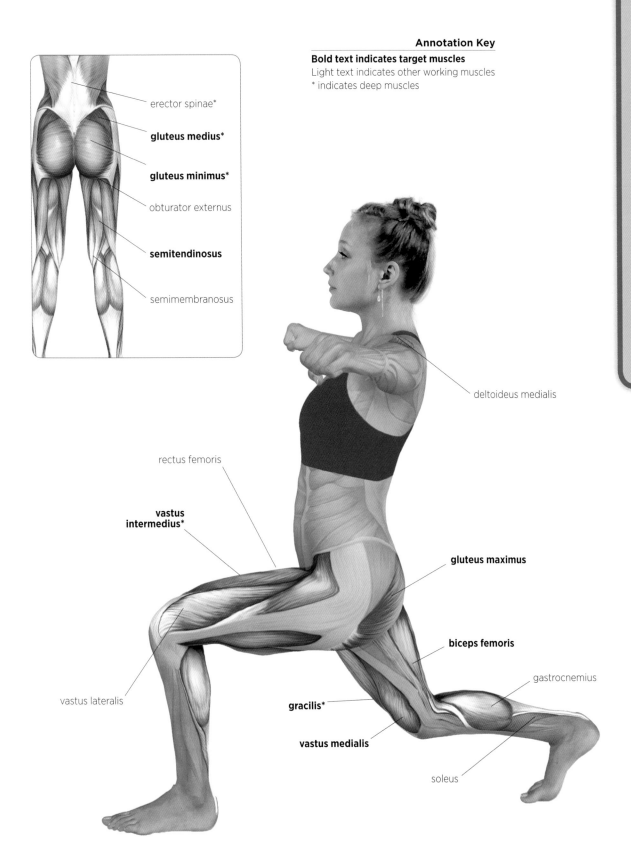

FACT FILE

TARGETS
• Quadriceps
• Glutes
• Inner thighs
• Hamstrings
• Calves

TYPE
• Dynamic

BENEFITS
• Stretches thighs
• Strengthens glutes and leg muscles
• Improves posture
• Enhances balance

CAUTIONS
• Arm or shoulder injuries
• Knee issues

Annotation Key

Bold text indicates target muscles
Light text indicates other working muscles
* indicates deep muscles

erector spinae*

gluteus medius*

gluteus minimus*

obturator externus

semitendinosus

semimembranosus

deltoideus medialis

rectus femoris

vastus intermedius*

gluteus maximus

biceps femoris

gastrocnemius

vastus lateralis

gracilis*

vastus medialis

soleus

Straight-Leg Lunge

This lunge stretch variation is modified to benefit people with tight calves and Achilles tendons. A proper straight-leg lunge can help you develop a more stable core, improve your balance, and strengthen your legs and glutes.

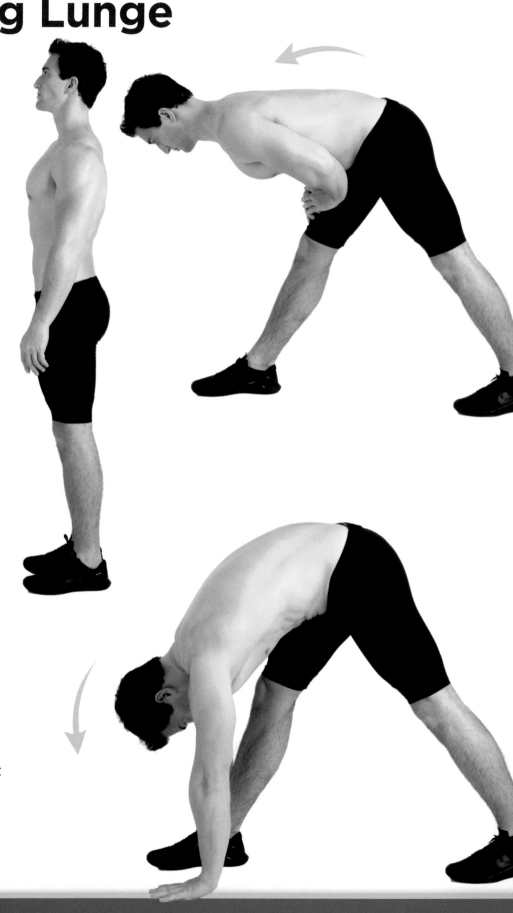

HOW TO DO IT

• Stand with your legs parallel and your feet shoulder-width apart.

• Bend your knees slightly and tuck your pelvis slightly forward. Lift your chest, and press your shoulders downward and back.

• Take one step forward with your right foot.

• Keeping your legs straight, hinge your torso forward as far as possible over your right leg.

• Allow the weight of your upper body to intensify the stretch.

• Hold for the recommended time, return to the starting position, and then repeat on the opposite side.

FACT FILE

TARGETS
• Hamstrings
• Calves

TYPE
• Dynamic

BENEFITS
• Helps to stabilize the core
• Improves balance
• Strengthens legs
• Improves spinal flexibility

CAUTIONS
• Hip pain
• Knee injury
• Lower-back pain

DO IT RIGHT

• Flex your front foot, lifting the ball of your foot off the floor, to maximize the intensity of the stretch.
• Press the heel of your back leg into the floor throughout the stretch.
• Avoid holding unnecessary tension in your upper body—relax and breathe naturally.

Annotation Key
Bold text indicates target muscles
Light text indicates other working muscles
* indicates deep muscles

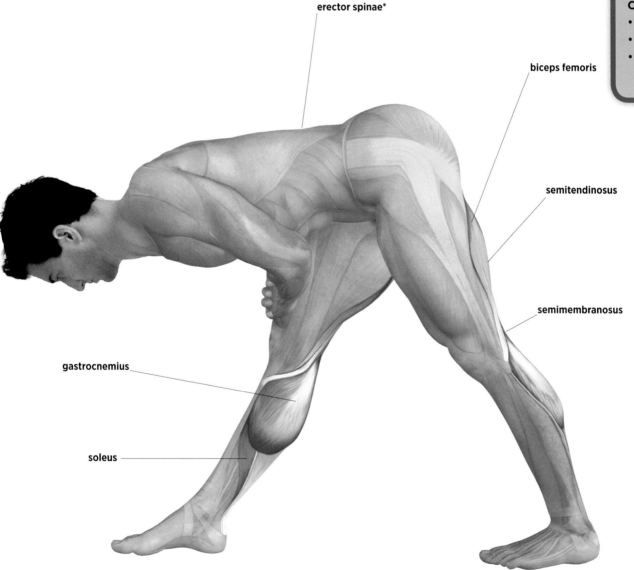

erector spinae*

biceps femoris

semitendinosus

semimembranosus

gastrocnemius

soleus

Deep Lunge

This version of a forward lunge is often called High Lunge in yoga, and is also known as a Low Forward Lunge. It is an effective leg and arm strengthener that targets your glutes and quadriceps, along with your hamstrings and calf muscles. The deep position also lengthens your groin muscles.

HOW TO DO IT

• Begin in Downward-Facing Dog (pages 72–73). Step your right foot forward in between your hands, with your right knee and shin in lined with your right ankle.

• With your fingertips resting on the floor, square your hips, grounding your right heel into the floor and drawing your right hip crease back.

• Extend your left leg straight behind you, resting the ball of your foot on the floor. Lengthen all the way from the crown of your head to your left heel. Gaze slightly ahead, keeping the back of your neck long.

• Hold for the recommended breaths, and then repeat on the opposite side.

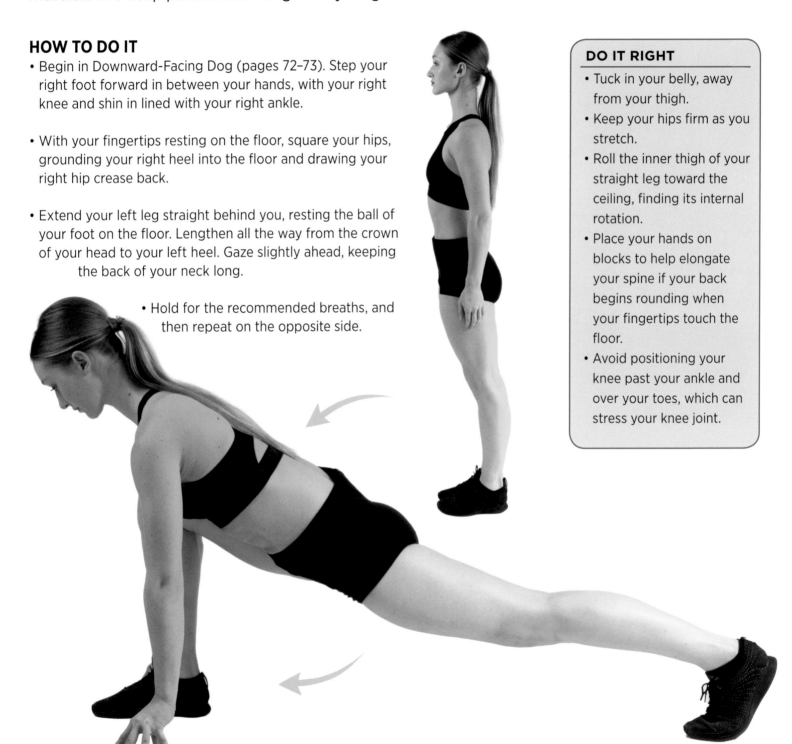

DO IT RIGHT

• Tuck in your belly, away from your thigh.
• Keep your hips firm as you stretch.
• Roll the inner thigh of your straight leg toward the ceiling, finding its internal rotation.
• Place your hands on blocks to help elongate your spine if your back begins rounding when your fingertips touch the floor.
• Avoid positioning your knee past your ankle and over your toes, which can stress your knee joint.

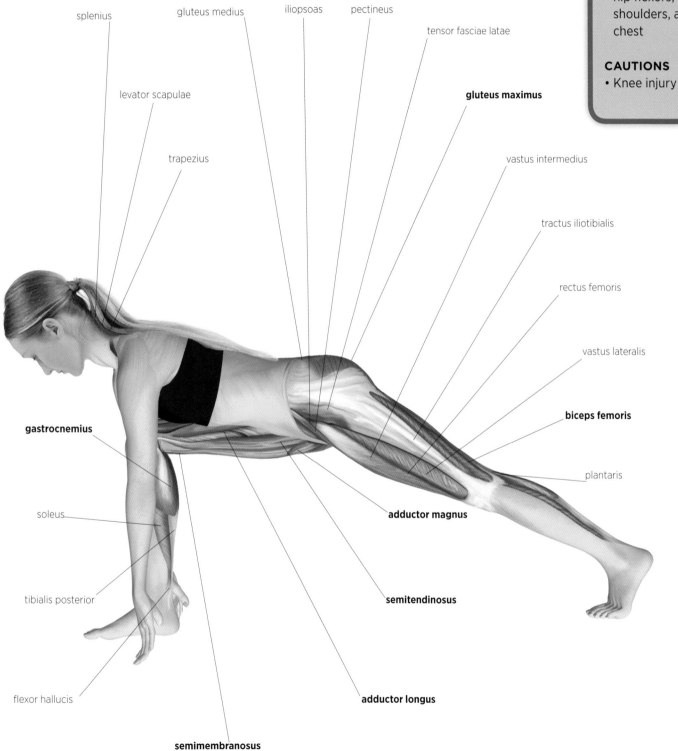

Annotation Key
Bold text indicates target muscles
Light text indicates other working muscles
* indicates deep muscles

FACT FILE

TARGETS
• Lower body

TYPE
• Dynamic

BENEFITS
• Strengthens
  thighs
• Stretches
  hip flexors,
  shoulders, and
  chest

CAUTIONS
• Knee injury

splenius

gluteus medius

iliopsoas

pectineus

tensor fasciae latae

levator scapulae

gluteus maximus

trapezius

vastus intermedius

tractus iliotibialis

rectus femoris

vastus lateralis

biceps femoris

gastrocnemius

plantaris

adductor magnus

soleus

tibialis posterior

semitendinosus

flexor hallucis

adductor longus

semimembranosus

Wide-Legged Forward Bend

The Wide-Legged Forward Bend is one of the most effective ways to lengthen your hamstrings and back muscles. This inversion stretch boosts your energy and circulation while improving hip mobility.

HOW TO DO IT

- Stand straight with your feet generously more than shoulder-width apart.

- Bend your knees slightly and tuck your pelvis slightly forward. Lift your chest, and press your shoulders downward and back.

- Hinge forward from your hips, keeping your back flat.

- Place your fingertips or palms on the floor.

- Hold for the recommended time, and release the stretch.

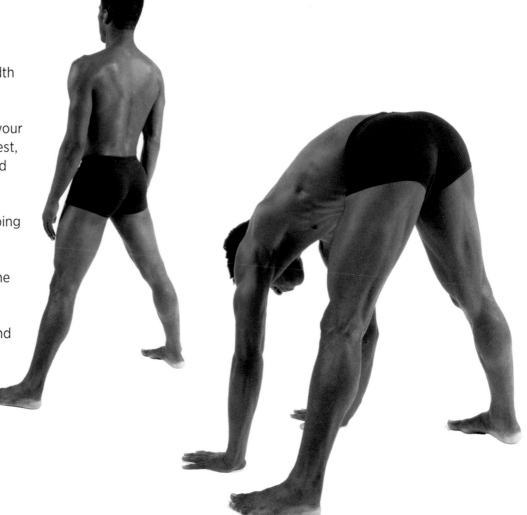

MODIFICATION

HARDER: Walk your hands in between your legs, bend your elbows, and gently place your forehead on the floor. Your hands should be available if necessary for balance.

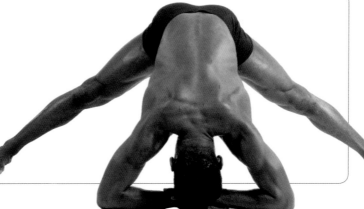

DO IT RIGHT

- Keep your chest elevated.
- Exhale as you bend forward from your hips.
- Avoid tensing your neck and shoulders.

MODIFICATION

EASIER: Widen your stance or place a yoga block on the floor for support.

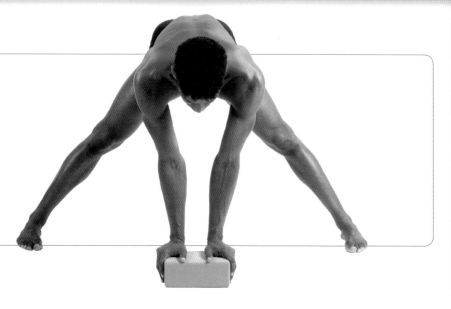

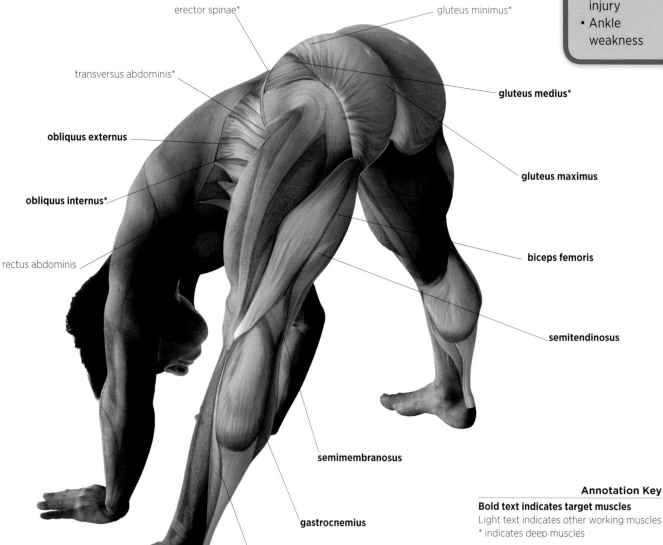

erector spinae*

gluteus minimus*

transversus abdominis*

gluteus medius*

obliquus externus

gluteus maximus

obliquus internus*

rectus abdominis

biceps femoris

semitendinosus

semimembranosus

gastrocnemius

soleus

Annotation Key

Bold text indicates target muscles
Light text indicates other working muscles
* indicates deep muscles

Iliotibial Band Stretch

Athletes, in particular distance runners, often struggle with tight iliotibial bands—the thick length of connective tissue that runs along the outside of your thigh from your hip joint down to your knee. This stretch improves mobility in your upper legs and helps prevent sports-related injuries.

HOW TO DO IT

- Stand straight with your arms at your sides.

- Cross your right leg in front of your left, and place your right foot along the outside of your left foot. Your toes should be pointing forward.

- Bend forward from your hips while keeping your back leg straight.

- Reach your fingertips toward the floor, and if you are able, rest your palms on the floor.

- Hold for the recommended time, release the stretch, and then repeat on the opposite side.

DO IT RIGHT
- Keep both feet flat on the floor.
- Maintain proper alignment by forming a straight line with your spine and your back leg.
- Avoid lifting your back heel off the floor.
- Avoid arching or rounding your back.

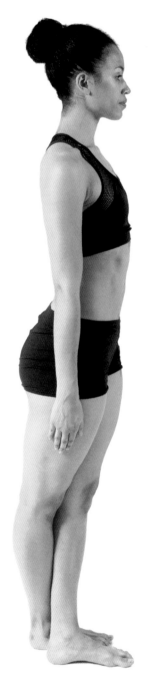
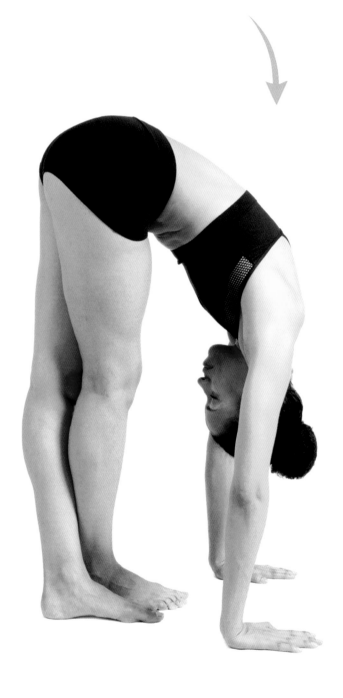

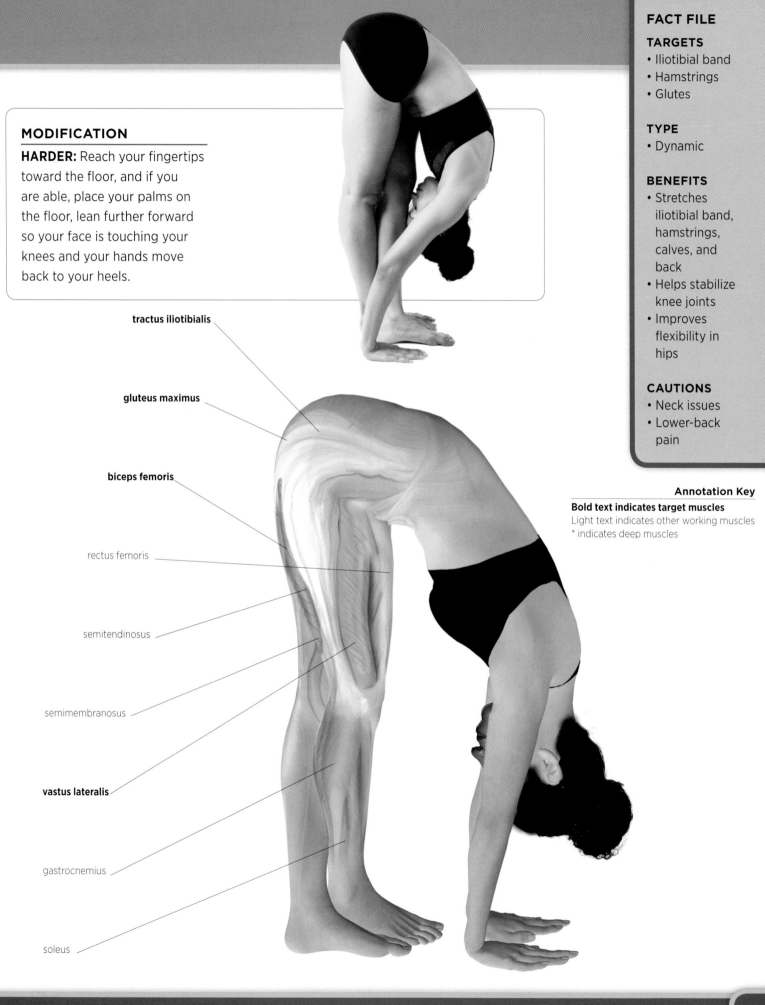

FACT FILE

TARGETS
• Iliotibial band
• Hamstrings
• Glutes

TYPE
• Dynamic

BENEFITS
• Stretches iliotibial band, hamstrings, calves, and back
• Helps stabilize knee joints
• Improves flexibility in hips

CAUTIONS
• Neck issues
• Lower-back pain

MODIFICATION

HARDER: Reach your fingertips toward the floor, and if you are able, place your palms on the floor, lean further forward so your face is touching your knees and your hands move back to your heels.

Annotation Key
Bold text indicates target muscles
Light text indicates other working muscles
* indicates deep muscles

tractus iliotibialis

gluteus maximus

biceps femoris

rectus femoris

semitendinosus

semimembranosus

vastus lateralis

gastrocnemius

soleus

Heel-Drop/Toe-Up Stretch

The Heel-Drop/Toe-Up Stretch targets the main muscles in your calves—the gastrocnemius and the soleus—and lengthens your Achilles tendon. Stretching the muscles and tendons of your calves should be a consistent part of your lower-body stretching regimen.

HOW TO DO IT

• Stand on an aerobic step, a riser, or a stair with your feet shoulder-width apart and your arms at your sides.

• Bend your knees very slightly and tuck your pelvis slightly forward. Lift your chest, and press your shoulders downward and back.

• Place the ball of your right foot on the edge of the step.

• Drop your right heel down while controlling the amount of weight you put on your right leg to increase or decrease the intensity of the stretch in your calf.

• Release the stretch, and then repeat on the opposite side.

• Step down from the riser, and stand with your feet shoulder-width apart. Tuck your pelvis slightly forward. Lift your chest, and press your shoulders downward and back.

• Position the ball of your right foot on the step.

• With your knees straight, bring your hips forward to feel the stretch in your right calf.

• Release the stretch, and then repeat on the opposite side.

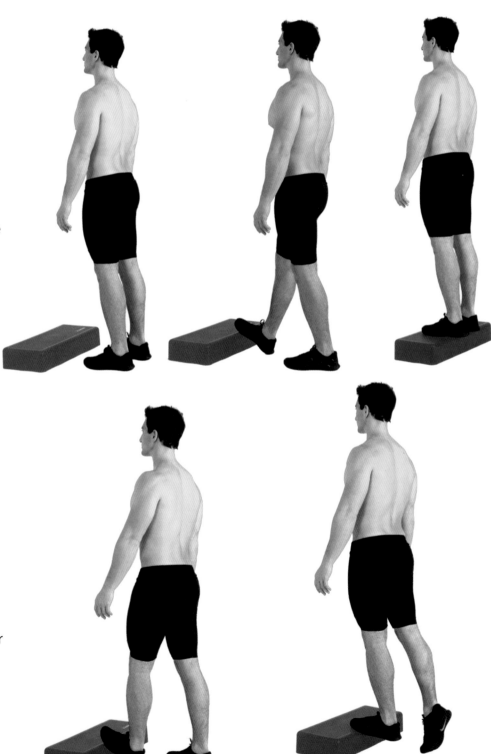

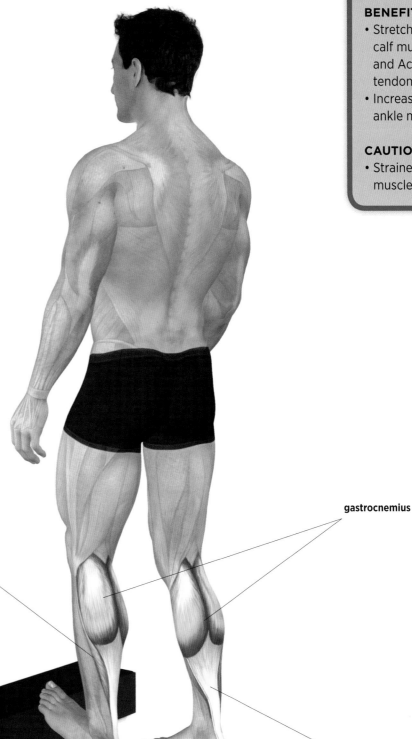

FACT FILE

TARGETS
- Calves
- Achilles tendon

TYPE
- Static

BENEFITS
- Stretches calf muscles and Achilles tendon
- Increases ankle mobility

CAUTIONS
- Strained calf muscle

Annotation Key

Bold text indicates target muscles
Light text indicates other working muscles
* indicates deep muscles

DO IT RIGHT

- Use a wall or other stable object to balance yourself if necessary.
- Engage all your calf muscles by gently and slowly rolling from your big toe to your pinky toe and back again, shifting your body weight over your toes as you stretch.
- Avoid bouncing to achieve a deeper stretch—all your movements should be subtle and performed carefully.

soleus

gastrocnemius

tendo calcaneus

Knee-Pull Plank

The aim of the Knee-Pull Plank is to build core strength, but it also deeply stretches your calves and Achilles tendon.

HOW TO DO IT

- Begin by assuming a standard plank, or push-up, position.

- Draw your right knee into your chest while leaning forward and flexing your foot. Keep your left foot flexed and balance on your toes.

- Extend your left leg through the heel and rock your body back, shifting your weight into your left foot.

- Keeping your spine aligned, straighten and extend your right leg toward the ceiling.

- Hold for the recommended time, release the stretch, and then repeat on the opposite side.

DO IT RIGHT
- Keep your body in a straight line throughout the exercise.
- Avoid bending the knee of your supporting leg.

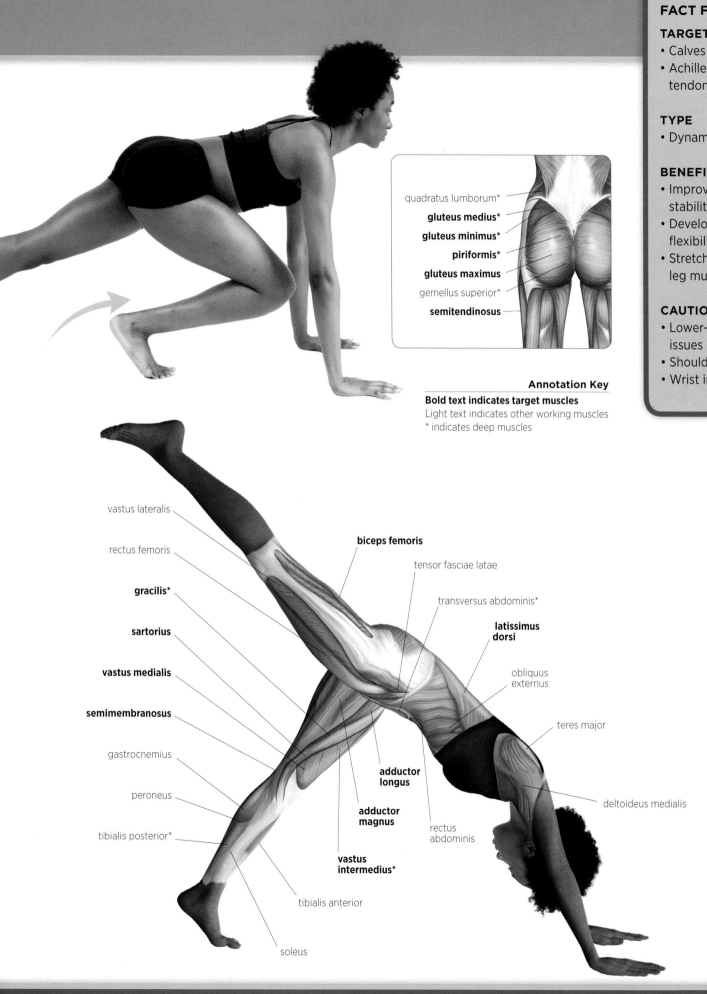

TARGETS
- Calves
- Achilles tendon

TYPE
- Dynamic

BENEFITS
- Improves core stability
- Develops flexibility
- Stretches all leg muscles

CAUTIONS
- Lower-back issues
- Shoulder pain
- Wrist injury

quadratus lumborum*
gluteus medius*
gluteus minimus*
piriformis*
gluteus maximus
gemellus superior*
semitendinosus

Annotation Key

Bold text indicates target muscles
Light text indicates other working muscles
* indicates deep muscles

vastus lateralis
rectus femoris
gracilis*
sartorius
vastus medialis
semimembranosus
gastrocnemius
peroneus
tibialis posterior*
vastus intermedius*
tibialis anterior
soleus

biceps femoris
tensor fasciae latae
transversus abdominis*
latissimus dorsi
obliquus externus
teres major
deltoideus medialis
rectus abdominis
adductor longus
adductor magnus

Mountain Climber Stretch

The Mountain Climber increases the endurance of the many muscles in your arms, legs, and core that must work in unison to execute this stretch. Although it is taxing, this exercise rewards you with more supple legs, stronger arms and core, and greater hip mobility.

HOW TO DO IT

- Begin in a high plank position with your arms straight, your hands shoulder-width apart, and your palms on the floor in line with your shoulders. Keep your feet together, and your back straight.

- Bring your left knee in toward your chest. Rest the ball of your left foot on the floor.

- Jump to switch your feet in the air, bringing your right foot forward and your left foot back.

- Continue quickly alternating your legs for the recommended repetitions.

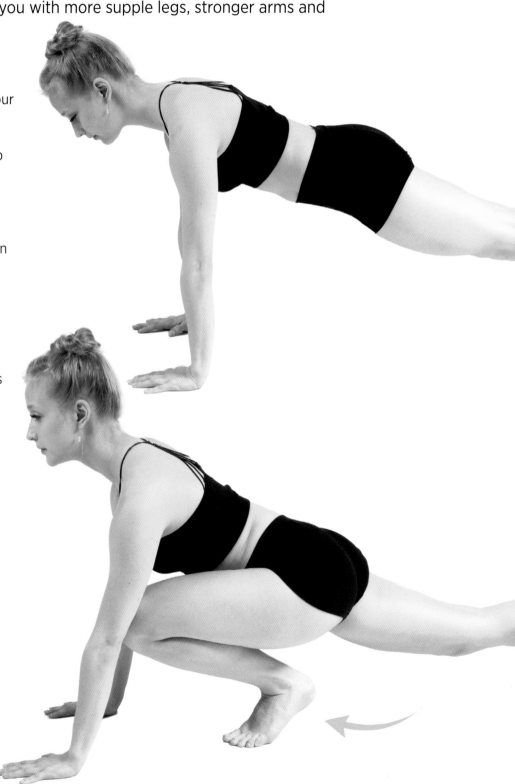

DO IT RIGHT
- Keep your back straight.
- Flare your hands out to ease shoulder stress.
- Avoid small leg movements; attempt to bring each knee safely to your chest.

FACT FILE

TARGETS
- Hip flexors
- Quadriceps
- Hamstrings
- Glutes
- Arms
- Shoulders

TYPE
- Dynamic

BENEFITS
- Warms up muscles
- Improves coordination
- Strengthens and tones abdominals, chest, arm, and leg muscles
- Increases cardiovascular endurance

CAUTIONS
- Wrist issues
- Knee injury

Annotation Key

Bold text indicates target muscles
Light text indicates other working muscles
* indicates deep muscles

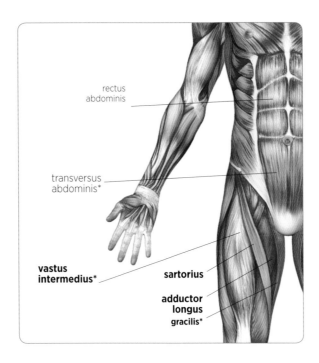

rectus abdominis

transversus abdominis*

vastus intermedius*

sartorius

adductor longus
gracilis*

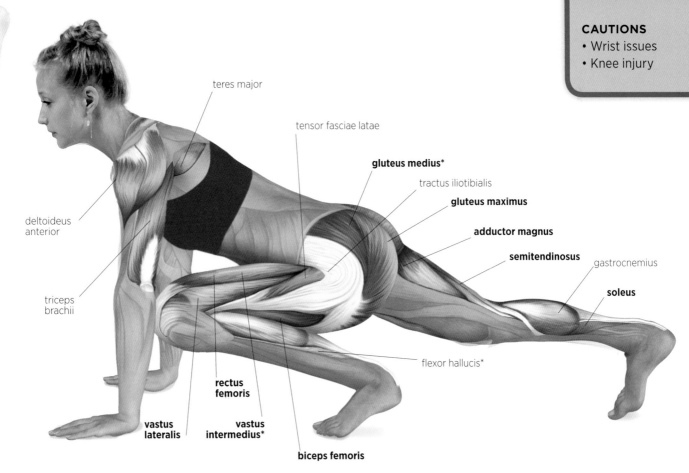

teres major

tensor fasciae latae

gluteus medius*

tractus iliotibialis

gluteus maximus

adductor magnus

semitendinosus

gastrocnemius

soleus

deltoideus anterior

triceps brachii

flexor hallucis*

rectus femoris

vastus lateralis

vastus intermedius*

biceps femoris

Unilateral Seated Forward Bend

The Unilateral Seated Forward Bend provides a deep stretch for the entire back of your body—from your heels to your neck. This seated forward bend focuses on one leg at a time, making it a great stretch for beginners.

HOW TO DO IT

• Sit on the floor as straight as possible, with your legs extended in front of you.

• Bend your right knee, letting it drop out to your side. Rest the sole of your right foot on your left inner thigh just above your knee.

• Rest your hands above your knee.

• Bend from your waist, and lean forward over your right leg. Open your forearms out to your sides.

• Hold for the recommended time, and then repeat on the opposite side.

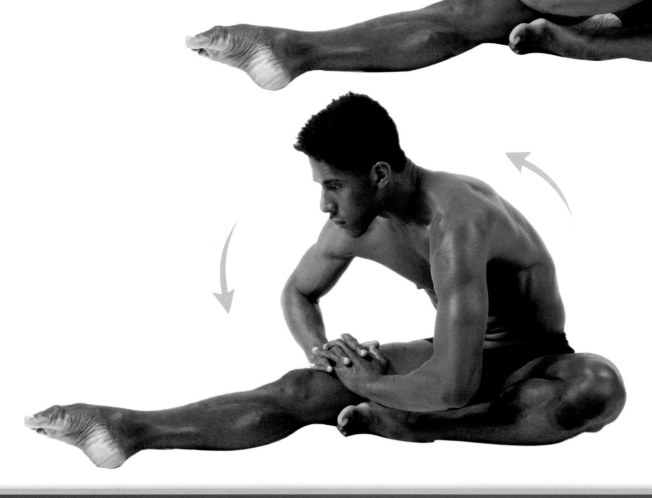

TARGETS
• Hamstrings
• Calves
• Back

TYPE
• Static

BENEFITS
• Stretches
  calves and
  hamstrings
• Reduces risk
  of knee injury

CAUTIONS
• Knee pain
• Lower-back
  pain

Annotation Key

Bold text indicates target muscles
Light text indicates other working muscles
* indicates deep muscles

DO IT RIGHT

• Drop your head to intensify
  the stretch and engage
  your rhomboid muscles
  between your shoulder
  blades.
• Avoid straining your back—
  if your back is tight, try
  performing this stretch
  with the support of a sofa
  or wall behind you. Be sure
  to position your lower back
  as close to the sofa or wall
  as possible.

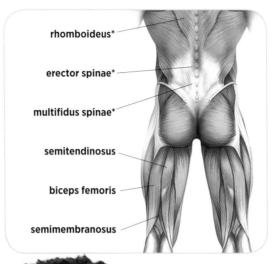

rhomboideus*

erector spinae*

multifidus spinae*

semitendinosus

biceps femoris

semimembranosus

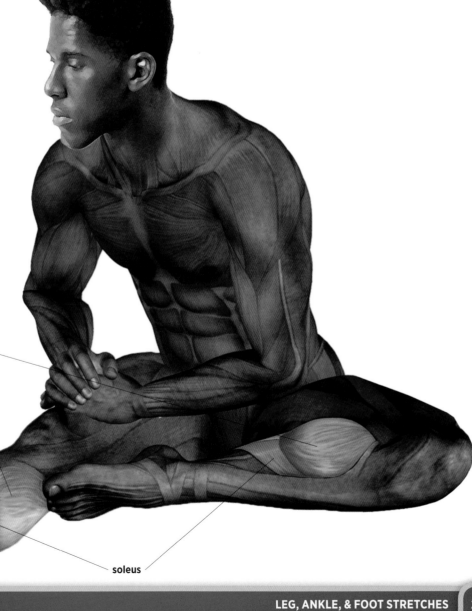

gastrocnemius

soleus

Bilateral Seated Forward Bend

The Bilateral Seated Forward Bend creates a deep stretch in the leg muscles. This position can indeed feel intense, but it's important to remember never to force the stretch or push too hard. The more you can learn to relax in this pose, the deeper your stretch will be.

HOW TO DO IT

• Sit on the floor as straight as possible with your back flat and your legs extended in front of you in parallel position.

• Your feet should be slightly flexed.

• Bend forward, lowering your abdominals over your thighs, forearms resting above your knees as you stretch.

• Hold for the recommended time, and slowly roll up to the starting position.

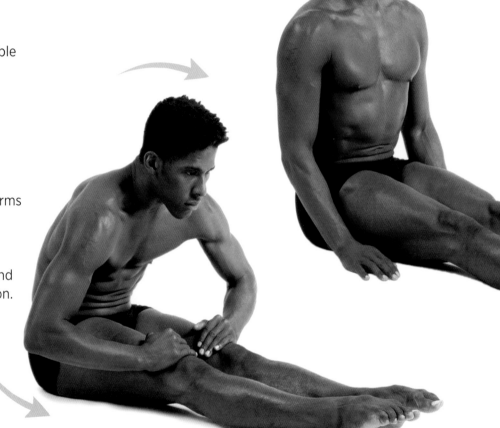

MODIFICATION

HARDER: For a deeper stretch in your hamstrings, place an elastic resistance band around the balls of your feet, using your hands to draw the band toward you.

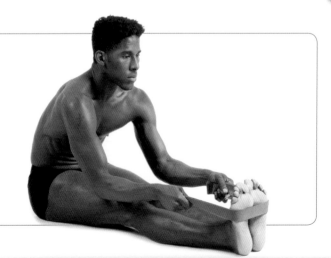

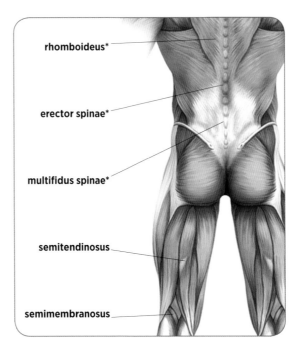

rhomboideus*

erector spinae*

multifidus spinae*

semitendinosus

semimembranosus

DO IT RIGHT

- Bend at the hips and keep your spine fairly straight as you stretch.
- Extend your torso as far forward over your legs as possible.
- Breathe naturally; avoid holding your breath.

FACT FILE

TARGETS
- Hamstrings
- Calves
- Back

TYPE
- Static

BENEFITS
- Lengthens and tones hamstrings
- Stretches tight calves
- Stretches Achilles tendon

CAUTIONS
- Knee injury
- Lower-back pain

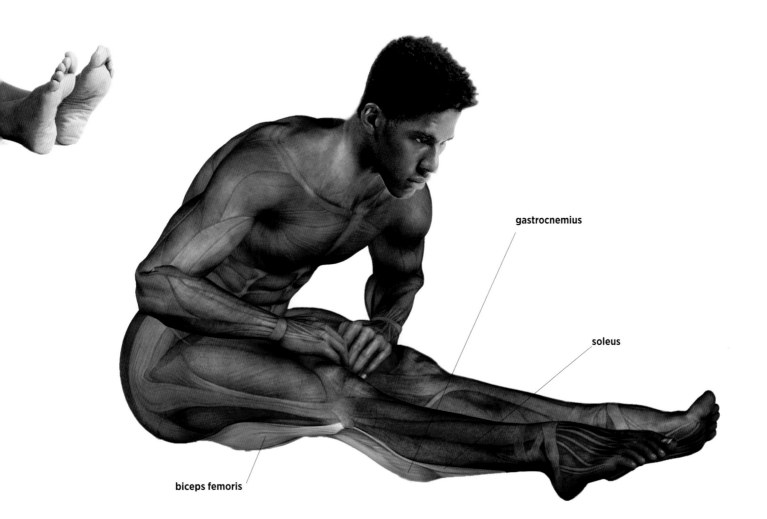

gastrocnemius

soleus

biceps femoris

Hip Stretch

Hip mobility affects your pelvic and spinal posture. Incorporate hip stretches in your daily exercise routine to maintain healthy body alignment and improve your balance.

HOW TO DO IT

• Sit on the floor with your legs extended in front of you and your feet flexed.

• Bend your right knee and cross it over your left thigh. Plant your right foot flat on the floor next to the outside of your left thigh.

• Wrap your left arm around your bent knee.

• Apply gentle pressure around your right knee to help rotate your torso. Keep your hips aligned as you pull your knee in toward your chest.

• Hold for the recommended time, and then slowly release.

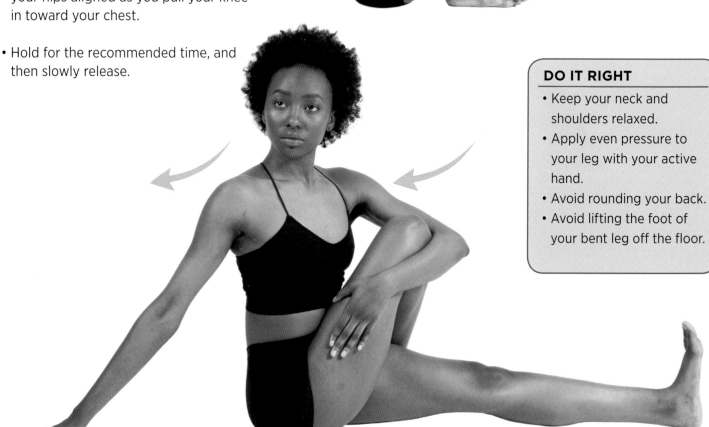

DO IT RIGHT
• Keep your neck and shoulders relaxed.
• Apply even pressure to your leg with your active hand.
• Avoid rounding your back.
• Avoid lifting the foot of your bent leg off the floor.

TARGETS
• Hips
• Back
• Shoulders
• Abdominal obliques

TYPE
• Static

BENEFITS
• Stretches hip extensors and flexors
• Mobilizes spine

CAUTIONS
• Lower-back issues
• Shoulder pain
• Hip problems

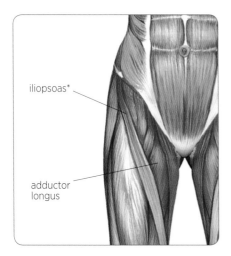

iliopsoas*

adductor longus

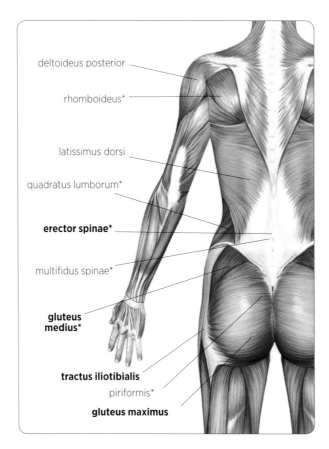

deltoideus posterior

rhomboideus*

latissimus dorsi

quadratus lumborum*

erector spinae*

multifidus spinae*

gluteus medius*

tractus iliotibialis

piriformis*

gluteus maximus

Annotation Key

Bold text indicates target muscles
Light text indicates other working muscles
* indicates deep muscles

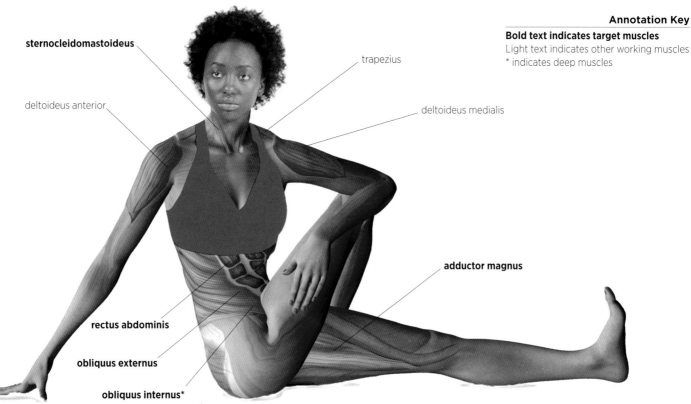

sternocleidomastoideus

trapezius

deltoideus anterior

deltoideus medialis

adductor magnus

rectus abdominis

obliquus externus

obliquus internus*

Side-Lying Knee Bend

This side-lying version of a quadriceps stretch allows you to target the tight or overworked muscles in your upper legs without having to stand while balancing on one leg. This means that you can pull into the stretch more deeply, without the fear of falling over.

HOW TO DO IT

- Lie on your left side, with your legs stacked and in line with your torso.

- Extend your left arm, and rest your head on your upper arm.

- Bend your right knee and grasp your ankle with your right hand.

- Pull your ankle in toward your buttocks as you stretch.

- Return to the starting position, and then repeat on the opposite side.

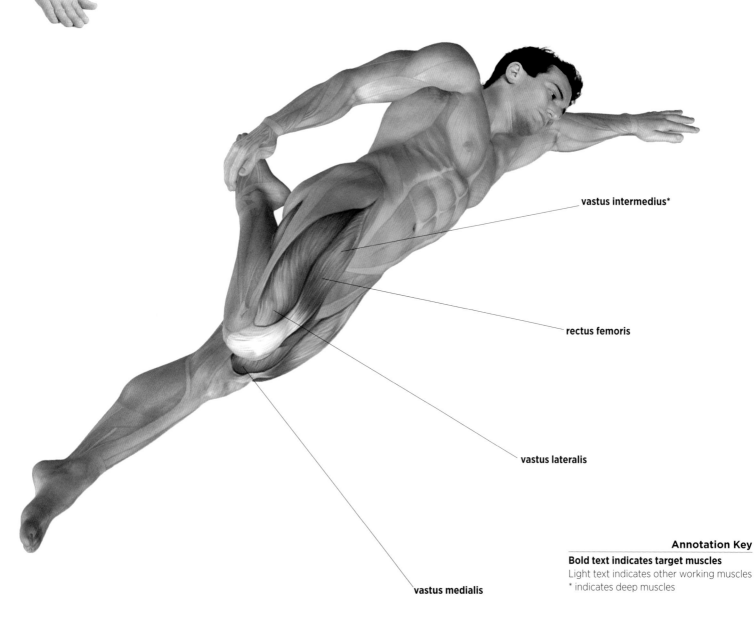

DO IT RIGHT

• Keep your knees together, stacked one on top of the other.
• Tuck your pelvis slightly forward and lift your chest to engage your core.
• Keep your toes pointed and your legs parallel to the floor throughout.
• Avoid rolling backward onto your gluteal muscles.

vastus intermedius*

rectus femoris

vastus lateralis

vastus medialis

Annotation Key
Bold text indicates target muscles
Light text indicates other working muscles
* indicates deep muscles

Iliotibial Band Roll

Many dancers, runners, cyclists, hikers, and other athletes experience a common outer-thigh injury called iliotibial band syndrome. Foam roller massage may be helpful in preventing and relieving the discomfort produced by this condition.

HOW TO DO IT

• Kneel upright facing a foam roller, with your knees a few inches behind the foam roller.

• Lean forward onto all fours, placing your hands about a foot in front of the foam roller.

• Lift your left knee and place as much of your left foot on the floor as possible. Lower your right hip onto the foam roller.

• Tilt your body slightly to the right, adjusting your body weight to achieve the desired pressure on your upper thigh, rolling slowly down to just above your knee.

• Pause over uncomfortable areas, gently rolling back and forth over them until you feel some relief.

• Return to the starting position, and then repeat on the opposite side.

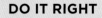

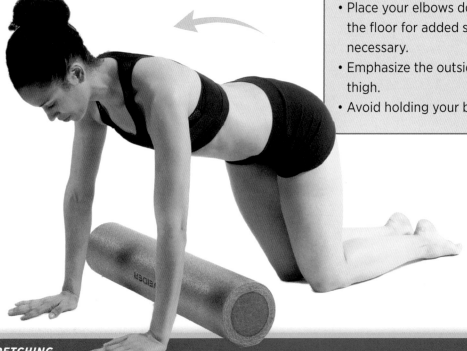

DO IT RIGHT

• Adjust the weight over your hands and feet to find the appropriate level of intensity.
• Place your elbows down on the floor for added support if necessary.
• Emphasize the outside of your thigh.
• Avoid holding your breath.

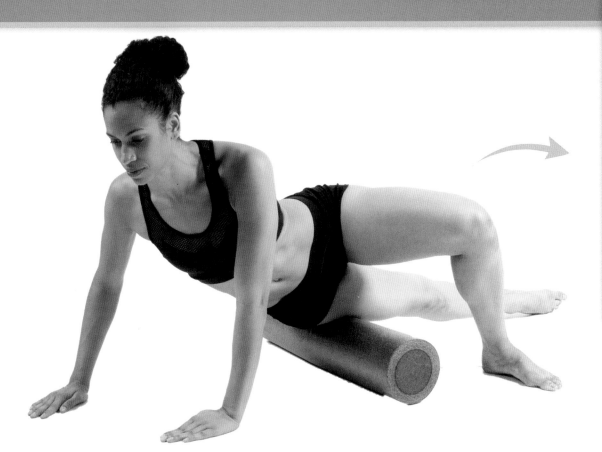

FACT FILE

TARGETS
• Iliotibial band

TYPE
• Dynamic

BENEFITS
• Stabilizes knees
• Relaxes tight hips

CAUTIONS
• Hip pain
• Knee injury

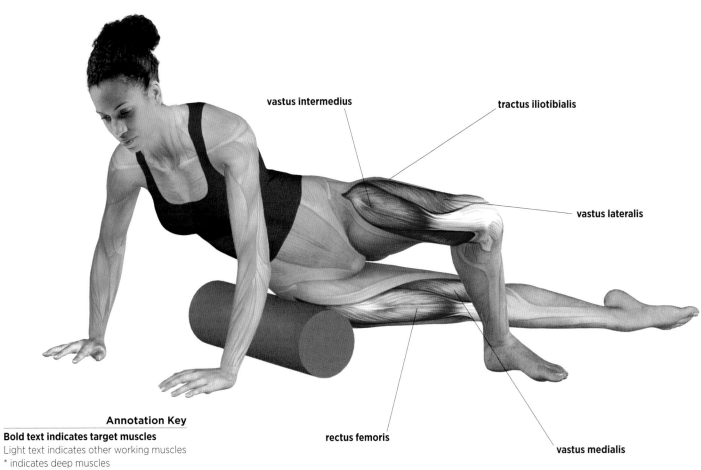

vastus intermedius

tractus iliotibialis

vastus lateralis

rectus femoris

vastus medialis

Annotation Key

Bold text indicates target muscles
Light text indicates other working muscles
* indicates deep muscles

Calf and Hamstrings Stretch

The straightforward Calf and Hamstrings Stretch relies on both the foam roller and the weight of your body to target the muscles in the back of your legs. By keeping your core engaged, you can adjust the amount of body weight placed on the roller and find a comfortable level of pressure.

HOW TO DO IT

- Kneel upright with the foam roller in your hands, and place it behind your knees.

- Carefully rock your pelvis slightly forward, just enough to place the foam roller deep behind your kneecaps.

- Lower your hips gently onto the foam roller.

- As you begin to sit, you will find that the foam roller naturally moves over your calf muscles.

- Guide the roller with your hands, moving the roller slowly down toward your heels.

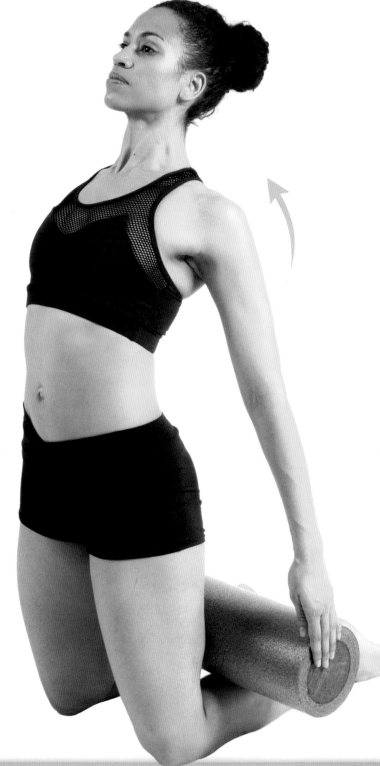

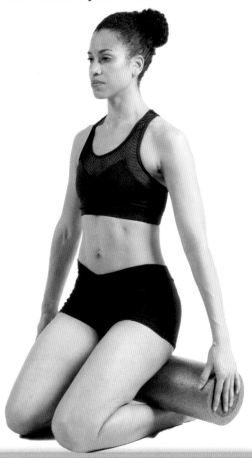

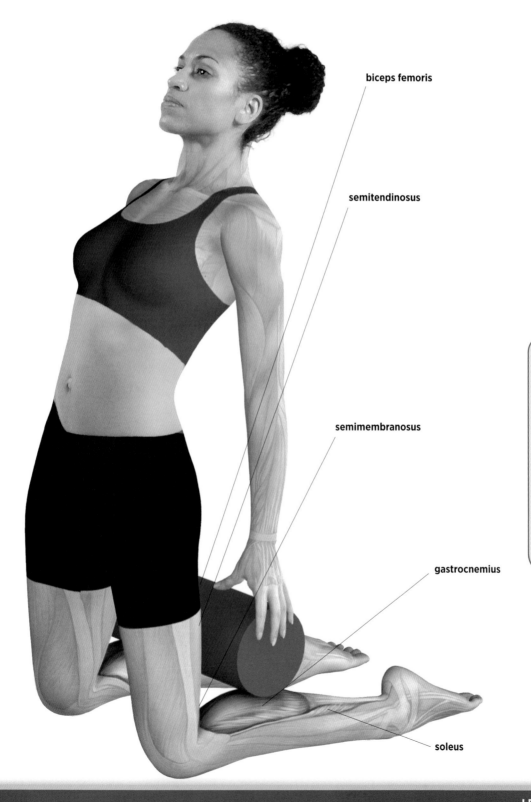

Annotation Key
Bold text indicates target muscles
Light text indicates other working muscles
* indicates deep muscles

biceps femoris

semitendinosus

semimembranosus

gastrocnemius

soleus

FACT FILE

TARGETS
• Back
• Spine
• Core

TYPE
• Dynamic

BENEFITS
• Relieves tight calves and hamstrings
• Improves mobility in lower legs

CAUTIONS
• Ankle pain
• Knee pain or weakness
• Hip pain

DO IT RIGHT
• Engage your core to adjust the body weight on the roller and on your legs.
• Avoid leaning forward; keep your upper body upright.
• Move slowly and deliberately.

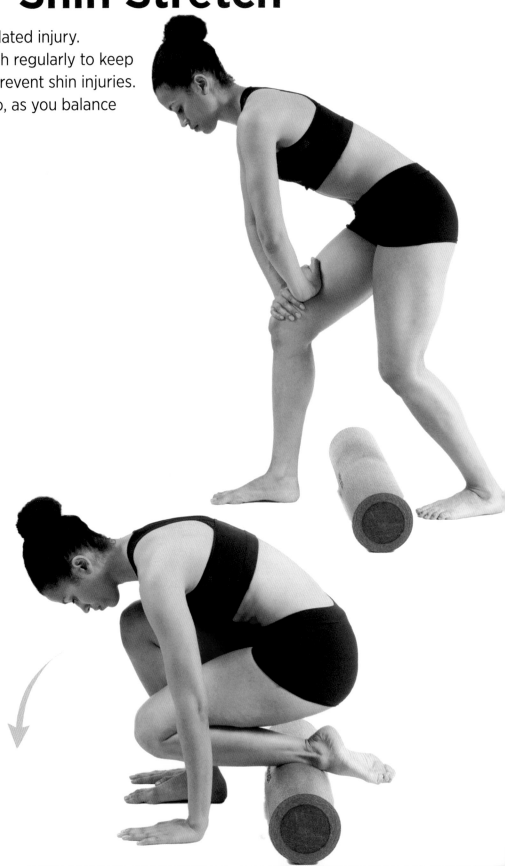

Foam Roller Shin Stretch

Shin splints are a common sports-related injury. Perform this Foam Roller Shin Stretch regularly to keep your shin muscles supple and help prevent shin injuries. Your core gets a bit of a workout too, as you balance over the foam roller.

HOW TO DO IT

• Stand over the foam roller in a slight lunge, with your right leg in front of the foam roller and your leg left behind it.

• Place your hands on your right thigh just above the knee for support.

• Lower your body downward, and place your hands on the floor on either side of your right foot.

• Lower your shin onto the foam roller and gently roll back and forth.

• Pause over uncomfortable areas, rolling over them several times, until you feel some relief.

• Return to the starting position, and then repeat on the opposite side.

DO IT RIGHT
• Control the amount of pressure you place on the foam roller by adjusting the amount of weight you place on your hands.
• Avoid holding your breath.

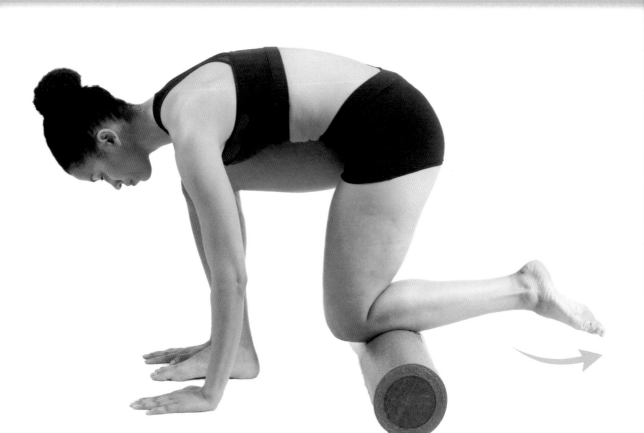

FACT FILE

TARGETS
• Shins

TYPE
• Static

BENEFITS
• Reduces shin
  pain and
  tightness
• Improves gait
  and posture

CAUTIONS
• Ankle pain
• Shin injury
• Wrist pain or
  weakness

Annotation Key

Bold text indicates target muscles
Light text indicates other working muscles
* indicates deep muscles

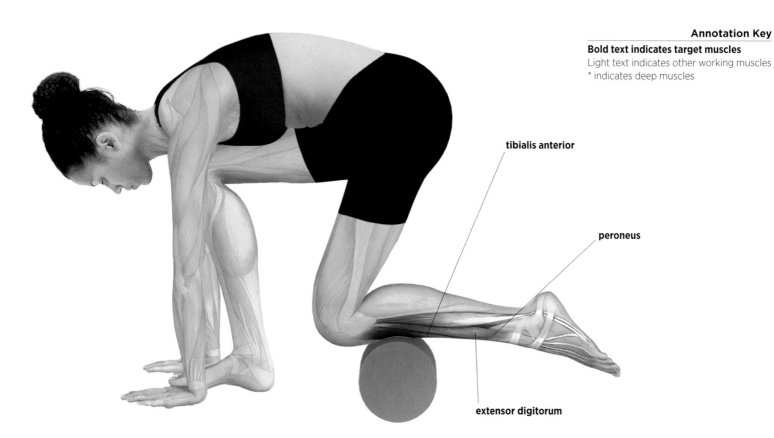

tibialis anterior

peroneus

extensor digitorum

Knee Squat

The Knee Squat integrates balance, coordination, resistance, and stretching to target your leg muscles. This exercise also strengthens the muscles of your feet.

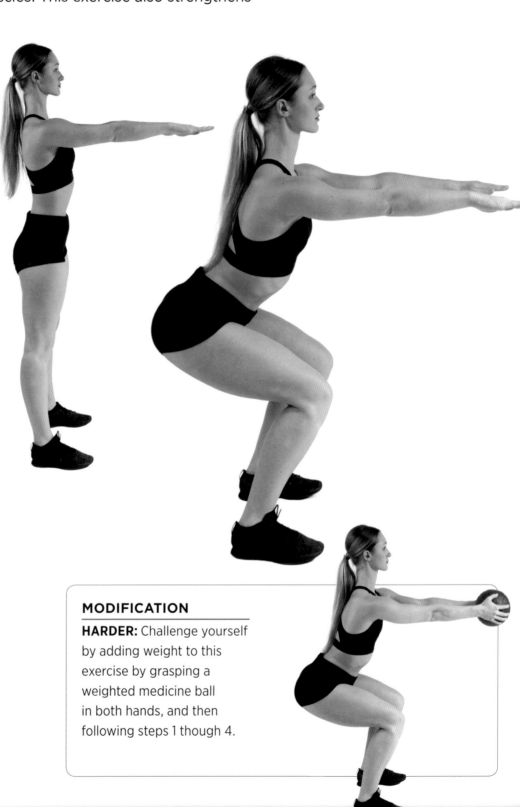

HOW TO DO IT

- Stand with your legs and feet parallel and shoulder-width apart, and your knees bent very slightly. Tuck your pelvis slightly forward, lift your chest, and press your shoulders downward and back.

- Extend your arms in front of your body for stability, keeping them even with your shoulders. Plant your feet firmly on the floor, and curl your toes slightly upward.

- Draw in your abdominal muscles and bend into a squat. Keep your heels planted on the floor and your chest as upright as possible, resisting the urge to bend too far forward.

- Exhale, and return to the original position. Repeat five to six times.

DO IT RIGHT
- Imagine pressing into the floor as you rise from the squat, creating your body's own resistance in your leg muscles.

MODIFICATION
HARDER: Challenge yourself by adding weight to this exercise by grasping a weighted medicine ball in both hands, and then following steps 1 though 4.

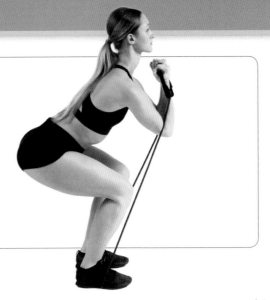

MODIFICATION

HARDER: To add resistance to this move, secure a resistance band under both feet. Stand with feet shoulder-width apart, and then with an end in each hand, bring your hands to shoulder level. Perform steps 3 and 4.

FACT FILE

TARGETS
• Hips
• Lower legs

TYPE
• Dynamic

BENEFITS
• Lengthens and strengthens calf muscles

CAUTIONS
• Foot pain

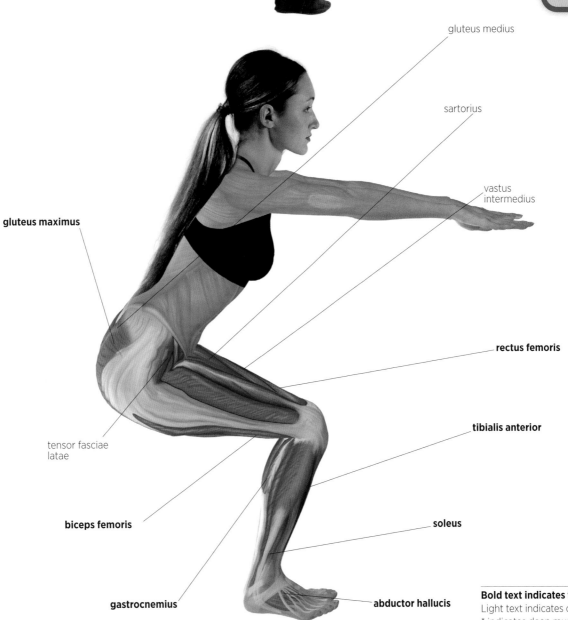

gluteus medius

sartorius

vastus intermedius

gluteus maximus

rectus femoris

tensor fasciae latae

tibialis anterior

biceps femoris

soleus

gastrocnemius

abductor hallucis

Annotation Key
Bold text indicates target muscles
Light text indicates other working muscles
* indicates deep muscles

Bilateral Quad Stretch

The quadriceps muscles are important for maintaining balance, strength, and flexibility. This reclining quad stretch is a deep and effective way to loosen up tight thighs.

HOW TO DO IT

• Kneel with your buttocks resting lightly on your heels.

• Reach your arms behind you and place your hands flat on the floor, with your fingers pointing forward.

• Keep a slight bend in your elbows.

• Lean slightly back to increase the intensity of the stretch.

• Continue to carefully lean backward until you are lying supine on the floor. Extend your arms away from your torso, palms faceup.

• Hold for the recommended time, and release the stretch.

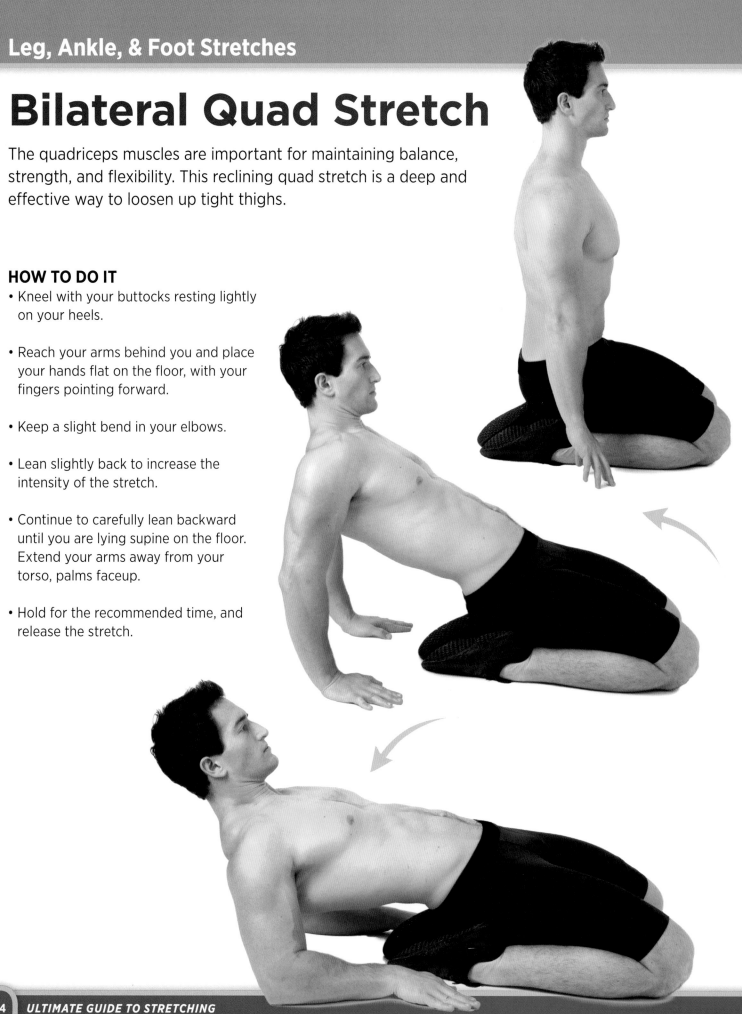

TARGETS
• Quadriceps

TYPE
• Dynamic

BENEFITS
• Stretches and strengthens quadriceps
• Improves gait and posture
• Improves muscle balance between quads and hamstrings

CAUTIONS
• Knee injury
• Hip pain
• Lower-back issues

DO IT RIGHT

• Contract and engage your gluteal muscles to avoid a curve in your lumbar spine.
• Avoid arching your back.

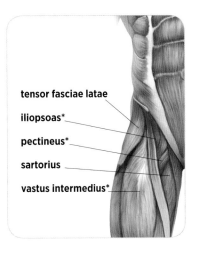

tensor fasciae latae

iliopsoas*

pectineus*

sartorius

vastus intermedius*

Annotation Key

Bold text indicates target muscles
Light text indicates other working muscles
* indicates deep muscles

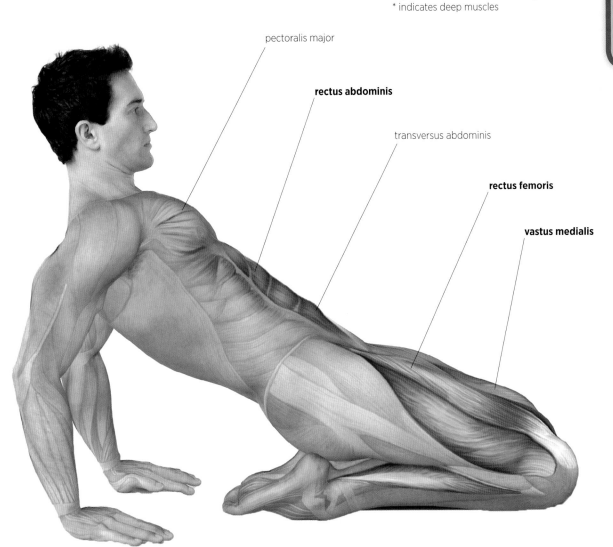

pectoralis major

rectus abdominis

transversus abdominis

rectus femoris

vastus medialis

Scissors Stretch

Improve your core stability while increasing your abdominal strength and endurance with the Scissors Stretch. This classic Pilates exercise also offers a good stretch for your hamstrings. When performed correctly, it helps mobilize your shoulders and upper arms.

HOW TO DO IT

• Lie on the floor with your arms at your sides and your legs raised in tabletop position.

• Draw in your abdominals.

• Extend your left leg straight up while lifting your head and shoulders off the floor.

• Hold the back of your left calf and pulse your leg toward you. Keep your shoulders relaxed.

• Lower your left leg to the floor, and repeat on the opposite side.

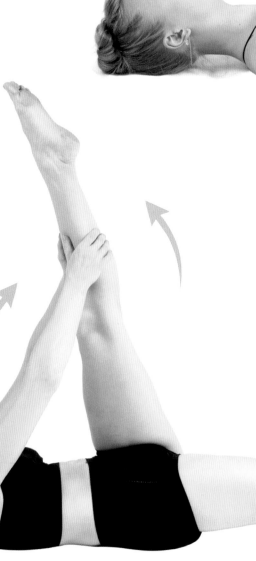

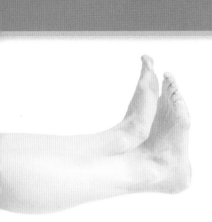

DO IT RIGHT

- Keep your pelvis stabilized and your spine straight.
- Avoid overextending your raised leg.

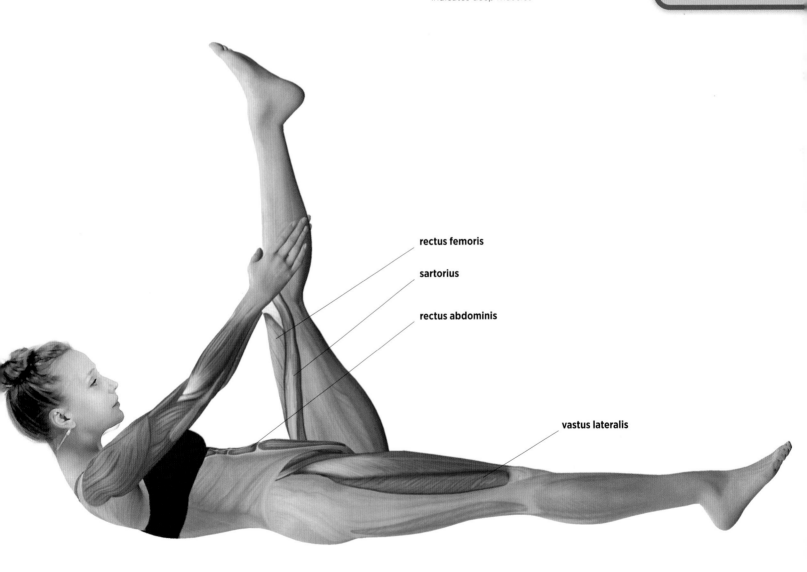

rectus femoris

sartorius

rectus abdominis

vastus lateralis

Point Foot Stretch

Properly stretching your feet helps you to maintain good balance and ankle mobility. Additionally, foot stretches improve flexibility in your lower-leg muscles, which can help prevent heel pain and Achilles tendon injuries.

FACT FILE

TARGETS
• Feet
• Calves
• Arch of the foot

TYPE
• Static

BENEFITS
• Strength in ankles
• Help with cardiovascular activities

CAUTIONS
• Stabilize ankle and foot

HOW TO DO IT

• Sit on a chair or on the floor, and cross your left leg over your right, placing your left ankle on top of your right thigh.

• Brace your left ankle with your left hand. Grasp the top of your left foot with your right hand. With your right palm, press down on the top of your foot and toes, so your toes point inward.

• Release the stretch, and then repeat on the opposite side.

DO IT RIGHT
• During the slope-down phase, push forcefully with your palms—the downward force must be stronger than the upward force of your pulling fingers.

plantar interosseous

flexor hallucis brevis*

flexor digitorum brevis

lumbricalis

flexor digiti minimi brevis

abductor hallucis

quadratus plantae

abductor digiti minimi

Flexion Foot Stretch

Regularly practicing foot stretches, such as the Flexion Foot Stretch, will strengthen your feet. As they become stronger and more flexible, you are less likely to suffer pain in the arches and tears in the tendons.

HOW TO DO IT

- Sit on a chair or on the floor, and cross your left leg over your right, placing your left ankle on top of your right thigh.

- Brace your right heel with your right hand. Grasp your toes and the ball of your foot with your left hand.

- Pull back on your toes until you feel a stretch in your arch.

- Release the stretch, and then repeat on the opposite side.

DO IT RIGHT
- Pull only until you feel a comfortable stretch.

FACT FILE

TARGETS
- Feet
- Calves
- Arches

TYPE
- Passive

BENEFITS
- Relieves ankle and heel pain
- Improves gait and posture
- Lengthens Achilles tendons and reduces risk of injury
- Improves range of motion in calves

CAUTIONS
- Ankle injury
- Heel pain

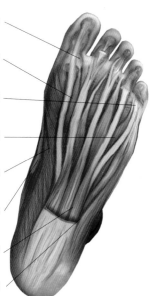

plantar interosseous
flexor hallucis brevis*
flexor digitorum brevis
lumbricalis
flexor digiti minimi brevis
abductor hallucis
quadratus plantae
abductor digiti minimi

Annotation Key

Bold text indicates target muscles
Light text indicates other working muscles
* indicates deep muscles

Slope-Up Foot Stretch

Use the Slope-Up Foot Stretch as a counterpose to the Slope-Down (page 321). It transfers more of the stretch from the top of the foot to the bottom.

HOW TO DO IT

- Sit on a chair or on the floor, and cross your left leg over your right, placing your left ankle on top of your right thigh.

- Grasp your foot so that the palm of your hand lies across the top of your foot and your fingers are wrapped around the bottom.

- Using your palm, push down on the top outside of your foot. At the same time, pull up the bottom of your foot with your fingers; this creates the "slope-up."

- Release the stretch, and then repeat on the opposite side.

DO IT RIGHT

- Push forcefully with your fingers—their upward force must be stronger than the downward force of your pushing palms.
- Avoid allowing your foot to shift; firmly stabilize your ankle and heel.

(page 321)

FACT FILE

TARGETS
- Feet
- Shins

TYPE
- Static

BENEFITS
- Relieves ankle and heel pain
- Improves gait and posture
- Lengthens Achilles tendon and reduces risk of injury
- Improves range of motion in calves

CAUTIONS
- Severe ankle or heel pain

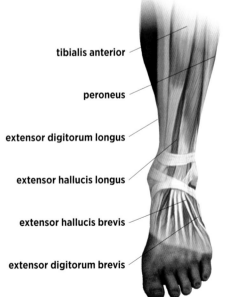

tibialis anterior

peroneus

extensor digitorum longus

extensor hallucis longus

extensor hallucis brevis

extensor digitorum brevis

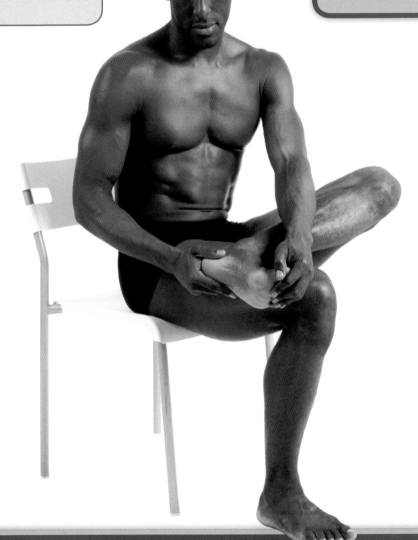

Slope-Down Foot Stretch

The isometric Slope-Down Foot Stretch uses your own resistance to create a soothing stretch for the top of your foot and your shin.

HOW TO DO IT

• Sit on a chair or on the floor, and cross your left leg over your right, placing your left ankle on top of your right thigh.

• Brace your right heel with your right hand.

• Grasp your foot so that the palm of your hand lies across the top of your foot and your fingers are wrapped around the bottom.

• Using your palm on the top outside of your foot, push down. At the same time, pull up the bottom of your foot with your fingers; this creates the "slope-down."

• Release the stretch, and then repeat on the opposite side.

DO IT RIGHT

• Push forcefully with your palms—their downward force must be stronger than the upward force of your pulling fingers.
• Avoid allowing your foot to shift—firmly stabilize your ankle and heel.

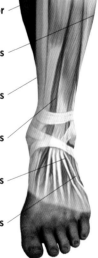

tibialis anterior

peroneus

extensor digitorum longus

extensor hallucis longus

extensor hallucis brevis

extensor digitorum brevis

Annotation Key

Bold text indicates target muscles
Light text indicates other working muscles
* indicates deep muscles

Band-Assisted Wing Stretch

Stretching your ankles can serve many benefits. The ankles carry your entire body weight and can easily become overexerted, causing cramping and pain. The Band-Assisted Wing Stretch can help keep your ankles strong and more limber.

HOW TO DO IT

• Sit on a chair with your feet flat on the floor and more than hip-width apart.

• Loop an elastic resistance band around the inside of your right foot, and hold both ends of the band with your right hand.

• Keeping your right leg stable, flex your right foot and pull the band to your right, stretching the inside of your ankle.

• Release the stretch, and then repeat on the opposite side.

DO IT RIGHT

• Use a towel if you don't have a resistance band.
• Avoid shifting your weight to the side you are stretching; your weight should be evenly balanced on your sit bones.

FACT FILE

TARGETS
• Ankles
• Calves

TYPE
• Static

BENEFITS
• Reduces ankle pain and tightness
• Increases mobility in ankles and surrounding tendons
• Improves gait and posture

CAUTIONS
• Ankle injury
• Foot pain

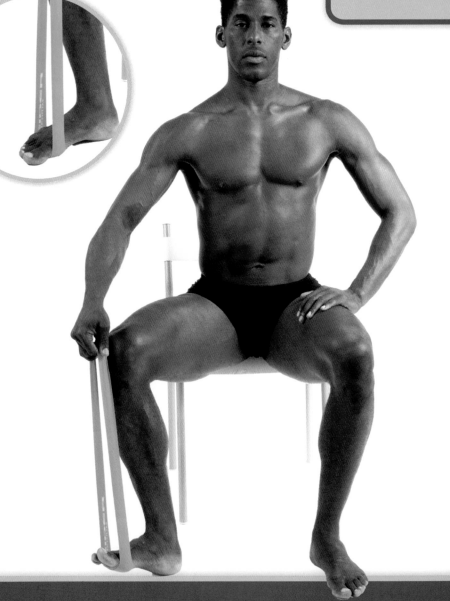

gastrocnemius

peroneus brevis

peroneus longus

soleus

tibialis posterior*

Band-Assisted Sickle Stretch

FACT FILE

TARGETS
• Ankles
• Calves

TYPE
• Static

BENEFITS
• Reduces ankle pain and tightness
• Increases mobility in ankles and surrounding tendons
• Improves gait and posture

CAUTIONS
• Severe ankle or foot pain

Practicing this Band-Assisted Sickle Stretch can be highly beneficial for athletes or anyone who performs aerobic activities. If you are constantly on your feet, you should add this ankle stretch to your exercise regimen.

HOW TO DO IT

• Sit on a chair with your feet flat on the floor and more than hip-width apart.

• Loop an elastic resistance band around the inside of your right foot, and hold both ends of the band with your right hand.

• Keeping your right leg stable, flex your right foot and pull the band to your left, stretching the outside of your ankle.

• Release the stretch, and then repeat on the opposite side.

DO IT RIGHT

• Use a towel if you don't have an elastic resistance band.
• Avoid shifting your weight to the side you are stretching; your weight should be evenly balanced on your sit bones.

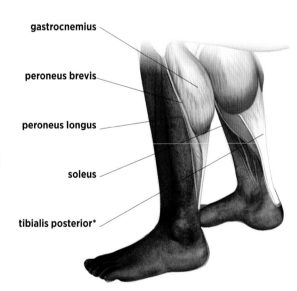

gastrocnemius

peroneus brevis

peroneus longus

soleus

tibialis posterior*

Annotation Key
Bold text indicates target muscles
Light text indicates other working muscles
* indicates deep muscles

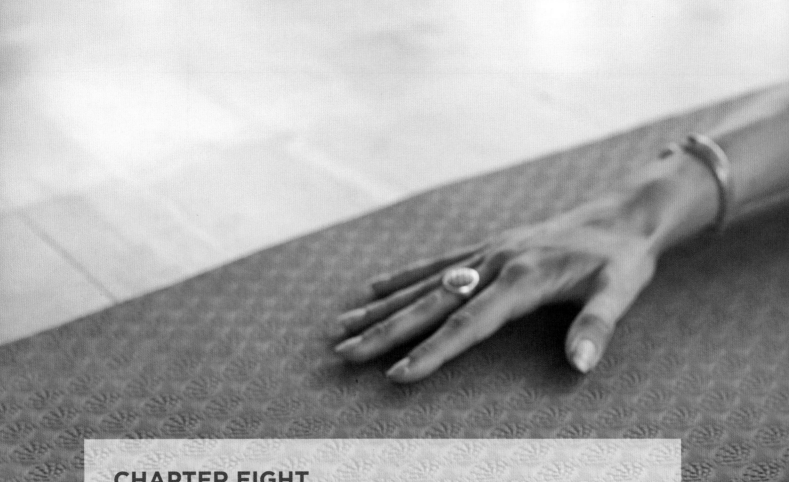

CHAPTER EIGHT

STRETCHING ROUTINES

Now that you have familiarized yourself with a variety of individual stretches, you're ready to perform combinations of stretches that target specific uses of your body. Here are 3 categories of stretching routines for you to try: Body, Sports, and Everyday routines. Go slow and steady, and your body will thank you.

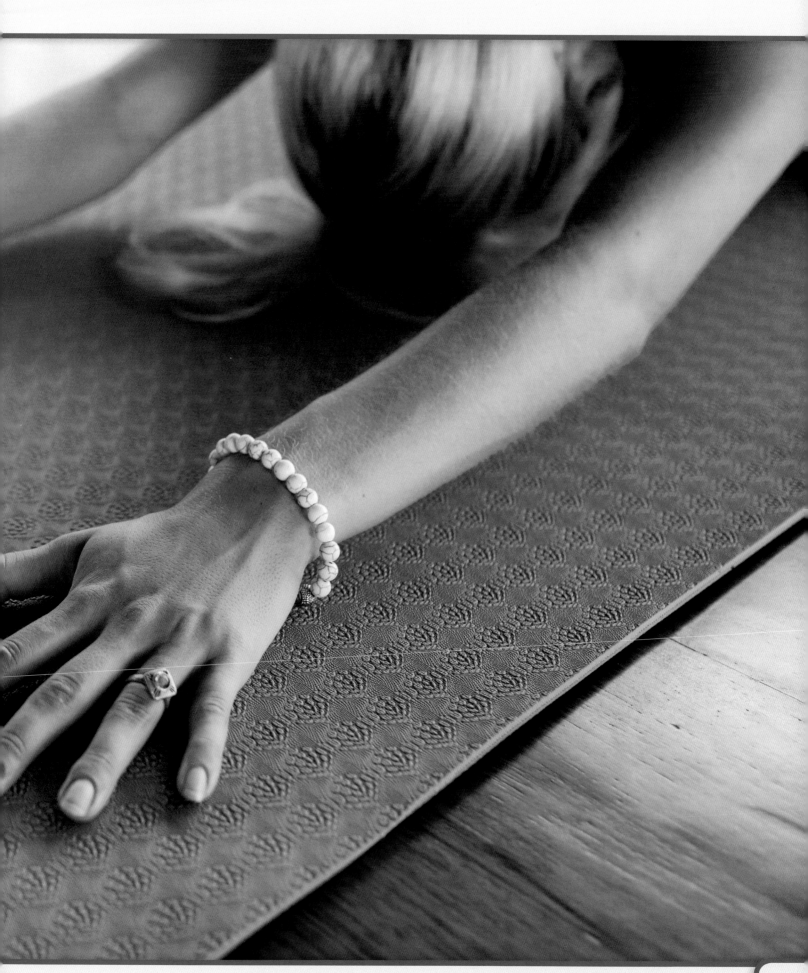

Full Body

This simple full-body series opens your chest and hips and helps improve your overall body alignment and range of motion.

1 WALL-ASSISTED CHEST STRETCH

Pages 104–5
• Perform 30–45 seconds per side

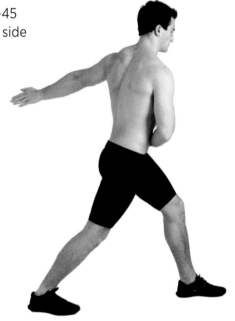

2 BOW YOGA STRETCH

Pages 122–23
• Perform 30–45 seconds

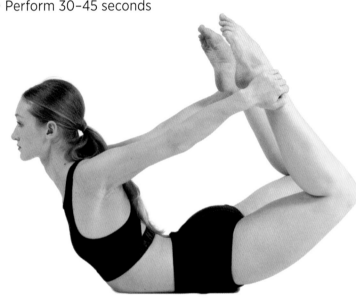

3 EXTENDED SIDE ANGLE YOGA STRETCH

Pages 132–33
• Perform 30–45 seconds per side

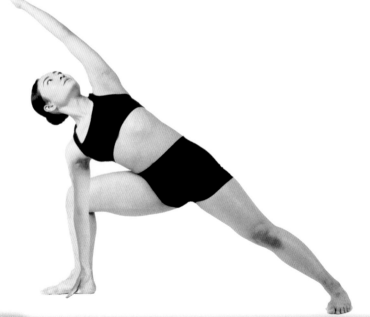

4 HALF MOON YOGA STRETCH

Pages 134–35
• Perform 30–45 seconds per side

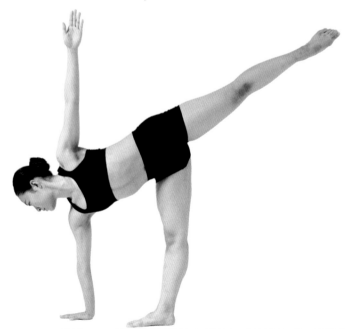

FACT FILE

TARGETS
• Full body

EQUIPMENT
• Body weight

BENEFITS
• Opens chest and hips and lengthens muscles in arms and legs

5 DOUBLE-LEG STRETCH

Pages 156–57
• Perform 30 seconds

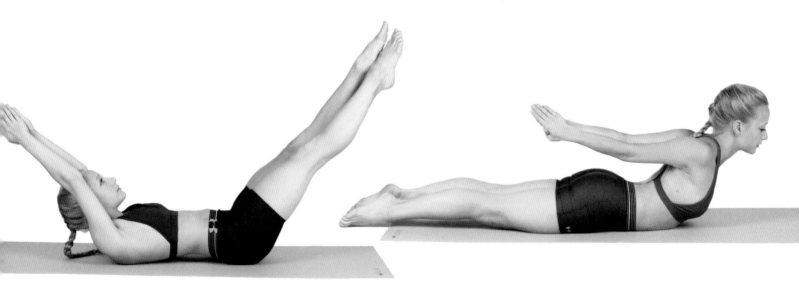

6 BREASTSTROKE STRETCH

Pages 84–85
• Perform 6 repetitions

7 STANDING QUADRICEPS STRETCH

Page 264
• Perform 30–45 seconds per side

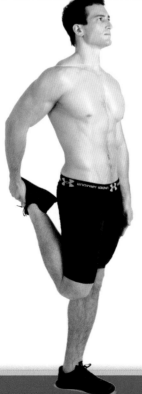

8 FORWARD LUNGE WITH TWIST

Pages 280–81
• Perform 30–45 seconds per side

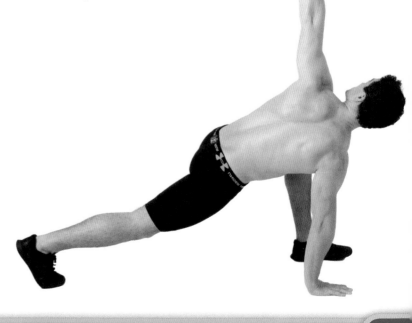

Neck

Loosen up those nasty morning cricks in your neck with this relaxing routine.
It targets all the muscles along the front, back, and sides of your neck.

1 SCALP STRETCH

Page 26
• Perform 30 seconds

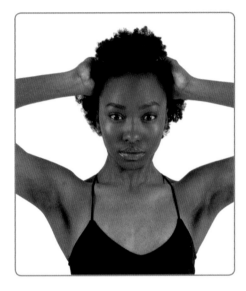

2 CERVICAL STARS

Pages 28–29
• Perform 30 seconds per direction

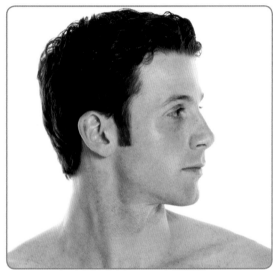

3 FLEXION STRETCH

Page 30
• Perform 30 seconds

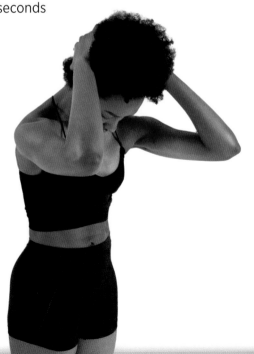

4 FLEXION ISOMETRIC

Page 31
• Perform 30 seconds

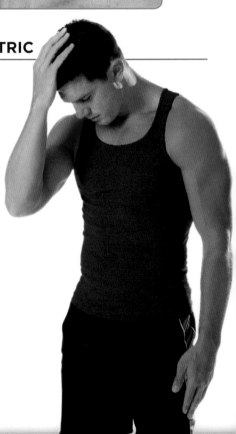

TARGETS
• Neck
• Upper back

EQUIPMENT
• Body weight

BENEFITS
• Loosens stiff
  neck muscles
  and reduces
  tension in
  upper back
  movement

5 LATERAL STRETCH

Page 32
• Perform 30 seconds per direction

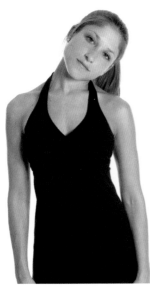

6 LATERAL ISOMETRIC

Page 33
• Perform 30 seconds per direction

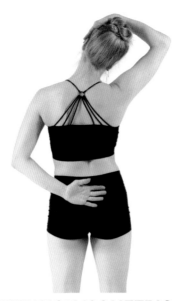

7 EXTENSION STRETCH

Page 36
• Perform 30 seconds

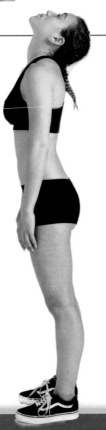

8 EXTENSION ISOMETRIC

Page 37
• Perform 30 seconds

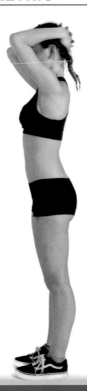

Arms

Lengthen your biceps and triceps and loosen your wrists after a long day at the computer or after a rigorous workout with this series of arm stretches.

1 CHAIR YOGA STRETCH

Pages 48–49
• Perform 30–45 seconds

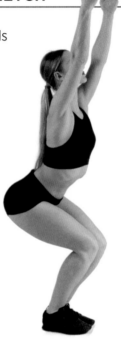

2 COW FACE YOGA STRETCH

Pages 58–59
• Perform 30 seconds per side

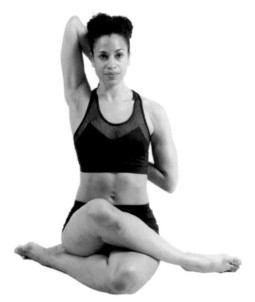

3 DOWNWARD-FACING DOG

Pages 72–73
• Perform 30–45 seconds

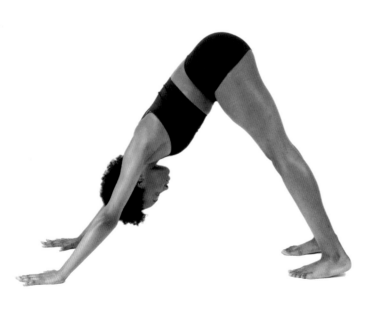

4 THREE-LEGGED DOG

Pages 74–75
• Perform 30 seconds per side

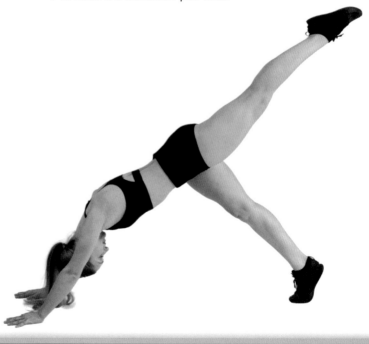

TARGETS
- Biceps
- Triceps
- Forearms
- Wrists

EQUIPMENT
- Body weight
- Chair

BENEFITS
- Reduces pain and stiffness in arms and wrists

5 TRICEPS STRETCH

Pages 96–97
- Perform 30 seconds per side

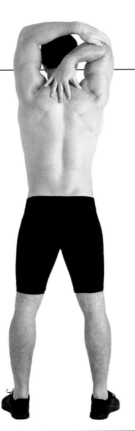

6 BICEPS STRETCH

Pages 98–99
- Perform six repetitions

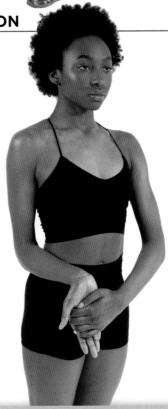

7 WRIST FLEXION

Page 100
- Perform 30 seconds per direction

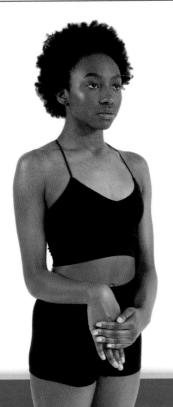

8 WRIST EXTENSION

Page 101
- Perform 30 seconds per direction

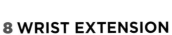

Chest

This chest-opening routine helps improve your posture and lung capacity and increases the range of motion in tight shoulders.

1 WALL-ASSISTED CHEST STRETCH

Pages 104–5
• Perform 30–45 seconds per side

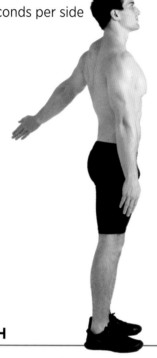

2 CAMEL YOGA STRETCH

Pages 106–7
• Perform 30–45 seconds

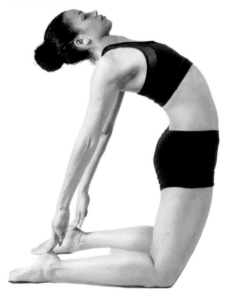

3 SAW STRETCH

Pages 108–9
• Perform 30–45 seconds

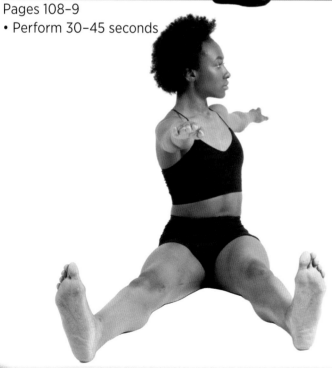

4 ONE-LEGGED ROYAL PIGEON YOGA STRETCH

Pages 110–11
• Perform 30 seconds per side

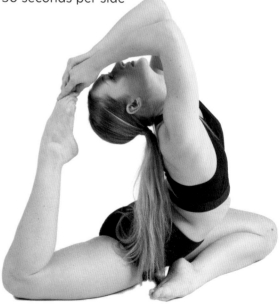

5 UPWARD-FACING PLANK STRETCH

Pages 112–13
• Perform 30–45 seconds

6 UPWARD-FACING DOG YOGA STRETCH

Pages 114–15
• Perform 30–45 seconds

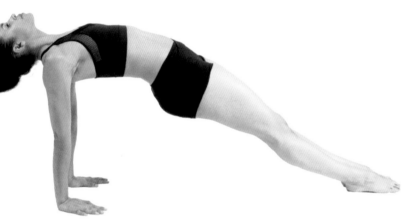

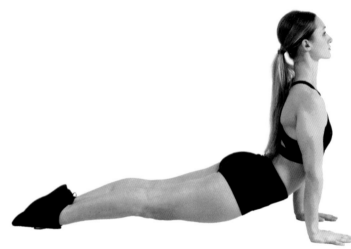

7 RISING SWAN STRETCH

Pages 116–17
• Perform 30–45 seconds

8 FISH YOGA STRETCH

Pages 118–19
• Perform 30–45 seconds

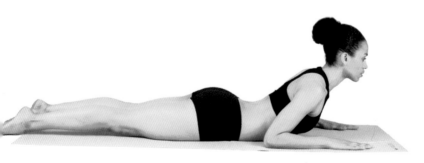

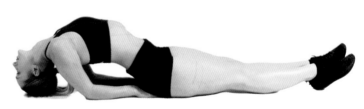

Abdominals

Try this ab-stretching routine to improve core stability and overall balance. It also reduces the risk of lower-back injury.

1 DIAGONAL REACH

Pages 128–29
• Perform 30 seconds per direction

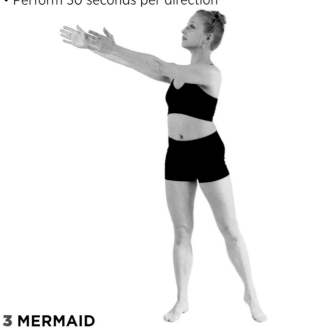

2 TRIANGLE YOGA STRETCH

Pages 130–31
• Perform 30 seconds per side

3 MERMAID

Pages 136–37
• Perform 30 seconds per side

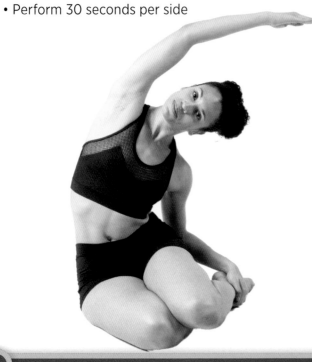

4 SIDE-LEANING HALF STRADDLE

Page 140
• Perform 30 seconds per side

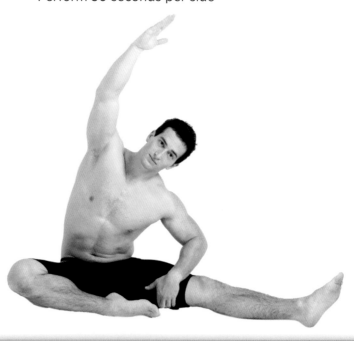

FACT FILE

TARGETS
• Abdominals
• Obliques
• Lower back

EQUIPMENT
• Body weight

BENEFITS
• Stabilizes abdominals and lower-back muscles while improving overall flexibility

5 LYING-DOWN ARCH STRETCH

Page 141
• Perform 30–45 seconds

6 SIDE-LYING RIB STRETCH

Pages 146–47
• Perform 30 seconds per side

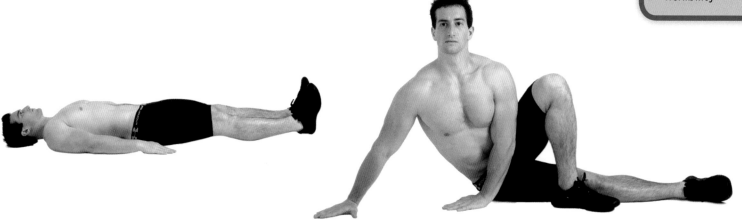

7 WHEEL YOGA STRETCH

Pages 152–53
• Perform 30–45 seconds

8 RECLINING HERO YOGA STRETCH

Pages 158–59
• Perform 30–45 seconds

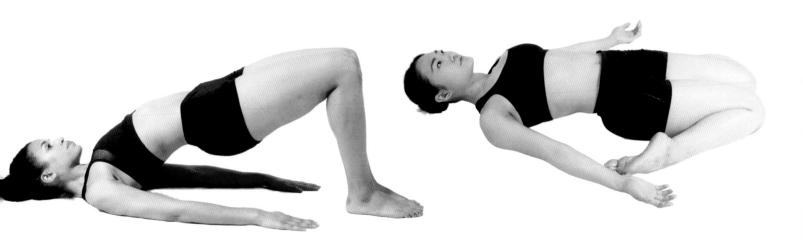

Lower Back

Improve your flexibility and alleviate lower back pain with this soothing routine. The extension stretches are a great counterpoint to long hours of sitting.

1 HALF LORD OF THE FISHES YOGA STRETCH
Pages 168–69
• Perform 30 seconds per side

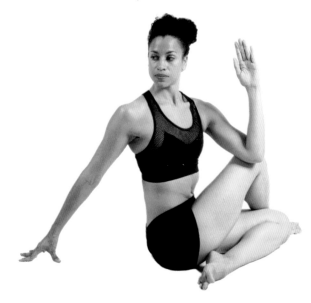

2 HIP CIRCLES
Pages 172–73
• Perform 30 seconds per direction

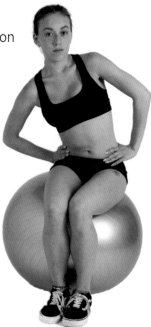

3 COBRA STRETCH
Pages 176–77
• Perform 30–45 seconds

4 PRONE TRUNK RAISE
Pages 178–79
• Perform 30–45 seconds

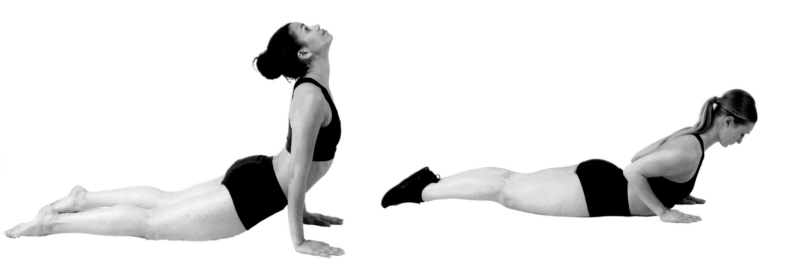

FACT FILE

TARGETS
• Lower back

EQUIPMENT
• Body weight
• Swiss Ball

BENEFITS
• Improves flexibility in lower back and reduces back pain movement

5 ARM-LEG EXTENSION

Pages 180–81
• Perform 30 seconds per side

6 ROTATED BACK EXTENSION

Pages 182–83
• Perform 30 seconds per side

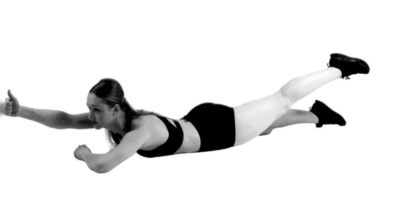

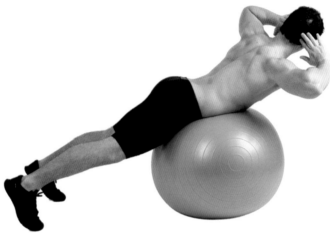

7 UNILATERAL KNEE-TO-CHEST STRETCH

Page 188
• Perform 30 seconds per side

8 LATISSIMUS DORSI STRETCH

Pages 190–91
• Perform 30 seconds per side

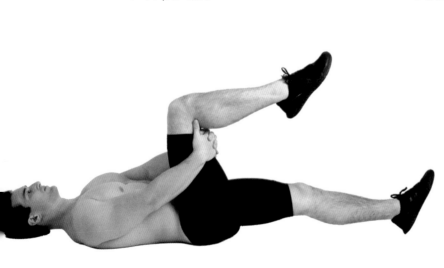

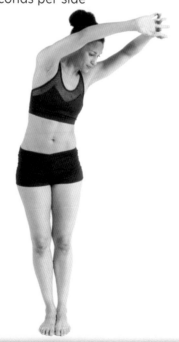

Hips

Add a little spring in your step with this hip-opening routine. It'll help address poor posture and muscle imbalances in your lower body.

1 HIP AND ILLIOTIBIAL BAND STRETCH

Pages 196–97
• Perform 30 seconds per side

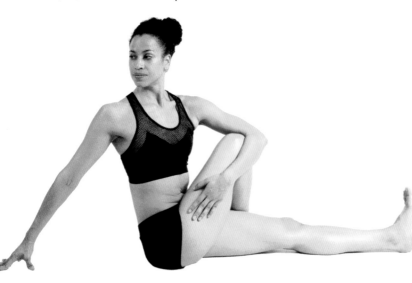

2 SUMO SQUAT

Pages 204–5
• Perform 30–45 seconds

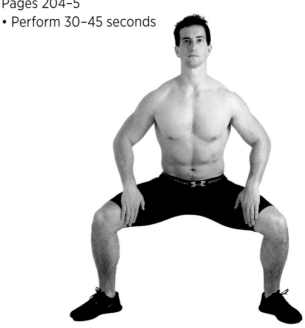

3 SIDE-LEANING SUMO SQUAT

Pages 206–7
• Perform 30 seconds per side

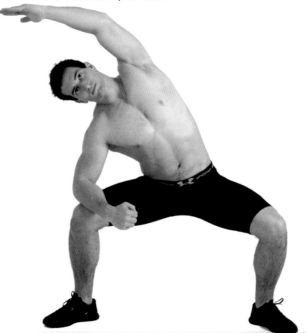

4 SIDE ADDUCTOR STRETCH

Pages 208–9
• Perform 30 seconds per side

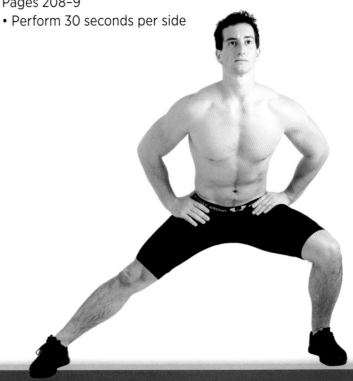

FACT FILE

TARGETS
• Lower body

EQUIPMENT
• Body weight

BENEFITS
• Enhances range of motion in hips and lower body and improves overall balance

5 GARLAND YOGA STRETCH

Pages 212–13
• Perform 30–45 seconds

6 QUADRUPED LEG LIFT

Pages 216–17
• Perform 30 seconds per side

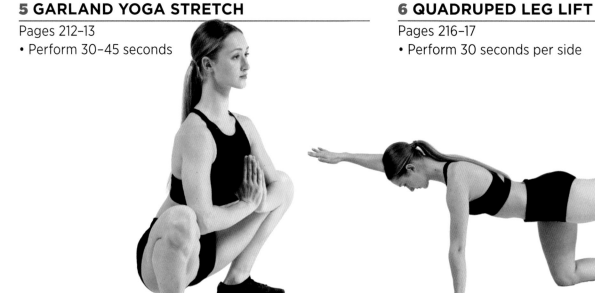

7 FROG STRADDLE

Pages 218–19
• Perform 30 seconds per side

8 PIGEON STRETCH

Pages 220–21
• Perform 30 seconds per side

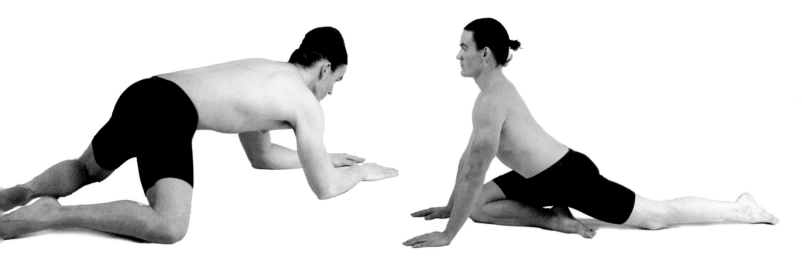

Legs

This all-around leg routine will loosen, ready, and lengthen tight hamstrings or calves.
Try this leg-stretching routine to increase your flexibility and reduce the risk of injury.

1 STANDING FORWARD BEND

Pages 258–59
• Perform 30–45 seconds

2 STANDING QUADRICEPS STRETCH

Pages 264
• Perform 30–45
  seconds per side

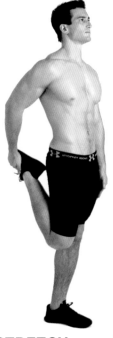

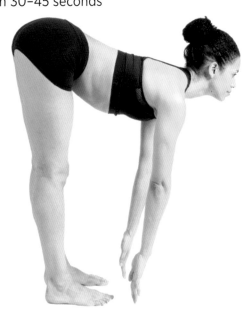

3 INVERTED HAMSTRING STRETCH

Pages 268–69
• Perform 30 seconds per side

4 HIP FLEXOR STRETCH

Pages 270–71
• Perform 30 seconds per side

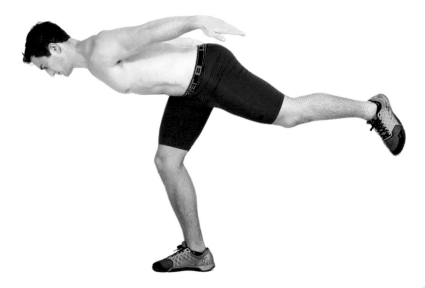

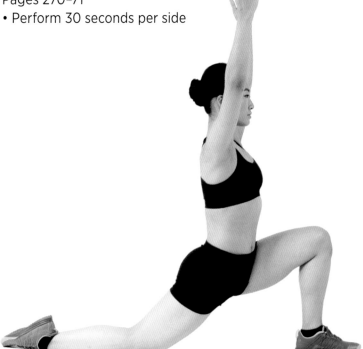

FACT FILE

TARGETS
• Quadriceps
• Hamstrings
• Calves
• Ankles

EQUIPMENT
• Body weight

BENEFITS
• Lengthens leg muscles, improves range of motion, and helps prevent injury

5 HIP-TO-THIGH STRETCH

Pages 272–73
• Perform 30 seconds per side

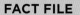

6 FORWARD LUNGE

Pages 278–79
• Perform 30 seconds per side

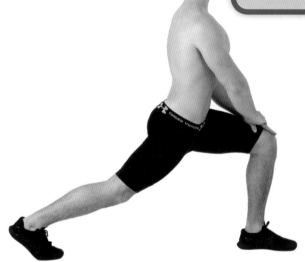

7 DEEP LUNGE

Pages 286–87
• Perform 30 seconds per side

8 KNEELING SPRINTER STRETCH

Page 265
• Perform 30 seconds per side

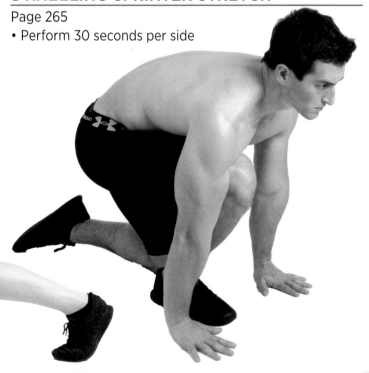

Shoulders

Melt away the tension in your shoulders with this stretching routine. It eases upper-body discomfort and improves shoulder mobility.

1 WARRIOR III YOGA STRETCH
Pages 52–53
• Perform 30 seconds per side

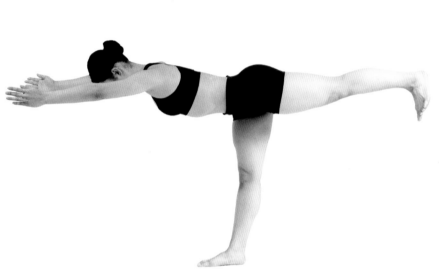

2 BHARADVAJA'S TWIST
Pages 62–63
• Perform 30 seconds per side

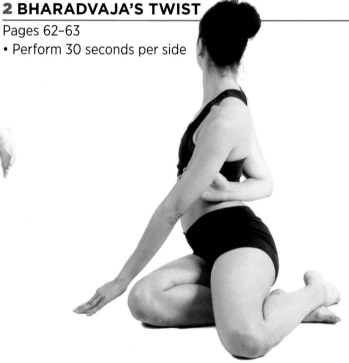

3 FRONT DELTOID TOWEL STRETCH
Page 68
• Perform 30 seconds

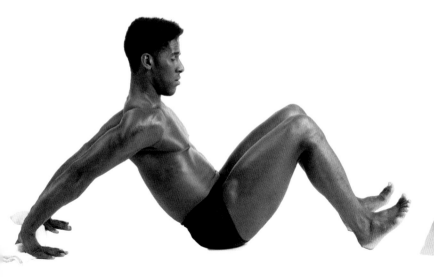

4 SPINE STRETCH REACHING
Page 69
• Perform 30–45 seconds

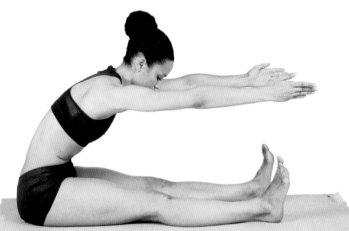

5 DOWNWARD-FACING DOG
Pages 72–73
• Perform 30–45 seconds

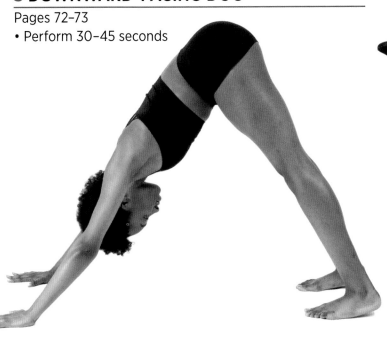

6 THREE-LEGGED DOG
Pages 74–75
• Perform 30 seconds per side

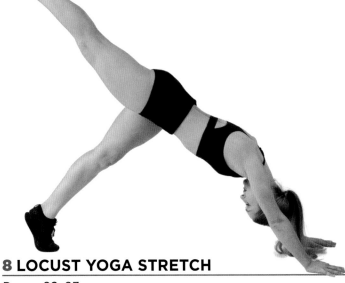

7 THREAD THE NEEDLE
Pages 80–81
• Perform 30 seconds per side

8 LOCUST YOGA STRETCH
Pages 82–83
• Perform 30–45 seconds

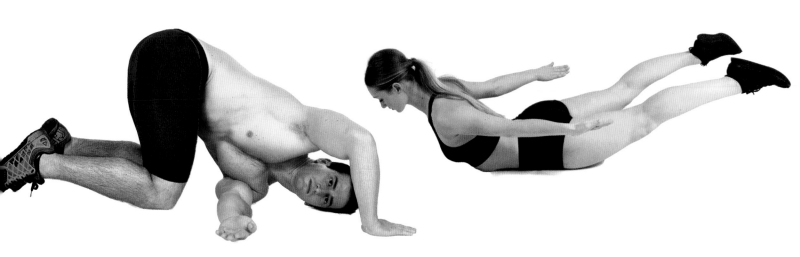

Baseball

Get ready to take the field with these all-around stretches. You'll improve your swing and overall athletic performance while reducing the risk of strains and other injuries.

1 LION STRETCH AND EYE BOX STRETCH COMBO

Page 27
• Perform 5 seconds

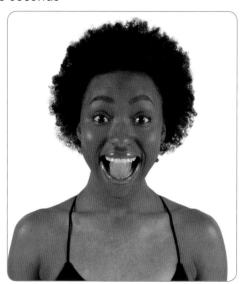

2 FRONT DELTOID TOWEL STRETCH

Page 68
• Perform 30 seconds

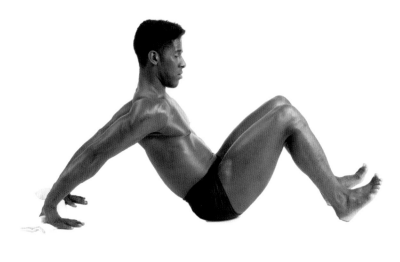

3 SIDE PLANK

Pages 144–45
• Perform 30 seconds per side

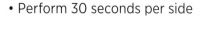

4 SEATED RUSSIAN TWIST

Pages 174–75
• Perform 30 seconds per side

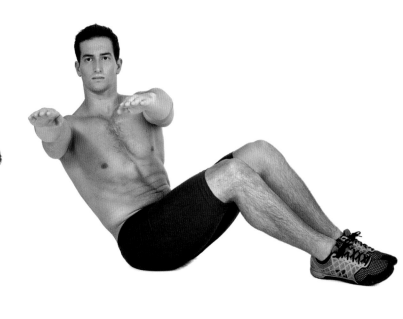

5 TRICEPS STRETCH

Pages 96–97
• Perform 30 seconds per side

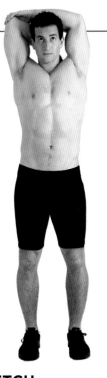

6 BICEPS STRETCH

Pages 98–99
• Perform
  30 seconds per side

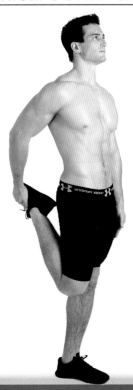

7 SIDE ADDUCTOR STRETCH

Pages 208–9
• Perform 30 seconds per side

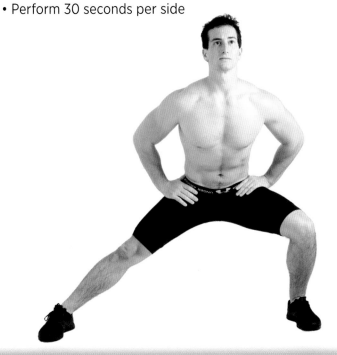

8 STANDING QUADRICEPS STRETCH

Page 264
• Perform 30–45
  seconds per side

Football

An essential part of every football player's routine, stretching activates the hips, glutes, and legs and improves muscle imbalances.

1 TURTLE NECK

Page 40
• Perform 10 repetitions

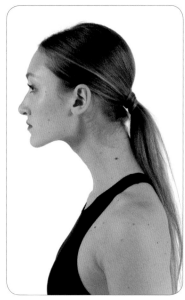

2 SHRUG

Page 41
• Perform 30–45 seconds

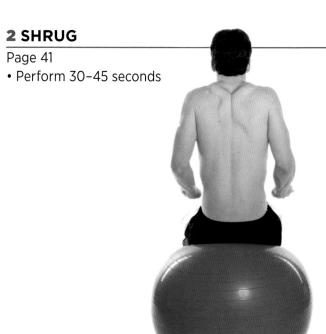

3 SCOOP RHOMBOIDS

Page 57
• Perform 10 repetitions

4 MARICHI'S YOGA STRETCH

Pages 60–61
• Perform 10 repetitions

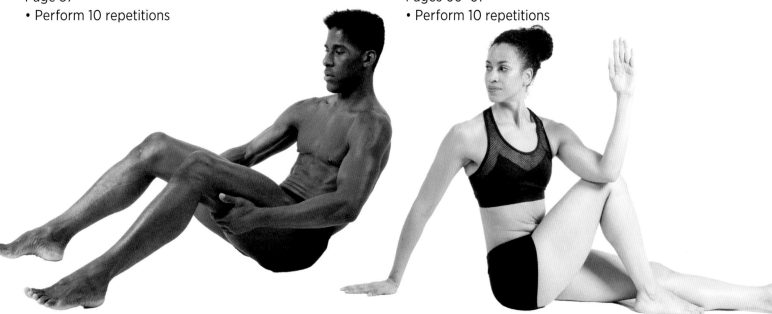

FACT FILE

TARGETS
- Back
- Core
- Legs

EQUIPMENT
- Body weight
- Swiss Ball

BENEFITS
- Increases mobility in shoulders, back, and legs

5 SIDE ADDUCTOR STRETCH

Pages 208–9
- Perform 30 seconds per side

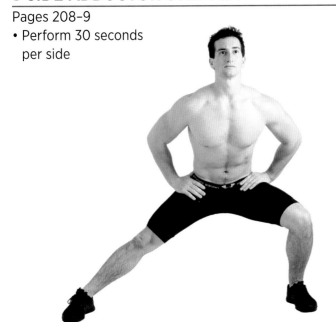

6 KNEELING SPRINTER STRETCH

Page 265
- Perform 30 seconds per side

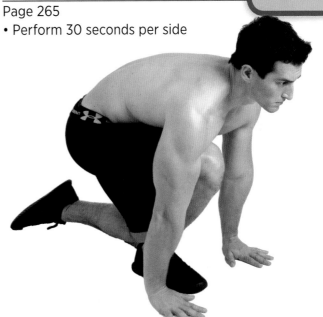

7 MOUNTAIN CLIMBER STRETCH

Pages 296–97
- Perform 30 seconds per side

8 RECLINING TWIST

Pages 92–93
- Perform 30 seconds per side

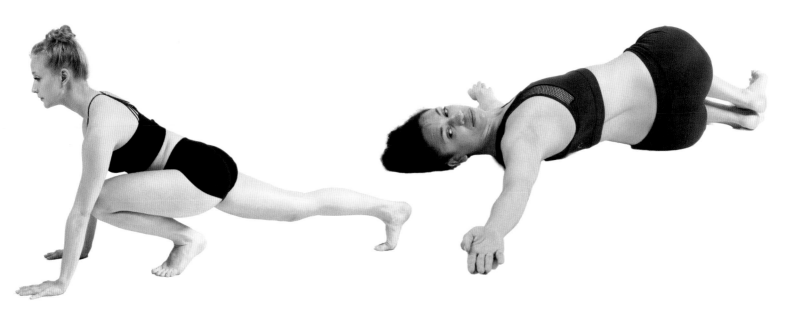

Tennis

Ace your next serve with this all-around routine. It stretches all the major muscle groups: arms, legs, and core.

1 SAW STRETCH

Pages 108–9
• Perform 30 seconds per side

2 SPINE TWIST

Pages 64–65
• Perform 30 seconds per side

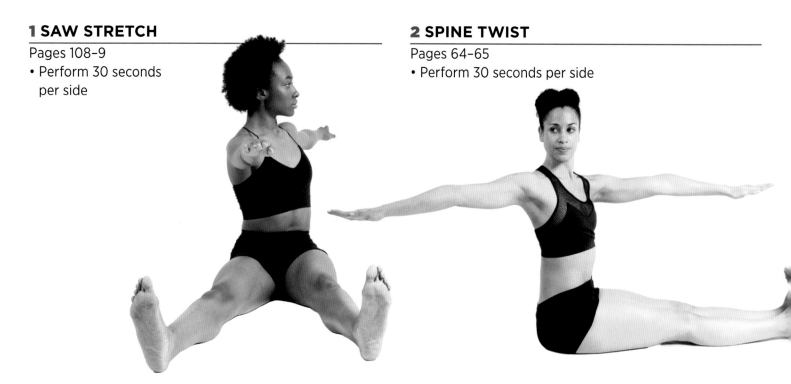

3 SPINE STRETCH FORWARD

Pages 66–67
• Perform 30–45 seconds

4 INVERTED HAMSTRING

Page 268–69
• Perform 30 seconds per side

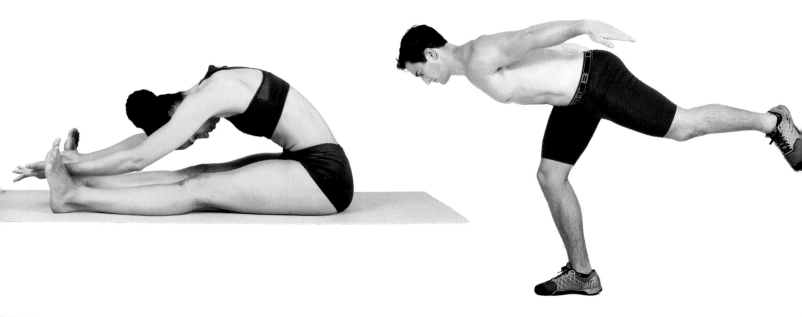

5 REVOLVED HEAD-TO-KNEE YOGA STRETCH
Pages 142–43
• Perform
  30 seconds per side

6 SIDE PLANK
Pages 144–45
• Perform
  30 seconds per side

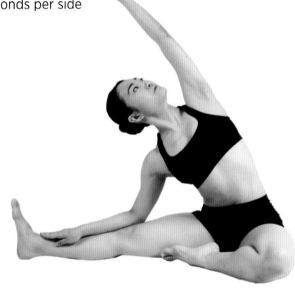

7 SEATED RUSSIAN TWIST
Pages 174–75
• Perform 30 seconds per side

8 SIDE-LYING KNEE BEND
Pages 304–5
• Perform 30 seconds per side

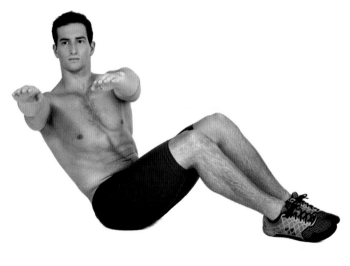
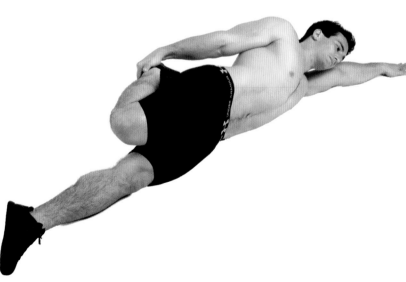

FACT FILE

TARGETS
• Chest
• Abdominals
• Hips
• Legs

EQUIPMENT
• Body weight

BENEFITS
• Develops core flexibility and improves range of motion in shoulders and hips

Soccer

Bring your game to the next level by developing your flexibility and range of motion with these soccer stretches.

1 SIDE ADDUCTOR STRETCH

Pages 208–9
• Perform 30 seconds per side

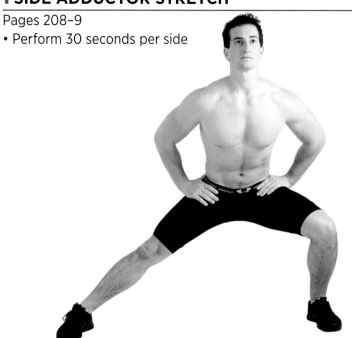

2 KNEE-PULL PLANK

Pages 294–95
• Perform 30 seconds per side

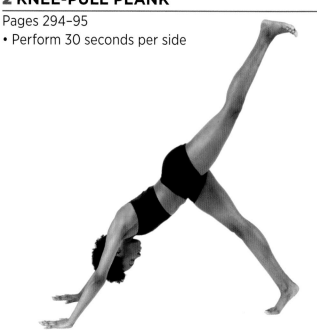

3 MOUNTAIN CLIMBER STRETCH

Pages 296–97
• Perform 30 seconds per side

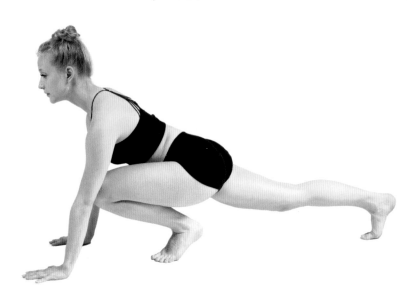

4 KNEE SQUAT

Pages 312–13
• Perform 30–45 seconds

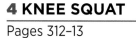
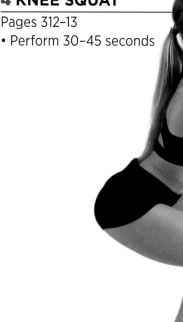

FACT FILE

TARGETS
• Core
• Hips
• Quadriceps
• Hamstrings

EQUIPMENT
• Body weight
• Swiss Ball

BENEFITS
• Improves
range of
motion in hips
and stretches
groin and leg
muscles

5 BILATERAL QUAD STRETCH

Pages 314–15
• Perform 30–45 seconds

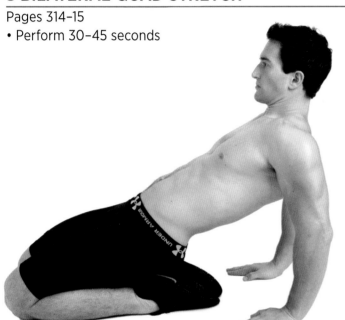

6 SINGLE-LEG STRETCH

Pages 154–55
• Perform 30 seconds per side

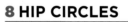

7 REVOLVED TRIANGLE YOGA STRETCH

Pages 170–71
• Perform 30 seconds per side

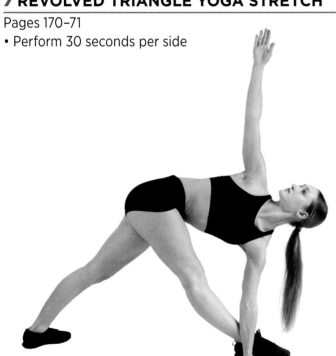

8 HIP CIRCLES

Pages 172–73
• Perform 30
seconds per direction

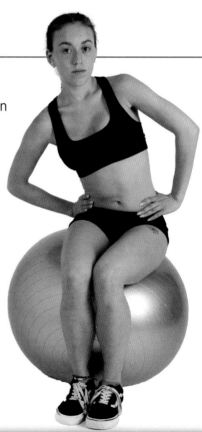

Swimming

These stretches will prepare you for the pool and help you master your swimming strokes with a better range of motion and greater flexibility.

1 LION STRETCH AND EYE BOX STRETCH COMBO

Page 27
• Perform 5 seconds per direction

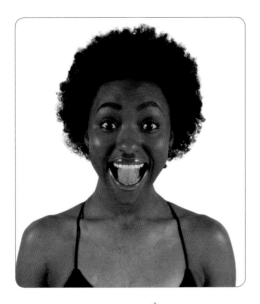

2 HIGH PLANK PIKE

Pages 42–43
• Perform 30–45 seconds

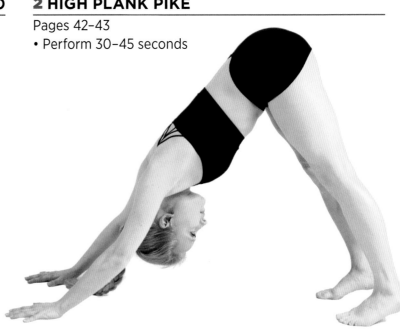

3 UPWARD SALUTE

Pages 54–55
• Perform 30–45 seconds

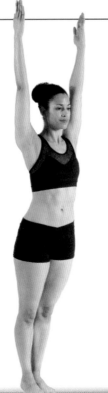

4 STANDING BACK ROLL

Page 56
• Perform 30 seconds

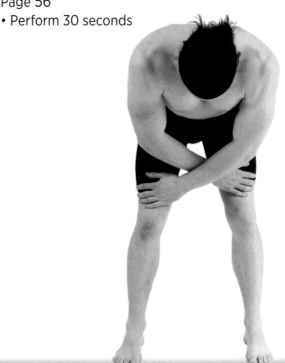

5 BREASTSTROKE STRETCH

Pages 84–85
• Perform 30 seconds

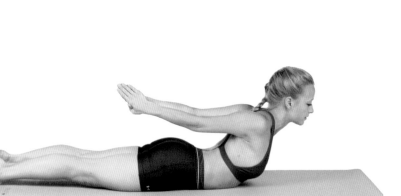

6 SCISSORS STRETCH

Pages 316–17
• Perform 30–45 seconds per side

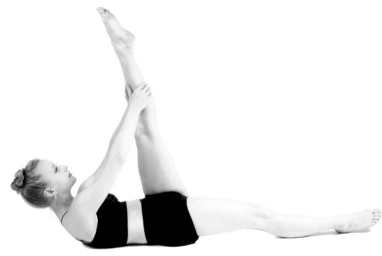

7 CORKSCREW STRETCH

Pages 160–61
• Perform 30–45 seconds

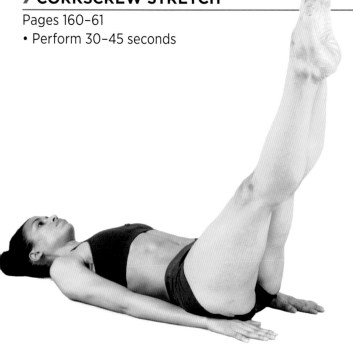

8 SEATED RUSSIAN TWIST

Pages 174–75
• Perform 30 seconds per side

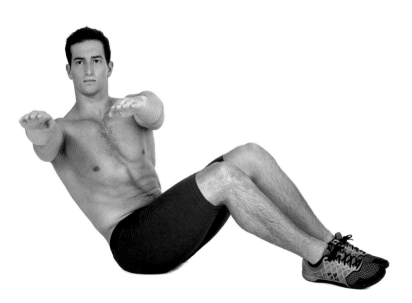

Martial Arts

These stretches will sharpen your focus and loosen your joints for your next martial arts class. You'll reduce the risk of injury and improve your range of motion.

1 ROTATION STRETCH

Page 34
• Perform 30 seconds per side

2 ROTATION ISOMETRIC

Page 35
• Perform 30 seconds per side

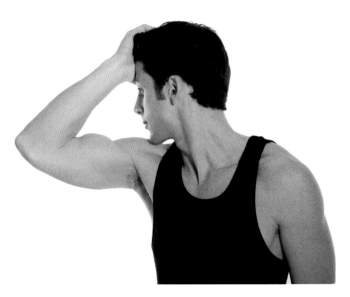

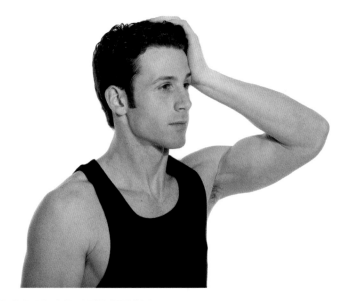

3 CAT-TO-COW STRETCH

Pages 78–79
• Perform 30–45 seconds

4 BRIDGE STRETCH

Pages 86–87
• Perform 30–45 seconds

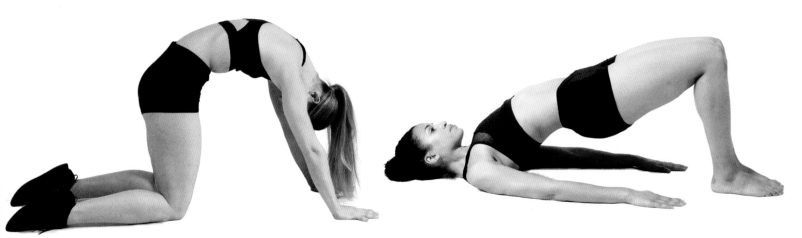

FACT FILE

TARGETS
• Neck
• Back
• Hips
• Legs

EQUIPMENT
• Body weight

BENEFITS
• Improves overall agility and flexibility in hips and legs

5 SEATED RUSSIAN TWIST

Pages 174–75
• Perform 30 seconds per side

6 KNEE-TO-CHEST HUG

Pages 88–89
• Perform 30 seconds per side

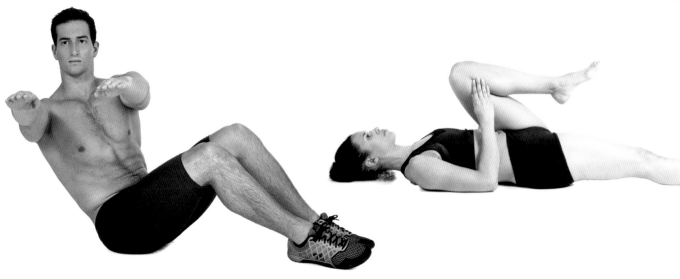

7 KNEE-PULL PLANK

Pages 294–95
• Perform 30 seconds per side

8 ROLLOVER STRETCH

Pages 192–93
• Perform 30–45 seconds

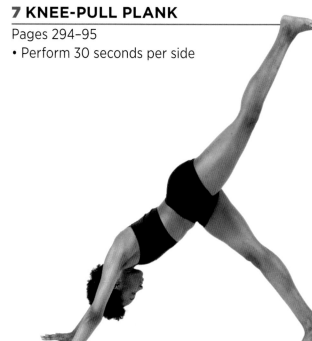

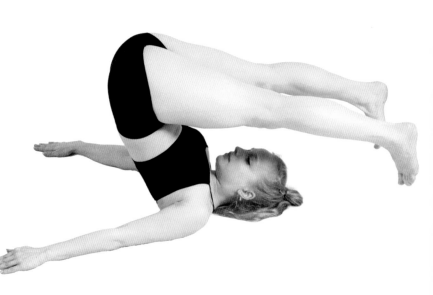

Running

Sprint across the finish line with smoother strides. You'll lengthen your hamstrings and quadriceps with this runner routine.

1 COBRA STRETCH

Pages 176–77
• Perform 30–45 seconds

2 ARM-LEG EXTENSION

Pages 180–81
• Perform 30 seconds per side

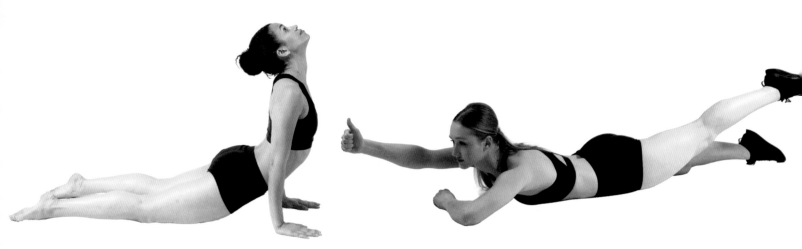

3 ABDOMINAL KICK

Pages 184–85
• Perform 30 seconds per side

4 INCHWORM STRETCH

Pages 186–87
• Perform 30 seconds per step

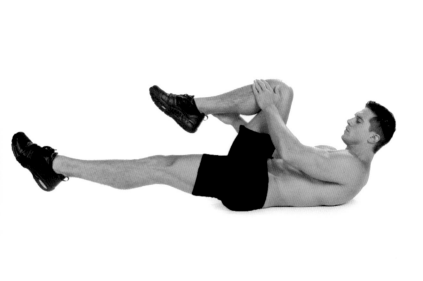

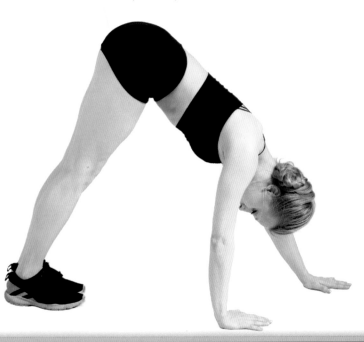

5 UNILATERAL LEG RAISE

Page 189
• Perform 30 seconds per side

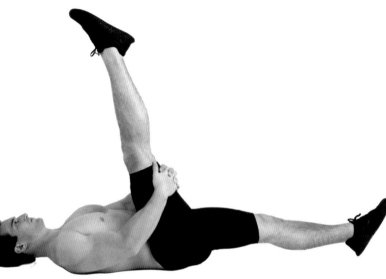

6 SIDE-LEANING SUMO SQUAT

Pages 206–7
• Perform 30 seconds per side

7 REVOLVED TRIANGLE YOGA STRETCH

Pages 170–71
• Perform 30 seconds per side

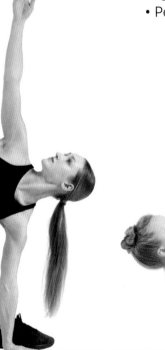

8 SCISSORS STRETCH

Pages 316–17
• Perform 30 seconds per side

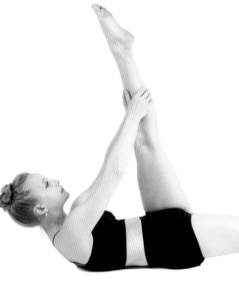

Sunrise Yoga

Namaste... Roll out your yoga mat and try this rejuvenating routine to get your blood flowing and get you ready for the day.

1 GOOD MORNING STRETCH

Pages 46–47
• Perform 30–45 seconds

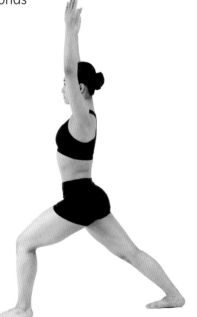

2 TWISTING CHAIR STRETCH

Pages 50–51
• Perform 30 seconds per side

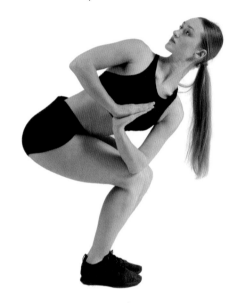

3 WARRIOR I YOGA STRETCH

Pages 266–67
• Perform 30 seconds per side

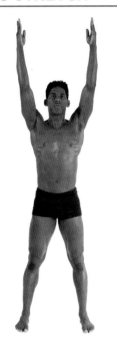

4 WARRIOR II YOGA STRETCH

Pages 198–99
• Perform 30 seconds per side

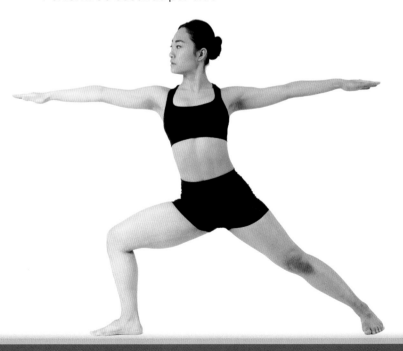

FACT FILE

TARGETS
• Full body

EQUIPMENT
• Body weight

BENEFITS
• Improves balance and flexibility and boosts circulation

5 WARRIOR III YOGA STRETCH

Pages 52–53
• Perform 30 seconds per side

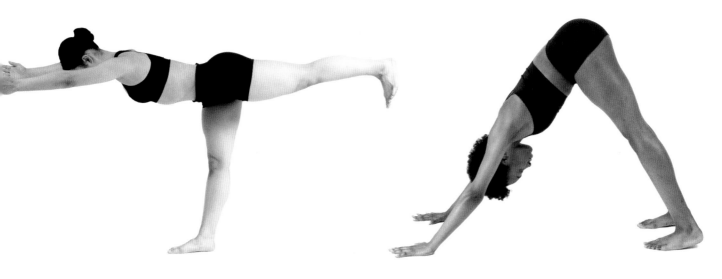

6 DOWNWARD-FACING DOG

Pages 72–73
• Perform 30–45 seconds

7 UPWARD-FACING DOG YOGA STRETCH

Pages 114–15
• Perform 30–45 seconds

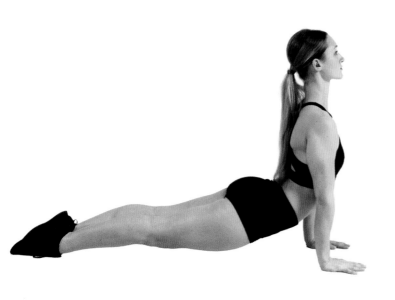

8 TREE YOGA STRETCH

Pages 200–201
• Perform 30 seconds per side

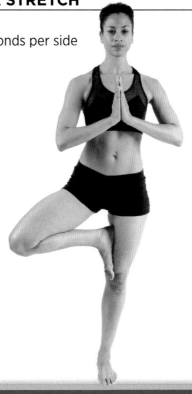

Morning Blast

Jump-start your day with this invigorating full-body series that deeply opens your chest and hips and targets all your main muscle groups.

1 HALF-FROG YOGA STRETCH

Pages 120–21
• Perform 30 seconds per side

2 LYING-DOWN PRETZEL STRETCH

Pages 124–25
• Perform 30 seconds per side

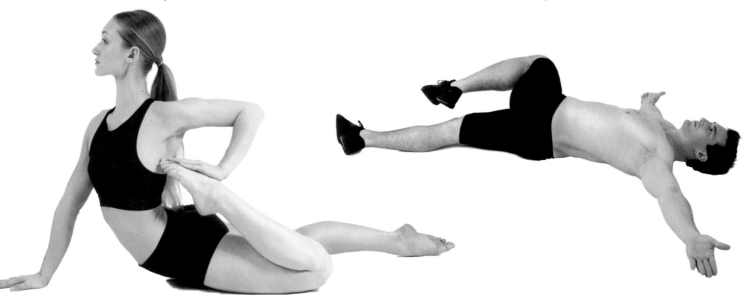

3 HALF STRADDLE STRETCH

Pages 138–39
• Perform 30 seconds per side

4 BREASTSTROKE STRETCH

Pages 84–85
• Perform 30 seconds

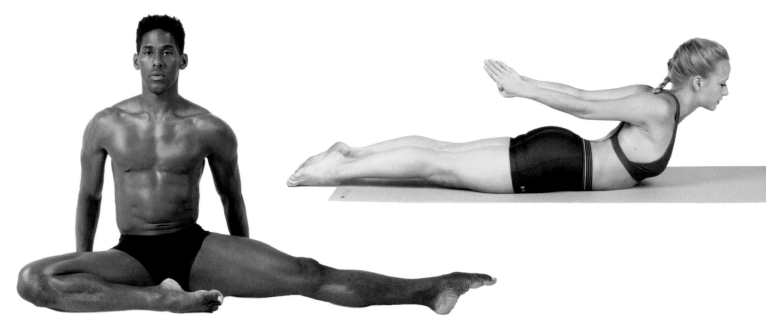

FACT FILE

TARGETS
• Full body

EQUIPMENT
• Body weight

BENEFITS
• Boosts circulation and opens hips and chest

5 REVERSE LUNGE WITH LATERAL EXTENSION

Pages 282–83
• Perform 30 seconds per side

6 DEEP LUNGE

Pages 286–87
• Perform 30 seconds per side

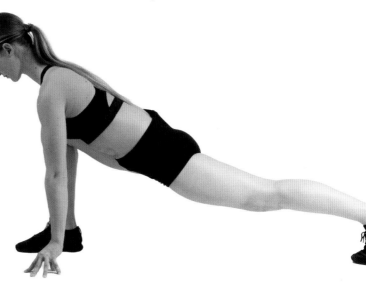

7 KNEE-PULL PLANK

Pages 294–95
• Perform 30 seconds per side

8 SIDE-LYING KNEE BEND

Pages 304–5
• Perform 30 seconds per side

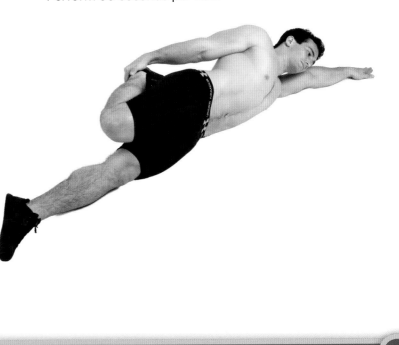

Evening Repose

Unwind at the end of a stressful day with this series of stretches that targets your lower-back and leg muscles.

1 KNEELING LAT STRETCH

Pages 70–71
• Perform 30 seconds per side

2 HEAD-TO-KNEE YOGA STRETCH

Pages 76–77
• Perform 30 seconds per side

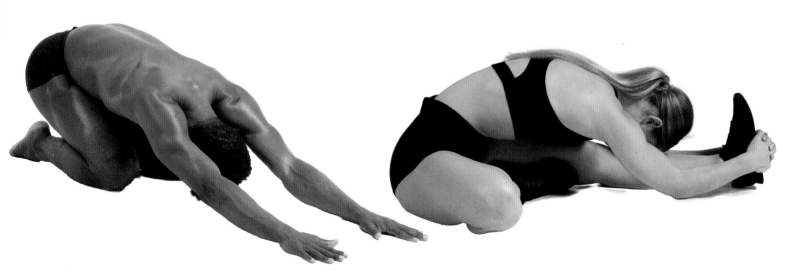

3 SEATED LEG CRADLE

Pages 222–23
• Perform 30 seconds per side

4 UNILATERAL KNEE-TO-CHEST STRETCH

Page 188
• Perform 30 seconds per side

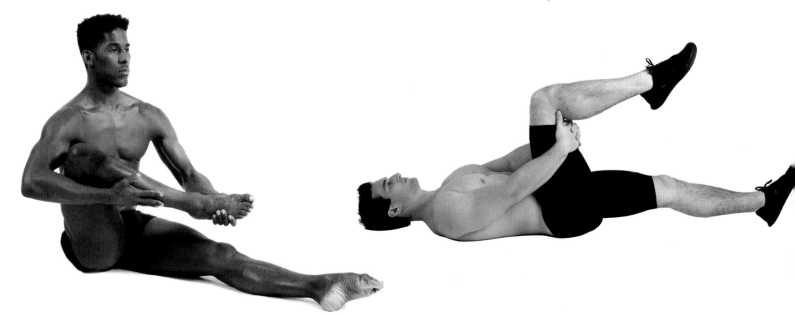

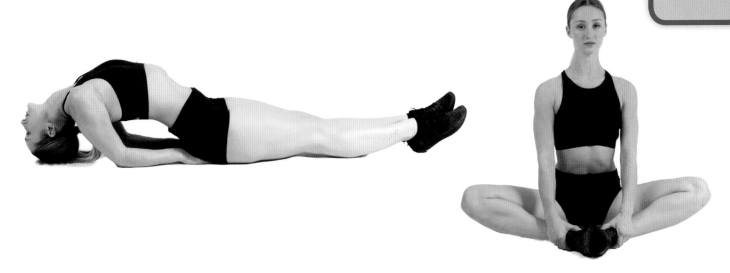

FACT FILE

TARGETS
• Hamstrings
• Quads
• Hip flexors
• Lower back

EQUIPMENT
• Body weight

BENEFITS
• Opens tight hips, relaxes lower-back, and lengthens leg muscles

5 FISH YOGA STRETCH

Pages 118–19
• Perform 30 seconds

6 BOUND ANGLE YOGA STRETCH

Pages 238–39
• Perform 30–45 seconds

7 UNILATERAL SEATED FORWARD BEND

Pages 298–99
• Perform 30 seconds per side

8 BILATERAL SEATED FORWARD BEND

Pages 300–301
• Perform 30 seconds per side

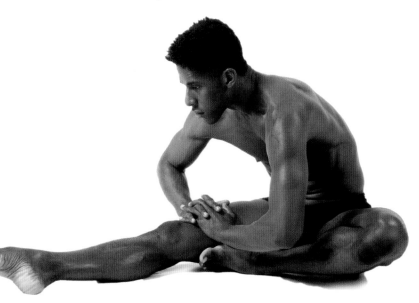

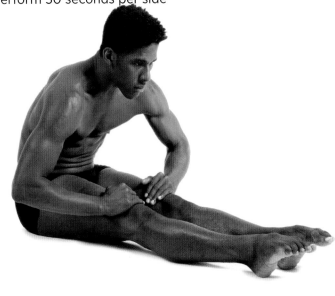

Take Five

Take a few minutes to perform this deep-tissue routine that targets some of the often-neglected areas such as the IT band, shins, and piriformis.

1 ILIOTIBIAL BAND ROLL
Pages 306–7
• Perform 30 seconds per side

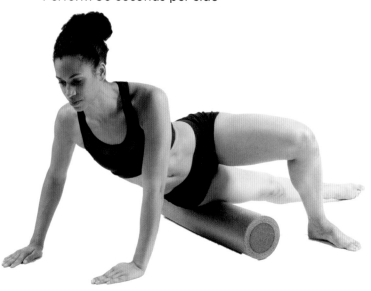

2 CALF AND HAMSTRINGS STRETCH
Pages 308–9
• Perform 30–45 seconds

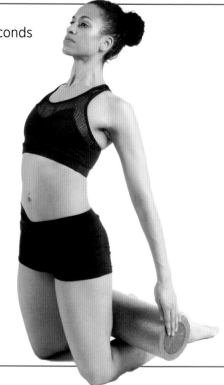

3 FOAM ROLLER SHIN STRETCH
Pages 310–11
• Perform 30 seconds per side

4 BACK ROLL
Pages 94–95
• Perform 30 seconds

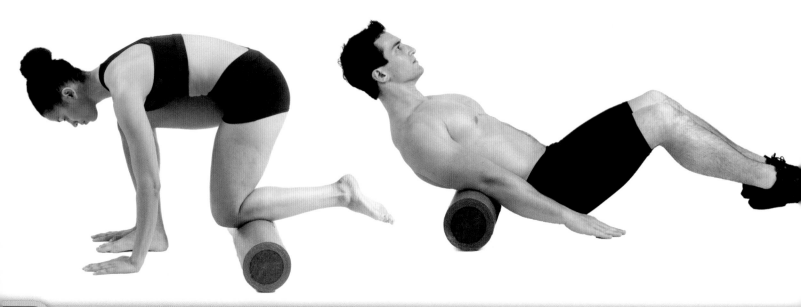

FACT FILE

TARGETS
- IT band
- Neck
- Piriformis
- Shins
- Ankles

EQUIPMENT
- Resistance band
- Foam roller
- Swiss Ball

BENEFITS
- Deeply stretches and massages hard-to-reach areas

5 BAND-ASSISTED WING STRETCH

Page 322
- Perform 30 seconds per side

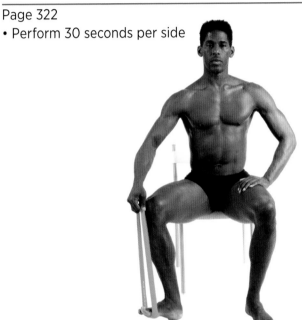

6 BAND-ASSISTED SICKLE STRETCH

Page 323
- Perform 30 seconds per side

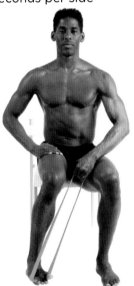

7 LYING-DOWN FIGURE 4 STRETCH

Pages 250–51
- Perform 30 seconds per side

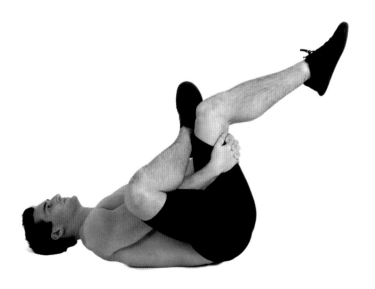

8 LEVATOR SCAPULAE STRETCH

Page 39
- Perform 30 seconds per direction

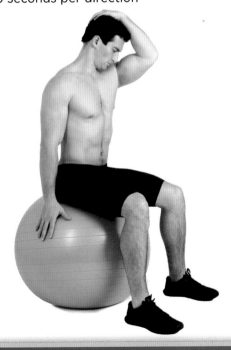

Midday

The perfect antidote to a noontime slump, the restorative Midday Routine features full-body stretches and invigorating inversions.

1 TOE TOUCH

Pages 260–61

• Perform 30–45 seconds

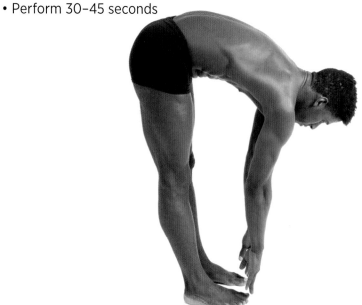

2 STANDING SPLITS

Pages 262–63

• Perform 30 seconds per side

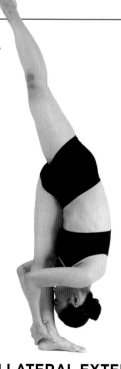

3 FORWARD LUNGE WITH TWIST

Pages 280–81

• Perform 30 seconds per side

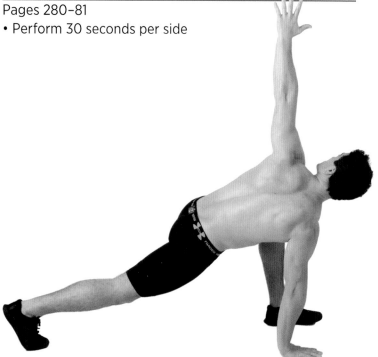

4 REVERSE LUNGE WITH LATERAL EXTENSION

Pages 282–83

• Perform 30 seconds per side

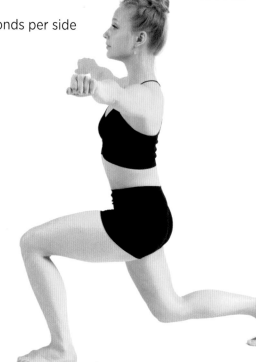

FACT FILE

TARGETS
• Lower body

EQUIPMENT
• Body weight
• Step

BENEFITS
• Boosts
circulation
and improves
balance and
core flexibility

5 STRAIGHT-LEG LUNGE

Pages 284–85
• Perform 30 seconds per side

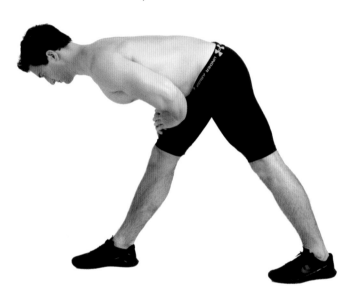

6 WIDE-LEGGED FORWARD BEND

Pages 288–89
• Perform 30–45 seconds

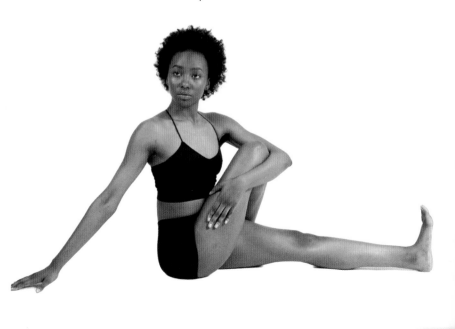

7 HEEL-DROP/TOE-UP STRETCH

Pages 292–93
• Perform 30 seconds per side

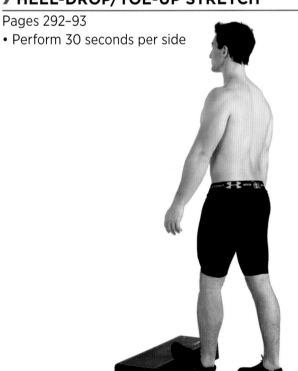

8 HIP STRETCH

Pages 302–3
• Perform 30 seconds per side

Sunset Straddle

If you've been on your feet all day, try this advanced series of stretches that deeply open your hips and ease tension in your lower body.

1 SIDE ADDUCTOR STRETCH

Pages 208–9
• Perform 30 seconds per side

2 HAPPY BABY STRETCH

Pages 254–55
• Perform 30 seconds per side

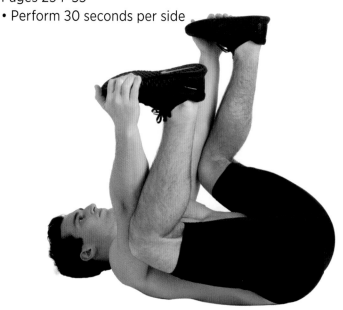

3 SEATED LEG CRADLE

Pages 222–23
• Perform 30 seconds per side

4 FRONT SPLIT

Pages 224–25
• Perform 30 seconds per side

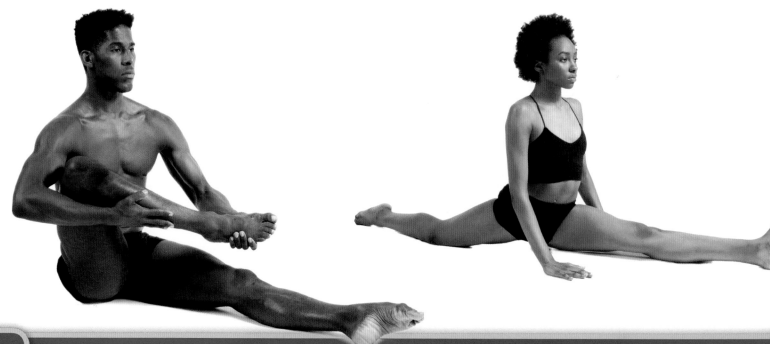

FACT FILE

TARGETS
• Lower body

EQUIPMENT
• Body weight

BENEFITS
• Eases tension
  in your lower
  body

5 LYING-DOWN GROIN STRETCH

Pages 246–47
• Perform 30 seconds

6 FROG STRADDLE

Pagse 218–19
• Perform 30–45 seconds

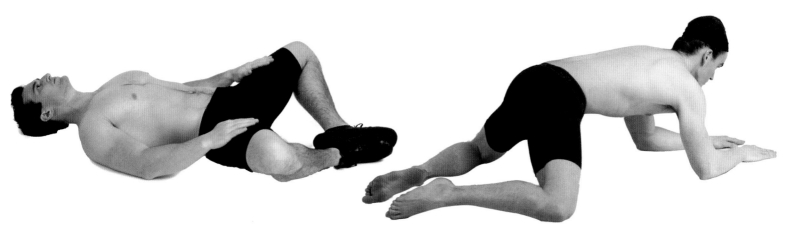

7 CHEST-TO-THIGH STRADDLE SPLIT

Page 230–31
• Perform 30 seconds per side

8 WIDE-ANGLE SEATED FORWARD BEND

Page 232–33
• Perform 30–45 seconds

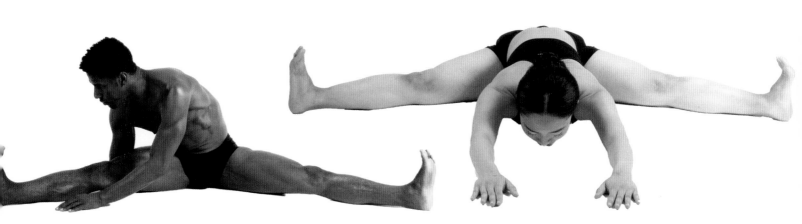

Coffee Break

Take a break from your computer and relieve tightness in your shoulders, chest, and back. Give your sore feet some love, too.

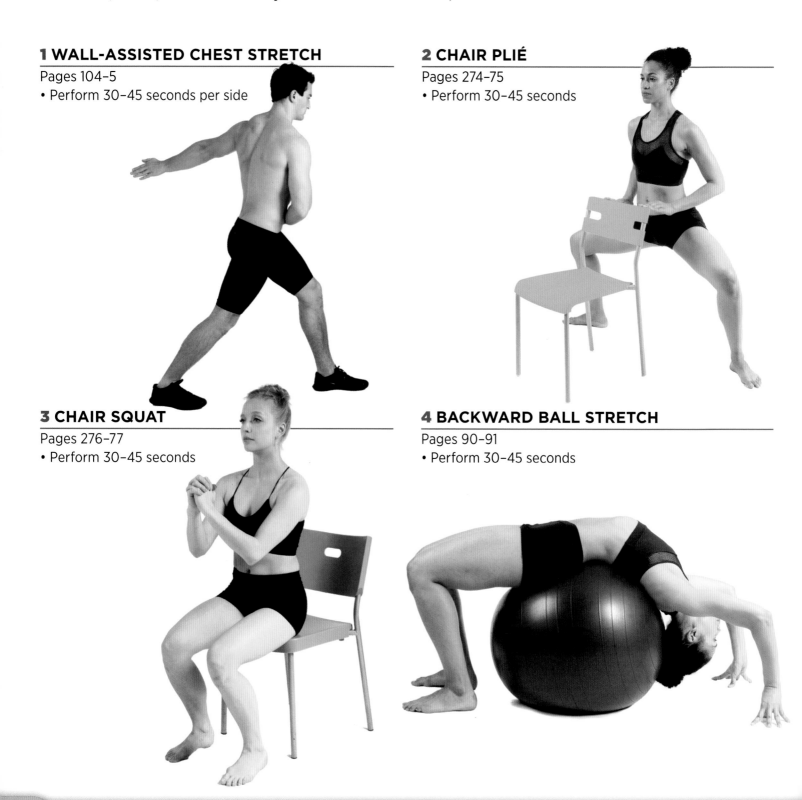

1 WALL-ASSISTED CHEST STRETCH
Pages 104–5
• Perform 30–45 seconds per side

2 CHAIR PLIÉ
Pages 274–75
• Perform 30–45 seconds

3 CHAIR SQUAT
Pages 276–77
• Perform 30–45 seconds

4 BACKWARD BALL STRETCH
Pages 90–91
• Perform 30–45 seconds

FACT FILE

TARGETS
• Full body

EQUIPMENT
• Body weight
• Swiss Ball
• Chair

BENEFITS
• Deeply opens chest and hips and eases tension in your shoulders and upper back

5 POINT FOOT STRETCH

Page 318
• Perform 30 seconds per side

6 FLEXION FOOT STRETCH

Page 319
• Perform 30 seconds per side

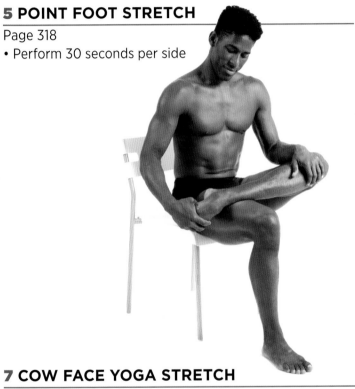

7 COW FACE YOGA STRETCH

Pages 58–59
• Perform 30–60 seconds

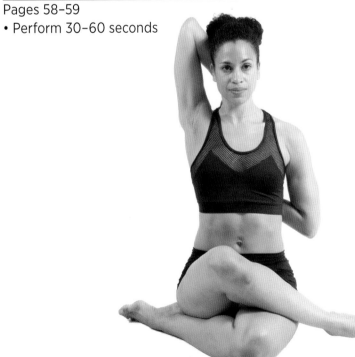

8 LATISSIMUS DORSI STRETCH

Pages 190–91
• Perform 3 repetitions per side

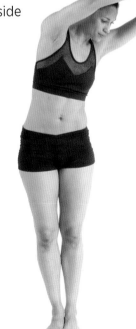

Happy Hour

Work on your balancing skills while flexing some muscle with this challenging routine that's great for stabilizing your core and realigning your spine.

1 HIP CIRCLES
Pages 172–73
• Perform 30 seconds per direction

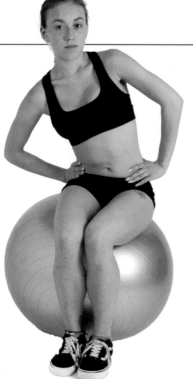

2 ROTATED BACK EXTENSION
Pages 182–83
• Perform 30 seconds per direction

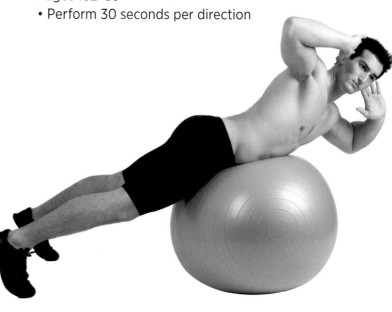

3 UPPER-TRAPEZIUS STRETCH
Page 28
• Perform 30–45 seconds

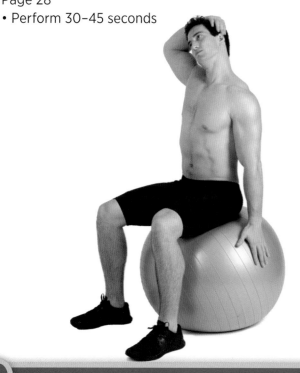

4 BACKWARD BALL STRETCH
Pages 90–91
• Perform 30–45 seconds

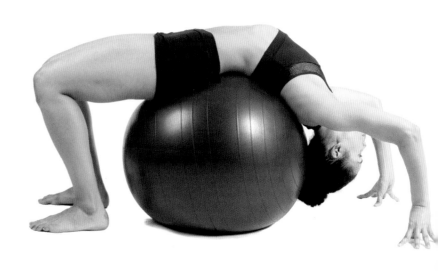

5 REVERSE BRIDGE ROTATION

Pages 148–49
• Perform 30 seconds per direction

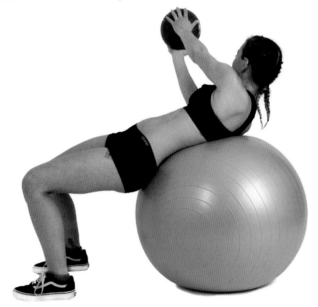

6 REVERSE BRIDGE BALL ROLL

Pages 150–51
• Perform 30 seconds per direction

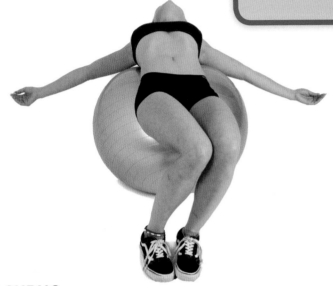

7 JACKKNIFE STRETCH

Pages 162–63
• Perform 30–45 seconds

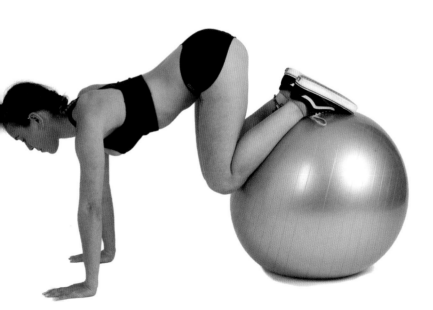

8 SHRUG

Page 41
• Perform 30–45 seconds

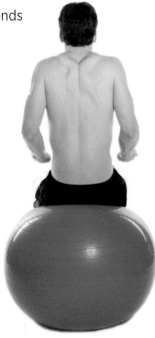

APPENDICES

Within this section you will find a glossary to help explain terms that may be unfamiliar to you; an icon index that shows the different stretches featured in the book; an index of all the topics covered by the book; and credits for the photos.

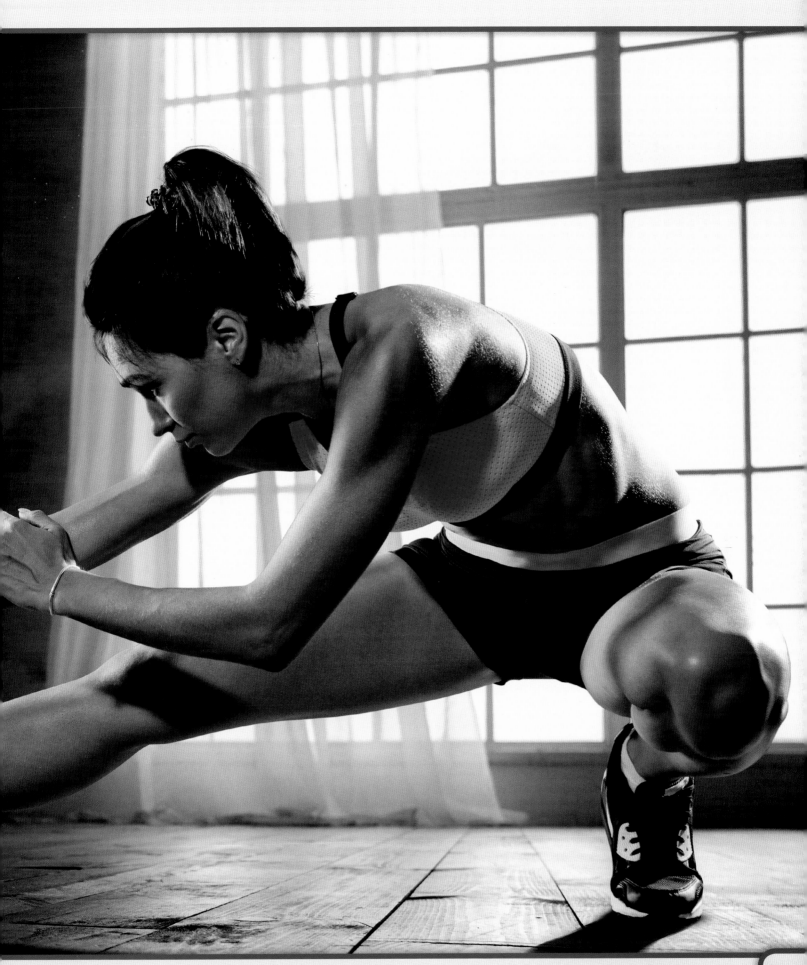

GENERAL TERMS

abduction: Movement away from your body.

active isolated stretching (AIS): A stretching technique in which the stretch is held for only a couple of seconds at a time and is performed in several repetitions, with the goal of exceeding the previous point of resistance by a few degrees in each ensuing repetition.

active stretching: A stretching technique in which added force is applied by the person stretching for greater intensity.

adduction: Movement toward your body.

aerobic exercise: A type of exercise involving aerobic metabolism in which your body uses oxygen to create energy; refers to sustained activity.

anaerobic exercise: A type of exercise involving anaerobic metabolism in which your muscles do not use oxygen to create energy; refers to short bursts of activity.

anterior: Located in the front of your body.

ballistic stretching: An active form of stretching that forces a part of your body to go beyond its normal range of motion by bouncing to a stretched position.

cardiovascular exercise: Any exercise that increases your heart rate, making oxygen and nutrient-rich blood available to working muscles.

cooldown: An exercise performed at the end of the workout session that works to cool and relax your body.

core: Refers to the deep muscle layers that lie close to your spine and provide structural support for your entire body. The core is divided into two groups: the major and the minor muscles. The major core muscles reside in the abdominal area and in the middle and lower back. This area encompasses the pelvic floor muscles (levator ani, pubococcygeus, iliococcygeus, puborectalis, and coccygeus), the abdominals (rectus abdominis, transversus abdominis, obliquus externus, and obliquus internus), the spinal extensors (multifidus spinae, erector spinae, splenius, longissimus thoracis, and semispinalis), and the diaphragm. The minor core muscles include the latissimus dorsi, gluteus maximus, and trapezius. The minor core muscles assist the major muscles when your body engages in activities or movements that require added stability.

core stabilizer: An exercise that calls for resisting motion along your lumbar spine through activation of your abdominal muscles and deep stabilizers; improves core strength and endurance.

core strengthener: An exercise that allows for motion in your lumbar spine, while working your abdominal muscles and deep stabilizers; improves core strength.

dynamic stretching: A stretching technique that requires the use of continuous movement patterns.

extension: The straightening of a joint.

extensor muscle: A muscle that extends a limb, or other body part, away from your body.

flexion: The bending of a joint.

flexor muscle: A muscle that decreases the angle between two bones, as when bending your elbow or raising your thigh toward your abdomen.

hamstrings: The three muscles at the back your thigh (semitendinosus, semimembranosus, and biceps femoris) that flexes your knee and extends your hip.

hyperextension: An exercise that works your lower back as well as your middle and upper back, specifically the erector spinae, which usually involves raising your torso and/or lower body from the floor while keeping your pelvis firmly anchored.

internal rotation: The act of moving a part of your body toward the center of your body.

interval: A period of activity or rest.

isolation exercise: A movement that focuses on only one muscle or muscle group.

iliotibial band (ITB): A thick band of fibrous tissue that runs down the outside of your thigh, beginning at your hip and extending to the outer side of your tibia just below your knee joint. The band functions in concert with several of your thigh muscles to provide stability to the outside of your knee joint.

lateral: Refers to the outer side of your body; the opposite of medial.

lunge: A group of lower-body exercise in which one leg is positioned forward with your knee bent and foot flat on the floor while your other leg is positioned behind you.

medial: Refers to the middle of your body; the opposite of lateral.

meditation: The focusing and calming of your mind, often through breath work to reach deeper levels of consciousness.

myofascial release stretching: A stretching technique that involves the use of applied force or an external stretching device to apply gentle, sustained pressure to specific points of muscle tightness or discomfort.

neutral: Describes the position of your legs, pelvis, hips, or other part of your body that is neither arched nor curved forward.

neutral position: A position in which the natural curve of your spine is maintained, typically adopted when lying on your back with one or both feet on the mat.

passive, or isometric, stretching: A stretching technique in which added force is applied by an external source (e.g., a partner or an assistive device) to increase intensity.

posterior: Refers to the back of your body.

posterior chain: Your gluteals, hamstrings, and back.

props: Tools such as mats, blocks, blankets, and straps used to extend your range of motion or facilitate achieving a pose.

pulling muscles: The primary muscle groups associated with pulling movements: abdominals, biceps, forearms, latissimus dorsi, hamstrings, obliques, and trapezius.

pushing muscles: The primary muscle groups associated with pushing movements: calves, deltoids, gluteals, pectorals, quadriceps, and triceps.

quadriceps: A large muscle group that includes the four prevailing muscles at the front of your thigh: rectus femoris, vastus intermedius, vastus lateralis, and vastus medialis; the main extensor muscles of your knee that surround the front and sides of your femur muscle.

range of motion: The distance and direction a joint can move between the flexed and the extended positions.

resistance: The weight your muscles are working against to complete a movement, whether your own body weight or added weight, such as dumbbells.

rotator muscle: One of a group of muscles that assists the rotation of a joint, such as your hip or shoulder.

scapula: The protrusion of bone in your middle to upper back known as your shoulder blade.

set: Refers to how many times you repeat a given number of repetitions of an exercise.

static stretching: A stretching technique in which the stretches are performed by extending the targeted muscle to its maximal point and then holding the that position for a particular length of time.

stretch: Refers to the straightening or extending of your body, or a part of your body, to full length.

ventral aspect: The front of your body.

warm-up: Any form of light exercise of short duration that prepares your body for more intense exercises.

yoga: From the Sanskrit *yug* ("yoke"), meaning "union." Yoga is an ancient discipline in which physical postures, breath practice, meditation, and philosophical study are used as tools for achieving liberation.

yogi: A male/female practitioner of yoga.

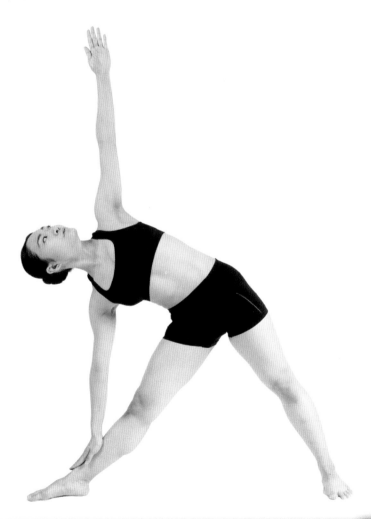

LATIN TERMS

The following glossary explains the Latin scientific terminology used to describe the muscles of the human body. Certain words are derived from Greek, which is indicated in each instance.

CHEST

coracobrachialis: Greek *korakoeidés*, "ravenlike," and *brachium*, "arm"

pectoralis (major and minor): *pectus*, "breast"

ABDOMEN

obliquus (externus and internus): *obliquus*, "slanting"

rectus abdominis: *rego*, "straight, upright," and *abdomen*, "belly"

serratus anterior: *serra*, "saw," and *ante*, "before"

transversus abdominis: *transversus*, "athwart," and *abdomen*, "belly"

NECK

scalenus: Greek *skalénós*, "unequal"

semispinalis: *semi*, "half," and *spinae*, "spine"

splenius: Greek *splénion*, "plaster, patch"

sternocleidomastoideus: Greek *stérnon*, "chest," Greek *kleís*, "key" and Greek *mastoeidés*, "breastlike"

BACK

erector spinae: *erectus*, "straight," and *spina*, "thorn"

latissimus dorsi: *latus*, "wide," and *dorsum*, "back"

multifidus spinae: *multifid*, "to cut into divisions," and *spinae*, "spine"

quadratus lumborum: *quadratus*, "square, rectangular," and *lumbus*, "loin"

rhomboideus: Greek *rhembesthai*, "to spin"

trapezius: Greek *trapezion*, "small table"

SHOULDERS

deltoideus (anterior, medialis, and posterior): Greek *deltoeidés*, "delta-shaped"

infraspinatus: *infra*, "under," and *spina*, "thorn"

levator scapulae: *levare*, "to raise," and *scapulae*, "shoulder [blades]"

subscapularis: *sub*, "below," and *scapulae*, "shoulder [blades]"

supraspinatus: *supra*, "above," and *spina*, "thorn"

teres (major and minor): *teres*, "rounded"

UPPER ARM

biceps brachii: *biceps*, "two-headed," and *brachium*, "arm"

brachialis: *brachium*, "arm"

triceps brachii: *triceps*, "three-headed" and *brachium*, "arm"

LOWER ARM

anconeus: Greek *anconad*, "elbow"

brachioradialis: *brachium*, "arm," and *radius*, "spoke"

extensor carpi radialis: *extendere*, "to extend," Greek *karpós*, "wrist" and *radius*, "spoke"

extensor digitorum: *extendere*, "to extend," and *digitus*, "finger, toe"

flexor carpi pollicis longus: *flectere*, "to bend," Greek *karpós*, "wrist," *pollicis*, "thumb" and *longus*, "long"

flexor carpi radialis: *flectere*, "to bend," Greek *karpós*, "wrist" and *radius*, "spoke"

flexor carpi ulnaris: *flectere*, "to bend," Greek *karpós*, "wrist" and *ulnaris*, "forearm"

flexor digitorum: *flectere*, "to bend," and *digitus*, "finger, toe"

palmaris longus: *palmaris*, "palm," and *longus*, "long"

pronator teres: *pronate*, "to rotate," and *teres*, "rounded"

HIPS

gemellus (inferior and superior): *geminus*, "twin"

gluteus maximus: Greek *gloutós*, "rump," and *maximus*, "largest"

gluteus medius: Greek *gloutós*, "rump" and *medialis*, "middle"

gluteus minimus: Greek *gloutós*, "rump" and *minimus*, "smallest"

iliopsoas: *ilium,* "groin," and Greek *psoa*, "groin muscle"

obturator externus: *obturare,* "to block" and *externus,* "outward"

obturator internus: *obturare*, "to block," and *internus*, "within"

pectineus: *pectin*, "comb"

piriformis: *pirum*, "pear," and *forma,* "shape"

quadratus femoris: *quadratus*, "square, rectangular," and *femur*, "thigh"

UPPER LEG

adductor longus: *adducere*, "to contract," and *longus*, "long"

adductor magnus: *adducere*, "to contract," and *magnus*, "major"

biceps femoris: *biceps*, "two–headed," and *femur*, "thigh"

gracilis: *gracilis*, "slim, slender"

rectus femoris: *rego*, "straight, upright," and *femur*, "thigh"

sartorius: *sarcio*, "to patch" or "to repair"

semimembranosus: *semi*, "half," and *membrum*, "limb"

semitendinosus: *semi*, "half," and *tendo*, "tendon"

tensor fasciae latae: *tenere*, "to stretch," *fasciae*, "band," and *latae*, "laid down"

vastus intermedius: *vastus*, "immense, huge," and *intermedius*, "between"

vastus lateralis: *vastus*, "immense, huge," and lateralis, "side"

vastus medialis: *vastus*, "immense, huge," and *medialis*, "middle"

LOWER LEG

adductor digiti minimi: *adducere*, "to contract," *digitus*, "finger, toe" and *minimum* "smallest"

adductor hallucis: *adducere*, "to contract," and *hallex*, "big toe"

extensor digitorum longus: *extendere*, "to extend," *digitus*, "finger, toe" and *longus*, "long"

extensor hallucis longus: *extendere*, "to extend," *hallex*, "big toe," and *longus*, "long"

flexor digitorum longus: *flectere*, "to bend," *digitus*, "finger, toe" and *longus*, "long"

flexor hallucis longus: *flectere*, "to bend," and *hallex*, "big toe" and *longus*, "long"

gastrocnemius: Greek *gastroknémía*, "calf [of the leg]"

peroneus: *peronei*, "of the fibula"

plantaris: *planta*, "the sole"

soleus: *solea*, "sandal"

tibialis (anterior and posterior): *tibia*, "reed pipe"

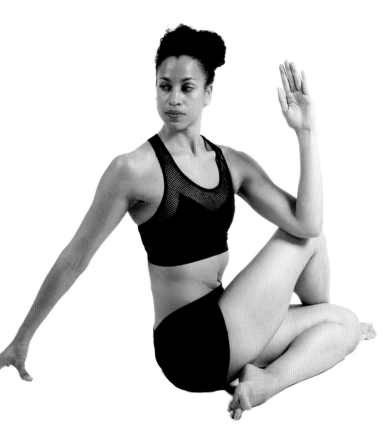

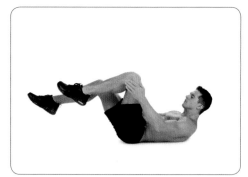

Abdominal Kick
Pages 184–85

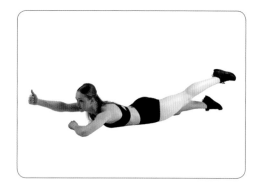

Arm-Leg Extension
Pages 180–81

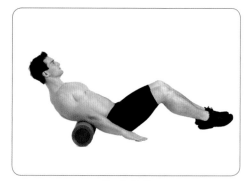

Back Roll
Pages 94–95

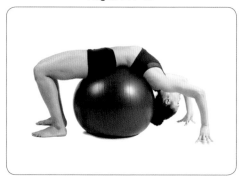

Backward Ball Stretch
Pages 90–91

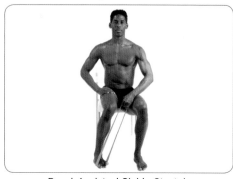

Band-Assisted Sickle Stretch
Page 323

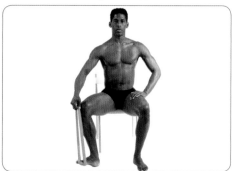

Band-Assisted Wing Stretch
Page 322

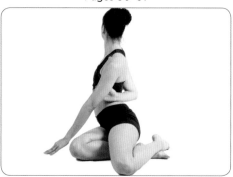

Bharadvaja's Twist
Pages 62–63

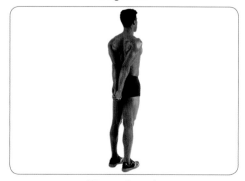

Biceps Stretch
Pages 98–99

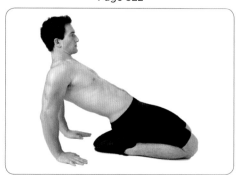

Bilateral Quad Stretch
Pages 314–15

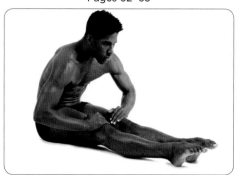

Bilateral Seated Forward Bend
Pages 300–1

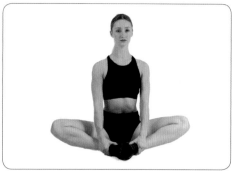

Bound Angle Yoga Stretch
Pages 238–39

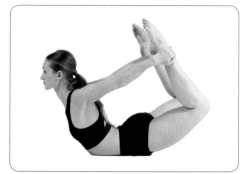

Bow Yoga Stretch
Pages 122–23

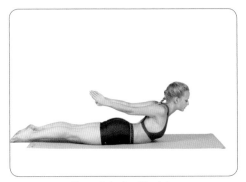

Breaststroke Stretch
Pages 84–85

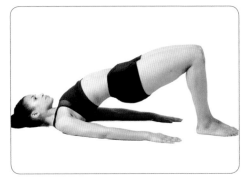

Bridge Stretch
Pages 86–87

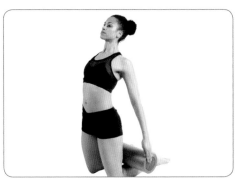

Calf and Hamstrings Stretch
Pages 308–9

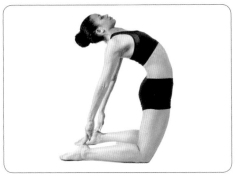

Camel Yoga Stretch
Pages 106–7

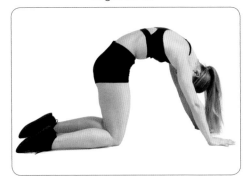

Cat-to-Cow Stretch
Pages 78–79

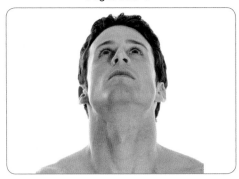

Cervical Stars
Page 28–29

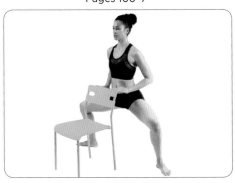

Chair Plié
Pages 274–75

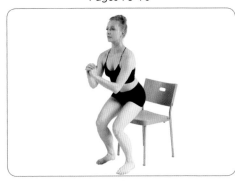

Chair Squat
Pages 276–77

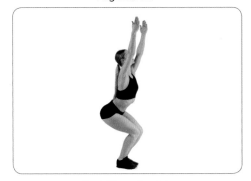

Chair Yoga Stretch
Pages 48–49

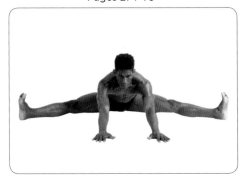

Chest-to-Floor Straddle Split
Pages 226–27

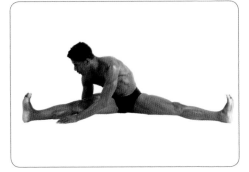

Chest-to-Thigh Straddle Split
Pages 230–31

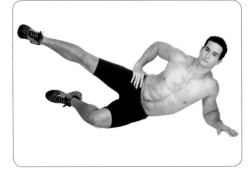

Clamshells
Pages 240–41

Icon Index

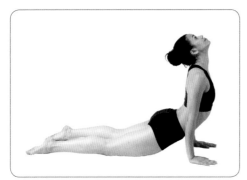

Cobra Stretch
Pages 176–77

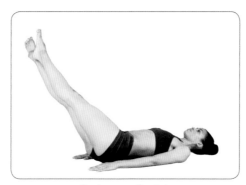

Corkscrew Stretch
Pages 160–61

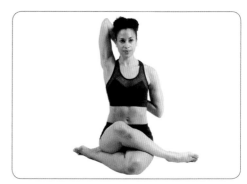

Cow Face Yoga Stretch
Pages 58–59

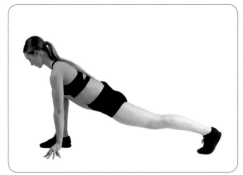

Deep Lunge
Pages 286–87

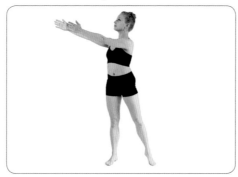

Diagonal Reach
Pages 128–29

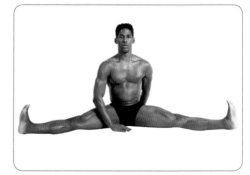

Double-Leg Straddle Split
Pages 228–29

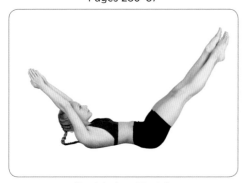

Double-Leg Stretch
Pages 156–57

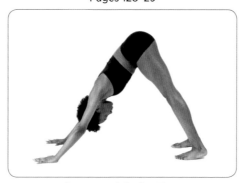

Downward-Facing Dog
Pages 72–73

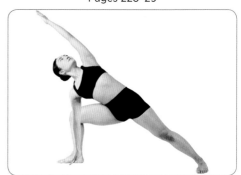

Extended Side Angle Yoga Stretch
Pages 132–33

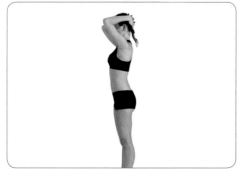

Extension Isometric
Page 37

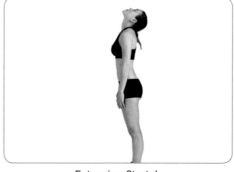

Extension Stretch
Page 36

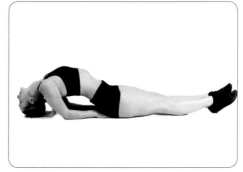

Fish Yoga Stretch
Pages 118–19

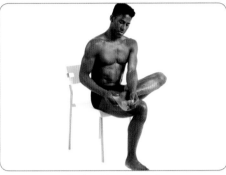

Flexion Foot Stretch
Page 319

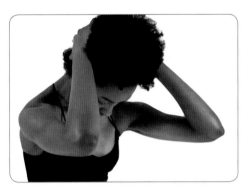

Flexion Stretch
Page 30

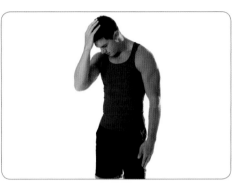

Flexion Isometric
Page 31

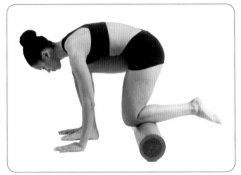

Foam Roller Shin Stretch
Pages 310–11

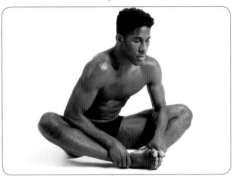

Folded Butterfly Stretch
Page 237

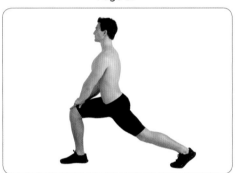

Forward Lunge
Pages 278–79

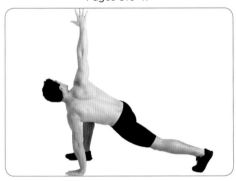

Forward Lunge with Twist
Pages 280–81

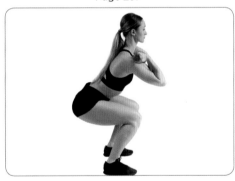

Forward Squat
Pages 202–3

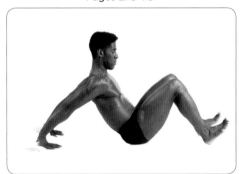

Front Deltoid Towel Stretch
Page 68

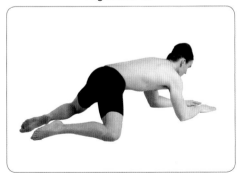

Frog Straddle
Pages 218–19

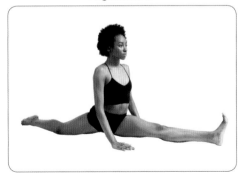

Front Split
Pages 224–25

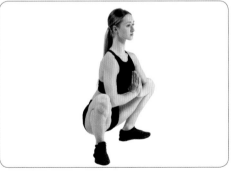

Garland Yoga Stretch
Pages 212–13

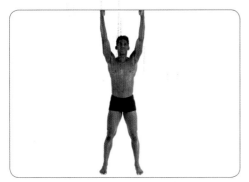

Good Morning Stretch
Pages 46–47

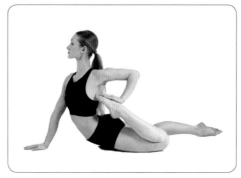

Half-Frog Yoga Stretch
Pages 120–21

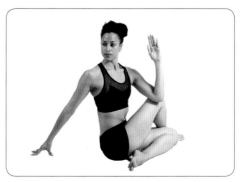

Half Lord of the Fishes Yoga Stretch
Pages 168–69

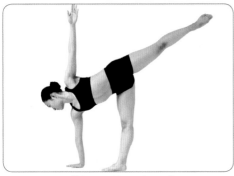

Half Moon Yoga Stretch
Pages 134–35

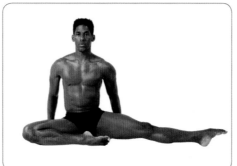

Half Straddle Stretch
Pages 138–39

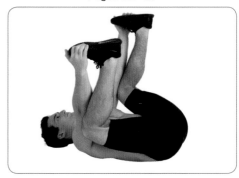

Happy Baby Stretch
Pages 254–55

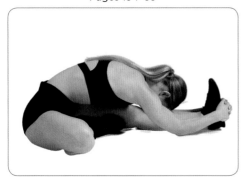

Head-to-Knee Yoga Stretch
Pages 76–77

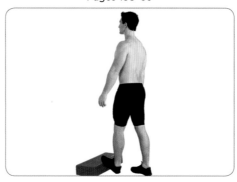

Heel-Drop/Toe-Up Stretch
Pages 292–93

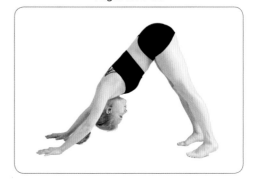

High Plank Pike
Pages 42–43

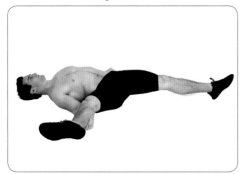

Hip Adductor Stretch
Pages 248–49

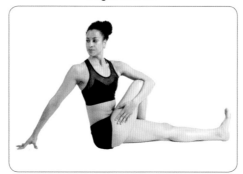

Hip and Iliotibial Band Stretch
Pages 196–97

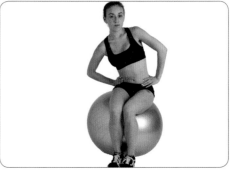

Hip Circles
Pages 172–73

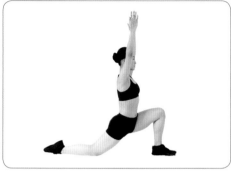

Hip Flexor Stretch
Pages 270–71

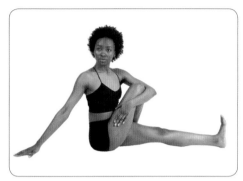

Hip Stretch
Pages 302–3

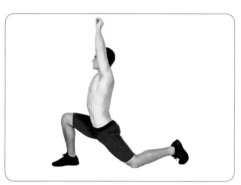

Hip-to-Thigh Stretch
Pages 272–73

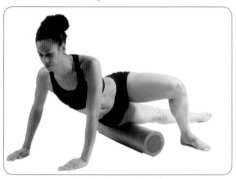

Iliotibial Band Roll
Pages 306–7

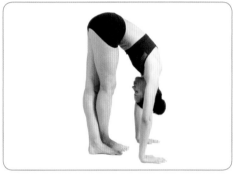

Iliotibial Band Stretch
Pages 290–91

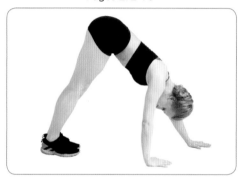

Inchworm Stretch
Pages 186–87

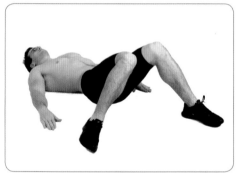

Internal Hip Rotator Stretch
Pages 252–53

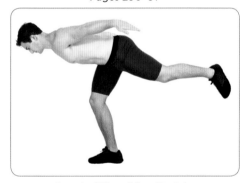

Inverted Hamstring Stretch
Pages 268–69

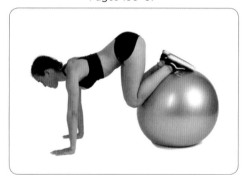

Jackknife Stretch
Pages 162–63

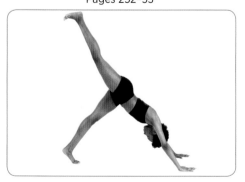

Knee-Pull Plank
Pages 294–95

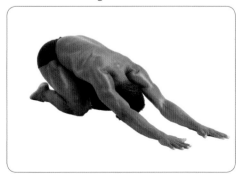

Kneeling Lat Stretch
Pages 70–71

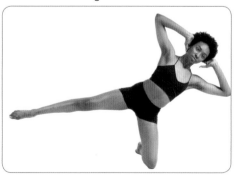

Kneeling Side Lift
Pages 214–15

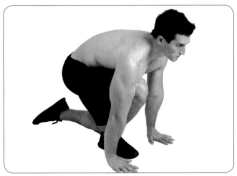

Kneeling Sprinter Stretch
Page 265

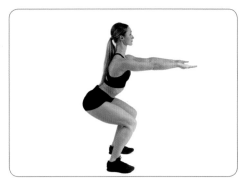

Knee Squat
Pages 312–13

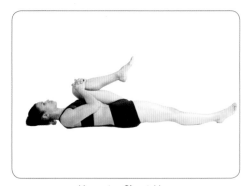

Knee-to-Chest Hug
Pages 88–89

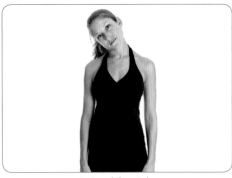

Lateral Stretch
Page 32

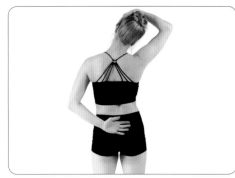

Lateral Isometric
Page 33

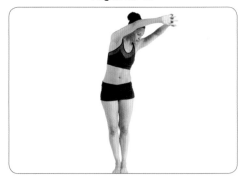

Latissimus Dorsi Stretch
Pages 190–91

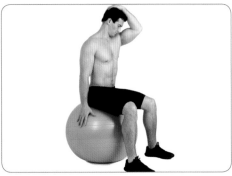

Levator Scapulae Stretch
Page 39

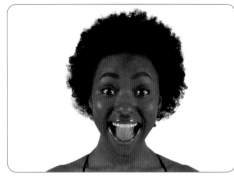

Lion Stretch and Eye Box Stretch Combo
Page 27

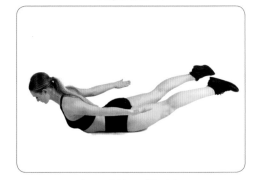

Locust Yoga Stretch
Pages 82–83

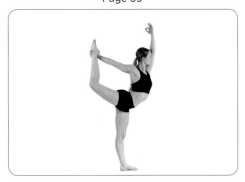

Lord of the Dance Yoga Stretch
Pages 166–67

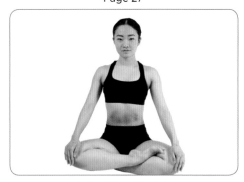

Lotus Yoga Stretch
Pages 234–35

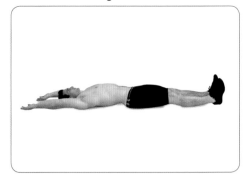

Lying-Down Arch Stretch
Page 141

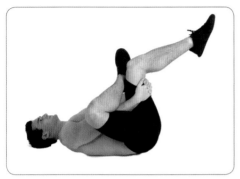

Lying-Down Figure 4 Stretch
Pages 250–51

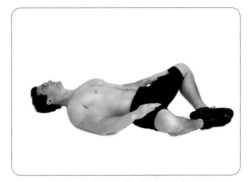

Lying-Down Groin Stretch
Pages 246–47

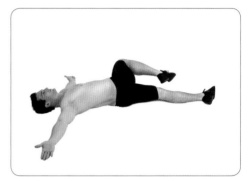

Lying-Down Pretzel Stretch
Pages 124–25

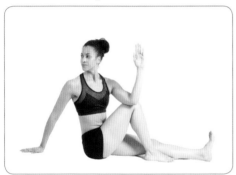

Marichi's Yoga Stretch
Pages 60–61

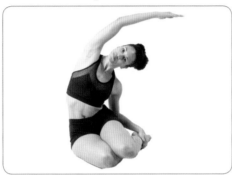

Mermaid Stretch
Pages 136–37

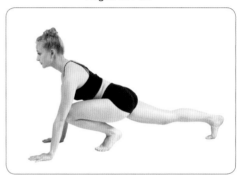

Mountain Climber Stretch
Pages 296–97

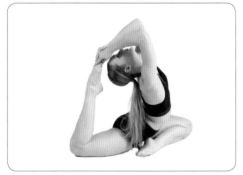

One-Legged Royal Pigeon Yoga Stretch
Pages 110–11

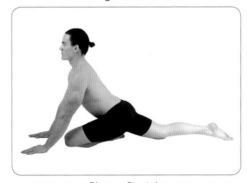

Pigeon Stretch
Pages 220–21

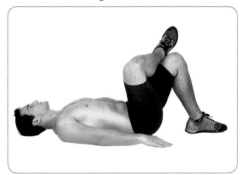

Piriformis Bridge
Pages 244–45

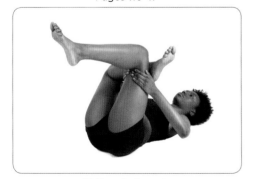

Piriformis Stretch
Pages 242–43

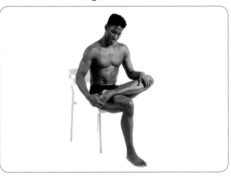

Point Foot Stretch
Page 318

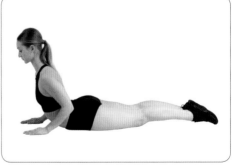

Prone Trunk Raise
Pages 178–79

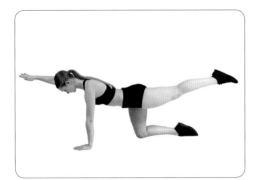

Quadruped Leg Lift
Pages 216–17

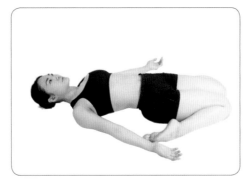

Reclining Hero Yoga Stretch
Pages 158–59

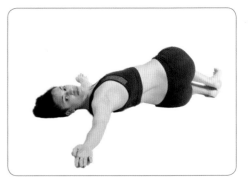

Reclining Twist
Pages 92–93

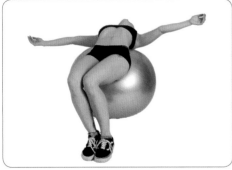

Reverse Bridge Ball Roll
Pages 150–51

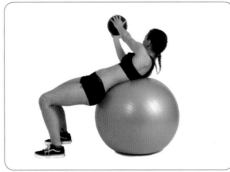

Reverse Bridge Rotation
Pages 148–49

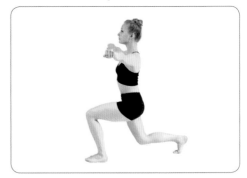

Reverse Lunge with Lateral Extension
Pages 282–83

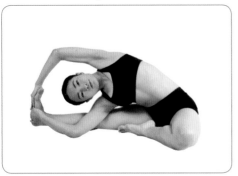

Revolved Head-to-Knee Yoga Stretch
Pages 142–43

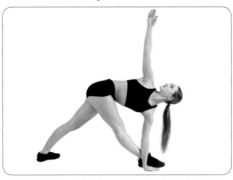

Revolved Triangle Yoga Stretch
Pages 170–71

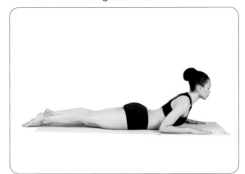

Rising Swan Stretch
Pages 116–17

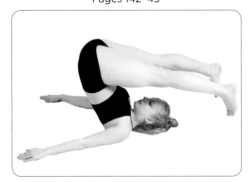

Rollover Stretch
Pages 192–93

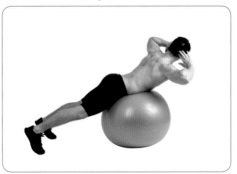

Rotated Back Extension
Pages 182–83

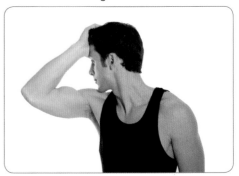

Rotation Stretch
Page 34

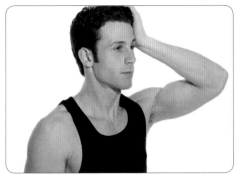

Rotation Isometric
Page 35

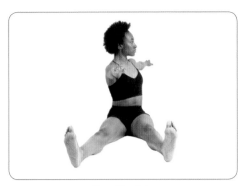

Saw Stretch
Pages 108–9

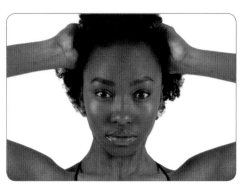

Scalp Stretch
Page 26

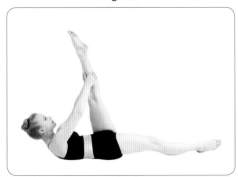

Scissors Stretch
Pages 316–17

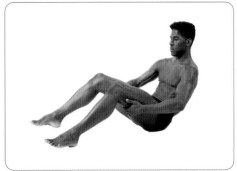

Scoop Rhomboids
Page 57

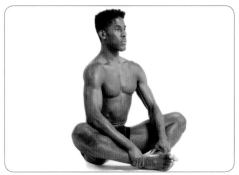

Seated ButterflyStretch
Page 236

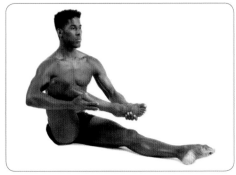

Seated Leg Cradle
Pages 222–23

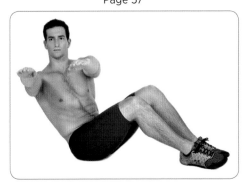

Seated Russian Twist
Pages 174–75

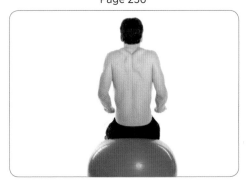

Shrug
Page 41

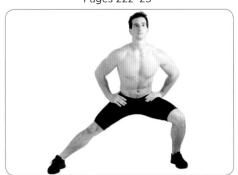

Side Adductor Stretch
Pages 208–9

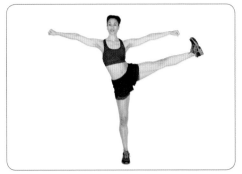

Side Kick
Pages 210–11

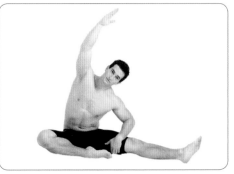

Side-Leaning Half Straddle
Page 140

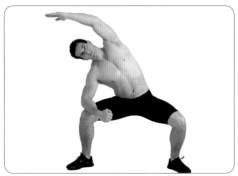

Side-Leaning Sumo Squat
Pages 206–7

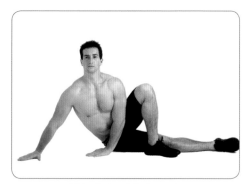

Side-Lying Knee Bend
Pages 304–5

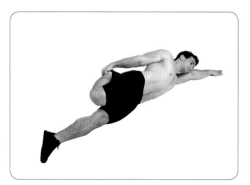

Side-Lying Rib Stretch
Pages 146–47

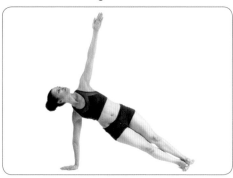

Side Plank
Pages 144–45

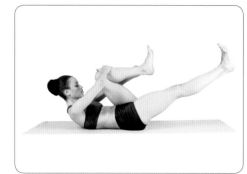

Single-Leg Stretch
Pages 154–55

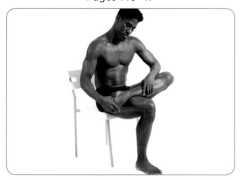

Slope-Down Foot Stretch
Page 321

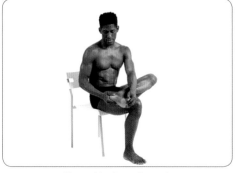

Slope-Up Foot Stretch
Page 320

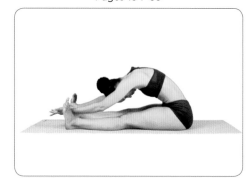

Spine Stretch Forward
Pages 66–67

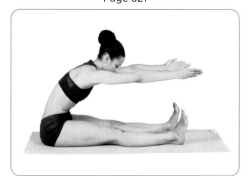

Spine Stretch Reaching
Page 69

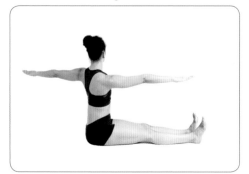

Spine Twist
Pages 64–65

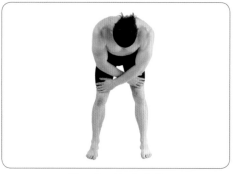

Standing Back Roll
Page 56

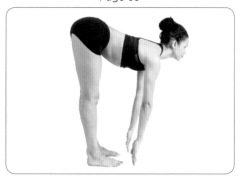

Standing Forward Bend
Pages 258–59

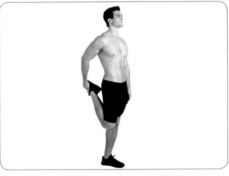

Standing Quadriceps Stretch
Page 264

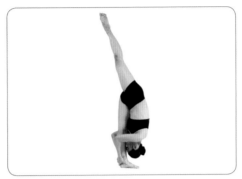

Standing Splits
Pages 262–63

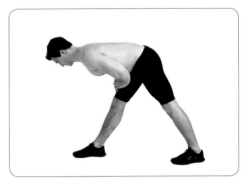

Straight-Leg Lunge
Pages 284–85

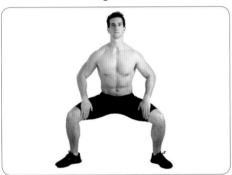

Sumo Squat
Pages 204–5

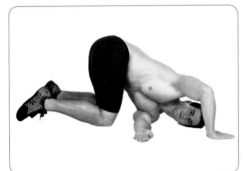

Thread the Needle
Pages 80–81

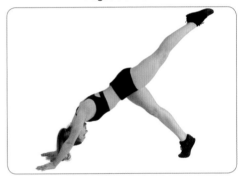

Three-Legged Dog
Pages 74–75

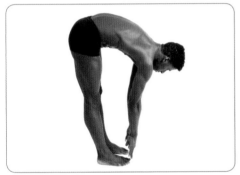

Toe Touch
Pages 260–61

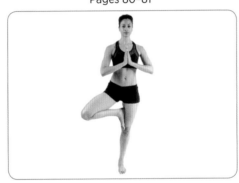

Tree Yoga Stretch
Pages 200–1

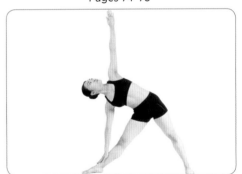

Triangle Yoga Stretch
Pages 130–31

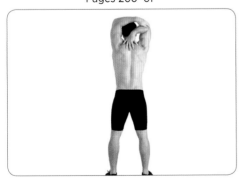

Triceps Stretch
Pages 96–97

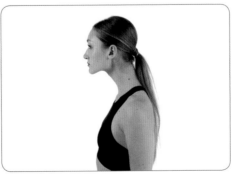

Turtle Neck
Page 40

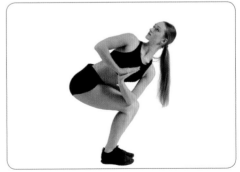

Twisting Chair Stretch
Pages 50–51

Icon Index

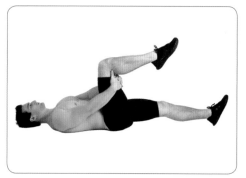

Unilateral Knee-to-Chest Stretch
Page 188

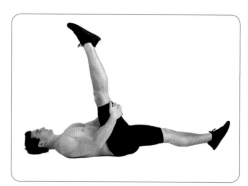

Unilateral Leg Raise
Page 189

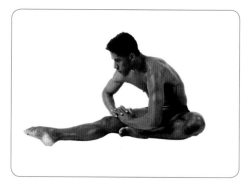

Unilateral Seated Forward Bend
Pages 298–99

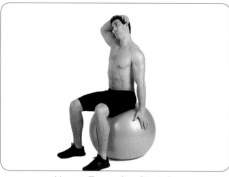

Upper-Trapezius Stretch
Page 38

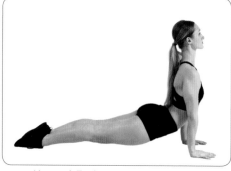

Upward-Facing Dog Yoga Stretch
Pages 114–15

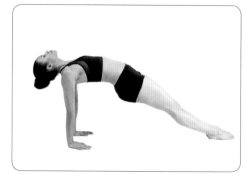

Upward-Facing Plank Stretch
Pages 112–13

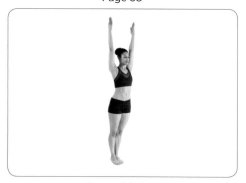

Upward Salute
Page 54–55

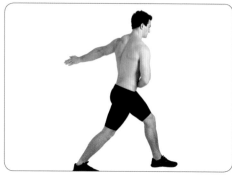

Wall-Assisted Chest Stretch
Pages 104–5

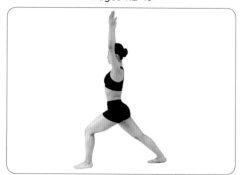

Warrior I Yoga Stretch
Pages 266–67

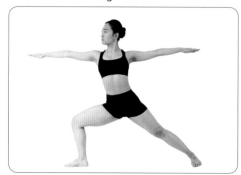

Warrior II Yoga Stretch
Pages 198–99

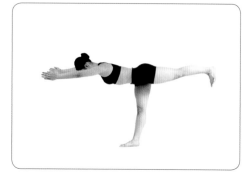

Warrior III Yoga Stretch
Pages 52–53

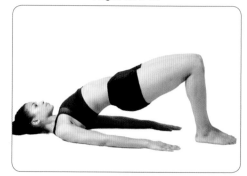

Wheel Yoga Stretch
Pages 152–53

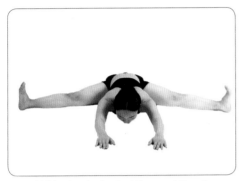

Wide-Angle Seated Forward Bend
Pages 232–33

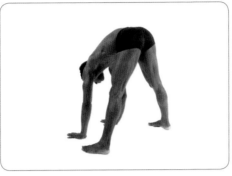

Wide-Legged Forward Bend
Pages 288–89

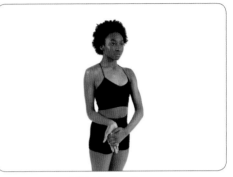

Wrist Extension
Page 101

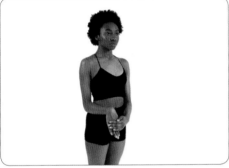

Wrist Flexion
Page 100

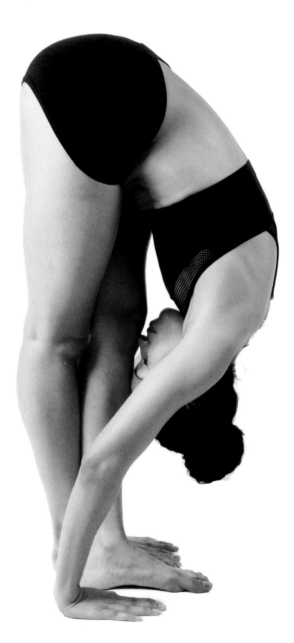

Index

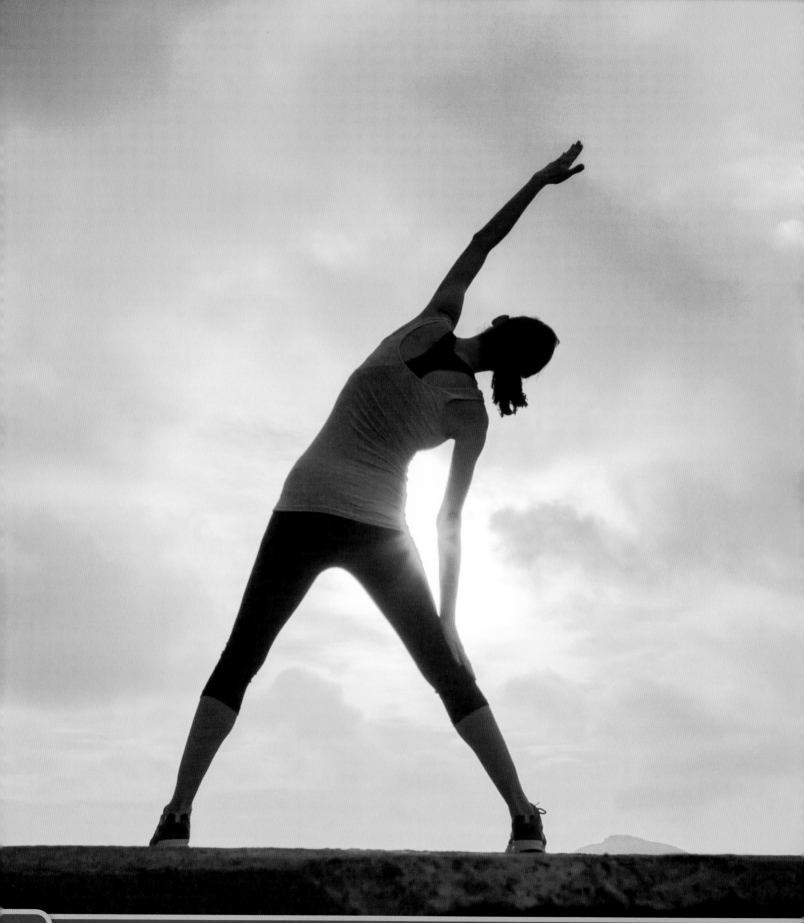

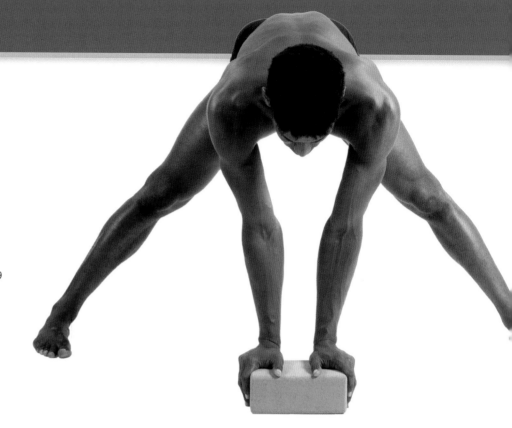

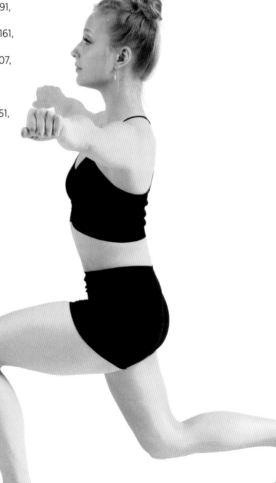

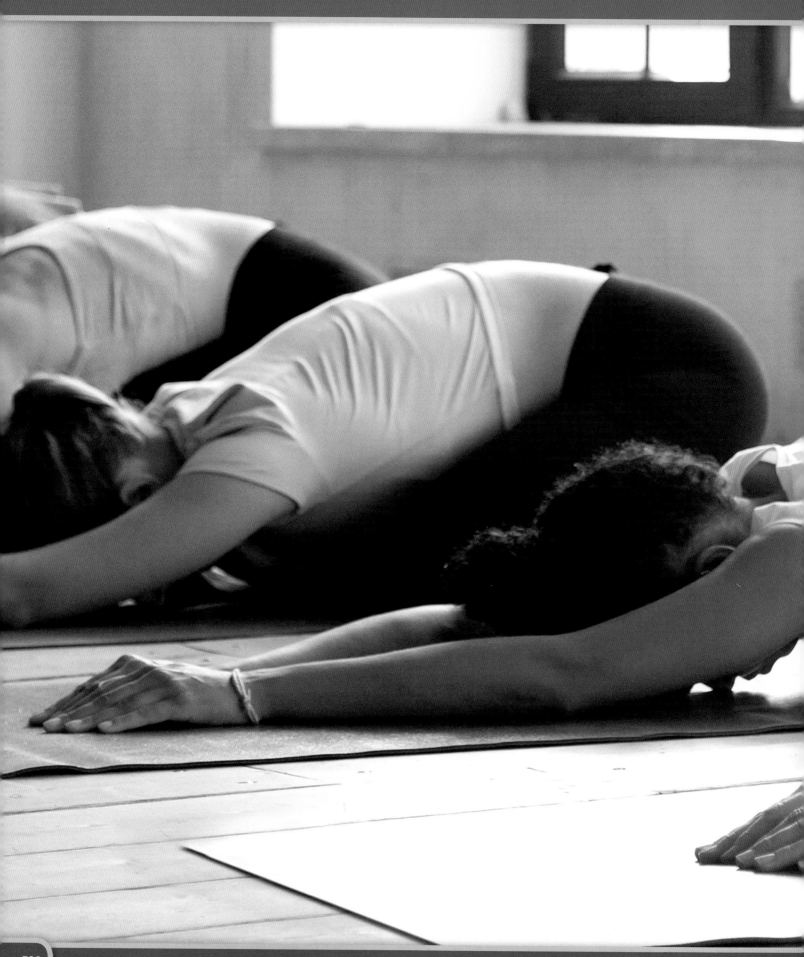

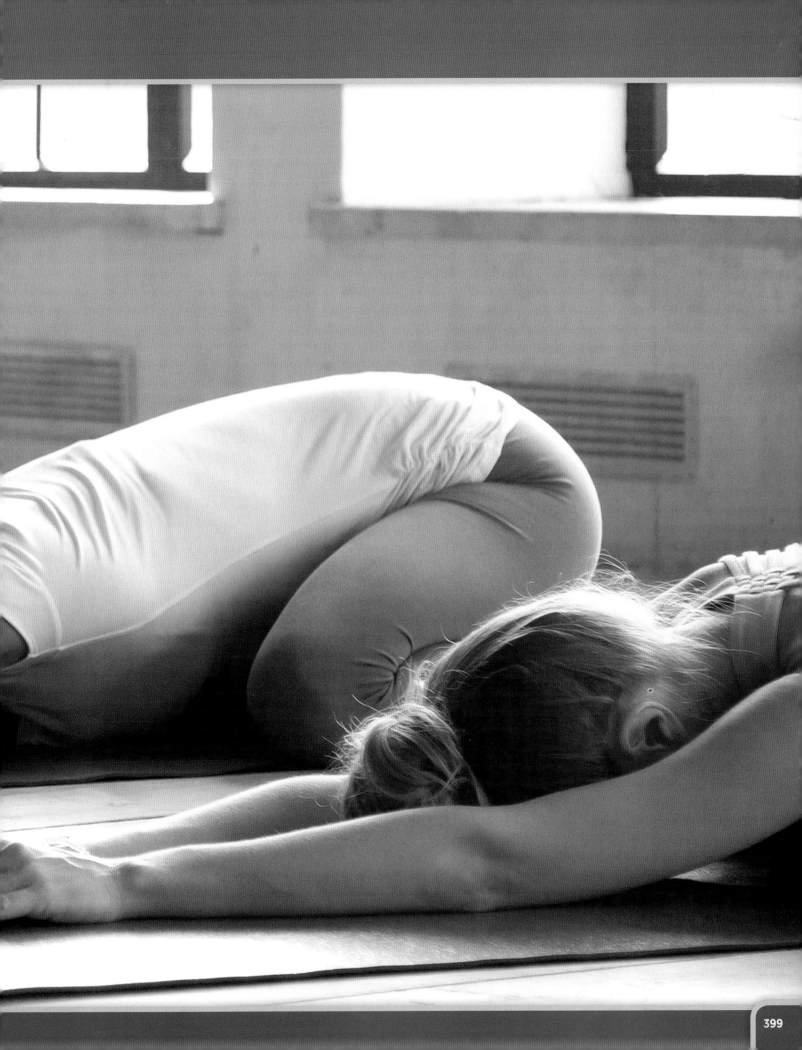

Credits

Photography

Naila Ruechel

Photography Assistant

Finn Moore

Models

Natasha Diamond-Walker
Jessica Gambellur
Lloyd Knight
Daniel Wright

Additional Photography

Page 4 spwidoff/Shutterstock.com
Page 7 Maridav/Shutterstock.com
Page 9 Syda Productions/Shutterstock.com
Page 10 kikovic/Shutterstock.com
Page 11 Zynatisg/Shutterstock.com
Page 12 Nomad_Soul/Shutterstock.com
Page 13 fizkes/Shutterstock.com
Page 15 bluedog studio/Shutterstock.com
Page 16 Rido/Shutterstock.com
Page 17 GP Studio/Shutterstock.com
Page 18 Goolia Photography/Shutterstock.com
Page 19 Jacob Lund/Shutterstock.com
Pages 24–25 Dean Drobot/Shutterstock.com
Pages 44–45 mavo/Shutterstock.com
Pages 102–3 Dusan Petkovic/Shutterstock.com
Pages 126–27 lenetstan/Shutterstock.com
Pages 164–65 Jacob Lund/Shutterstock.com
Pages 194–95 fizkes/Shutterstock.com
Pages 256–57 djile/Shutterstock.com
Pages 374–75 Rocksweeper/Shutterstock.com
Page 394 KieferPix/Shutterstock.com
Pages 398–99 fizkes/Shutterstock.com

Illustration

All anatomical illustrations by Adam Moore, Hector Diaz/3DLabz Animation Limited

Full-body anatomy and Insets by Linda Bucklin/Shutterstock.com